Therapists on the Front Line

*Psychotherapy With
Gay Men in the Age of AIDS*

Therapists
on the
Front Line

Psychotherapy With
Gay Men in the Age of AIDS

Edited by
Steven A. Cadwell, Ph.D.,
Robert A. Burnham, Jr., Ph.D., and
Marshall Forstein, M.D.

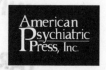

American
Psychiatric
Press, Inc.

Washington, DC
London, England

Copyright © 1994 American Psychiatric Press, Inc.
ALL RIGHTS RESERVED
Manufactured in the United States of America on acid-free paper
97 96 95 94   4 3 2 1
First Edition

American Psychiatric Press, Inc.
1400 K Street, N.W., Washington, DC   20005

Library of Congress Cataloging-in-Publication Data
Therapists on the front line : psychotherapy with gay men in the age
 of AIDS / edited by Steven A. Cadwell, Robert A. Burnham, Jr., and
 Marshall Forstein.
    p. cm.
  Includes bibliographical references and index.
  ISBN 0-88048-558-2
  1. Gay men—Mental health.   2. HIV infections—Patients—Mental
health.   3. AIDS (Disease)—Patients—Mental health.
4. Psychotherapy.   5. Psychotherapist and patient.   I. Cadwell,
Steven A., 1950–   . II. Burnham, Robert A., 1951–   .
III. Forstein, Marshall, 1949–   .
  [DNLM: 1. Acquired Immunodeficiency Syndrome—psychology.
2. Psychotherapy—methods. 3. Homosexuality—psychology. WD 308
T398 1994]
RC451.4.G39T48   1994
616.89′14′086642—dc20
DNLM/DLC
for Library of Congress   93-46269
                                                                        CIP

British Library Cataloguing in Publication Data
A CIP record is available from the British Library.

Editors' Dedication

---

*To Joe, Jim, and Carrie,
the man in each of our lives
who has helped, cajoled, and
supported us through the
process of this volume.*

Authors' Dedication

*To our patients, past and present,
many who have died
and many who have learned to
live and love in the Age of AIDS.*

and

*To our colleagues who have been with us
on the front lines
of this epidemic and have since died
from AIDS-related illnesses.
We miss them.*

Peter Alpert, Ph.D., San Francisco, California,
died 1991

Bruce Binette, M.S.W., Boston, Massachusetts,
died 1993

Donald Brown, M.D., San Francisco, California,
died 1989

Tony Candeloro, M.S.W., New York, New York,
died 1988

Jeffrey Cohen, M.D., San Francisco, California,
died 1990

Jeffrey Drennan, M.D., Providence, Rhode Island,
died 1993

Francis Giambroni, M.S.W., Boston, Massachusetts,
died 1991

David Lourea, Ph.D., San Francisco, California,
died 1992

Diego Lopez, M.S.W., New York, New York,
died 1987

Thomas D. Mackey, L.I.C.S.W., Boston, Massachusetts,
died 1992

Leon McKusick, Ph.D., San Francisco, California,
died 1993

Luis Palacios-Jiminez, M.S.W., New York, New York,
died 1989

Sam Serino, M.S.W., Boston, Massachusetts,
died 1992

Neil Seymour, M.F.C.C., San Francisco, California,
died 1989

Gary Walsh, L.C.S.W., San Francisco, California,
died 1984

Stephen Woo, M.D., Toronto, Canada,
died 1992

Contents

Section I
General Issues

Section II
Treatment Modalities

Individual Treatment

Group Treatment

Couples and Family Treatment

Section III
Specific Treatment Populations

Section IV
Impact on the Therapist

Section V
When the Therapist Is HIV Infected

Editors

Steven A. Cadwell, Ph.D.

Steven Cadwell received his B.A. from Amherst College, his M.S.W. from the University of Texas at Austin, and his Ph.D. from the Smith College School of Social Work. Dr. Cadwell has done research on burnout, empathy, and countertransference in clinical work with gay men with AIDS. He has lectured and given workshops at local, national, and international conferences. Dr. Cadwell provides consultation to agency, clinic, and hospital staffs who work with people with AIDS. He has led support groups for both patients and professionals affected by HIV and has been involved in treatment and service development for these individuals for the past 9 years. He is currently in private practice in Boston, Massachusetts, treating a predominantly gay population. He also serves as adjunct clinical faculty for the Smith College of Social Work.

Robert A. Burnham, Jr., Ph.D.

Robert Burnham received his A.B. from Stonehill College and his Ph.D. in counseling psychology from the University of Notre Dame. He completed his internship in clinical psychology at the Veterans Administration Outpatient Medical Center in Boston, Massachusetts, where he began his specialized training in psychological trauma. He was formerly on the teaching faculties of the Massachusetts School of Professional Psychology, where he taught family therapy, and Antioch/New England Graduate School, where he taught hypnotherapy. He is currently on the training faculty of the Family Institute of Cambridge, and is Visiting Lecturer on Ministry at Harvard Divinity School, teaching the psychology of pastoral care. Dr. Burnham studied hypnotherapy with the late Milton H. Erickson, M.D. He has trained students and conducted lectures internationally on Ericksonian hypnotherapeutic approaches, and he specializes in the areas of hyp-

notic strategies with trauma patients and the use of hypnotic techniques in family and couples therapy. Dr. Burnham provides consultation and supervision to clinical staff on HIV-related issues in family
and couples therapy. He established a network of family therapists in
the Boston metropolitan area who were trained and willing to treat
people with AIDS, their life partners, and their families of origin. He
also consults to clergy and pastoral counselors on countertransference
issues in clinical work with gay people with AIDS. He maintains a
private psychotherapy practice in Brookline, Massachusetts.

Marshall Forstein, M.D.

Marshall Forstein received his B.A. from Middlebury College and his
M.D. from the University of Vermont College of Medicine. He completed his internship in San Francisco, California, and residency in
psychiatry at the Massachusetts General Hospital in Boston, Massachusetts. Currently he is on the faculty of Harvard Medical School
through the Department of Psychiatry at the Cambridge Hospital in
Cambridge, Massachusetts, where he is Director of HIV Mental Health
Services. He is Medical Director of Mental Health and Addiction Services at the Fenway Community Health Center in Boston, which
serves a predominantly gay and lesbian population. Dr. Forstein developed and implemented the Alternative HIV Testing Program for the
Department of Public Health in Massachusetts, and continues to consult in the area of HIV to that department. He has been a member of
the steering committee of the American Psychiatric Association–National Institute of Mental Health AIDS Education Project and currently chairs the American Psychiatric Association's Commission on
AIDS. He is the immediate past president of the Association of Gay
and Lesbian Psychiatrists, an affiliate of the American Psychiatric Association. He has written and lectured extensively on the neuropsychiatric and psychosocial aspects of HIV infection and the
psychodynamic development of gay men. He has served on the Board
of Director of the AIDS Action Committee of Massachusetts and the
Steering Committee of the Boston AIDS Consortium.

Contributors

Sharone Abramowitz, M.D.

Sharone Abramowitz is on the clinical faculty of the Department of Psychiatry, University of California at San Francisco; adjunct faculty at the California School of Professional Psychology; and behavioral science faculty within the Department of Medicine, Division of Primary Care, at Highland General Hospital in Oakland, California. She has extensive experience with HIV and gay and lesbian issues.

Michael D. Baum, M.A., M.F.C.C.

Michael Baum is a psychotherapist in private practice in San Francisco, California, where he works with individuals, couples, and groups. He is a staff therapist in the Men's Clinical Program at Operation Concern, a gay and lesbian outpatient mental health clinic. In addition to teaching and presenting on issues related to AIDS and sexual compulsivity in gay men, he has been a counselor for the Shanti Project.

Alexandra Beckett, M.D.

Alexandra Beckett is an instructor in psychiatry at Harvard Medical School and Director of HIV Mental Health Services at the Beth Israel Hospital in Boston, Massachusetts. She is also a member of the American Psychiatric Association's Commission on AIDS. Involved with research and clinical care, Dr. Beckett has written and lectured on the neuropsychiatric aspects of HIV.

Shelley B. Brauer, Ph.D.

Shelley Brauer is a clinical social worker in private practice in Brookline and Hingham, Massachusetts. As a volunteer for the AIDS Action Committee of Massachusetts, she helped develop the 3-week psychoeducational groups for people infected with HIV. Her psychodynamically oriented practice includes individual and couples work with gay men affected by HIV.

Robert P. Cabaj, M.D.

Robert Cabaj is Medical Director of the Substance Abuse Consultation Service at San Francisco General Hospital and AIDS Health Project. He is an assistant clinical professor of psychiatry at the University of California at San Francisco, and a member of the American Psychiatric Association's Commission on AIDS. He has worked extensively in many aspects of HIV-related health care and in the area of substance abuse within the gay and lesbian community.

Jeffrey Cohen, M.D.

Jeffrey Cohen was an assistant clinical professor of psychiatry and Associate Director of Residency Training within the Department of Psychiatry at the University of California, San Francisco. He was involved extensively in AIDS-related work, and coauthored the first version of this book prior to his death from an AIDS-related illness.

Shani A. Dowd, L.C.S.W.

Shani Dowd is a member of the faculty of the Center for Training in Multicultural Psychology at Boston City Hospital, Boston, Massachusetts, where she teaches cross-cultural psychotherapy. She currently practices as a clinical social worker at a health maintenance organization—the Harvard Community Health Plan, Cambridge, Massachusetts—where she has been a member of the AIDS treatment team since 1984. She is a long-time volunteer with the AIDS Action Committee of Massachusetts, and has lectured widely to professional audiences on AIDS-related subjects.

Abraham Feingold, Psy.D.

Abraham Feingold is presently Mental Health Services Director of the Adult Clinical AIDS Program at Boston City Hospital, Boston, Massachusetts, through which he directs a Ryan White C.A.R.E. Act special project providing family-focused HIV mental health services within the Boston Department of Health and Hospitals. He has served as staff psychologist and Acting Clinical Director of the Gay and Lesbian Counseling Service in Boston. He is a clinical instructor in psychiatry (psychology) at Boston University School of Medicine, and maintains a private psychotherapy practice in Boston.

James M. Fishman, L.I.C.S.W.

James Fishman is a psychotherapist in private practice and Director of Men's Services at Operation Concern, Pacific Presbyterian Medical Center, in San Francisco, California. He has presented on AIDS- and gay-related issues for more than a decade and was a founding member of the Boston AIDS Action Committee.

Joel C. Frost, Ed.D.

Joel C. Frost is an associate in psychology (psychiatry) at the Beth Israel Hospital, Boston, Massachusetts, and instructor in the Department of Psychiatry, Harvard Medical School. He has written and lectured widely in the area of HIV and stress in health care workers and has been active in establishing a gay and lesbian presence in the American Group Psychotherapy Association. In his private psychotherapy practice, he works with gay and lesbian people individually and in groups.

Linda E. Hutton, Psy.D.

Linda Hutton is a clinical psychologist in private practice in Cambridge, Massachusetts. She is a staff member in the Department of Psychiatry, Behavioral Medicine Program, at the Cambridge Hospital and is a clinical faculty member at the Harvard Medical School. She began working with HIV-positive gay men in 1987 in both inpatient and outpatient settings, including the Hospice at Mission Hill in Boston. Dr. Hutton is a consultant for psychotherapists who have HIV or other serious or life-threatening medical illnesses. Her clinical specializations include working with the psychosocial aspects of medical illnesses, anxiety disorders, depression and loss; she is also interested in the integration of psychodynamic and behavioral psychotherapy.

Peter Kassel, Psy.D.

Peter Kassel is Associate Director of Medical Psychology and Director of Inpatient Psychology at Beth Israel Hospital in Boston, Massachusetts, where he teaches psychodynamic psychotherapy and psychotherapy with gay men and lesbians. He is also an instructor in psychiatry at Harvard Medical School. His research interests include psychological and neuropsychological aspects of HIV disease; suicide and the hardships experienced by HIV-infected individuals; the effects of caring for HIV-infected individuals on medical and mental health caregivers; and the development of sexual identity and orientation and its impact on body image. Dr. Kassel has been working with HIV-infected individuals since 1984; in 1989 he began facilitating support groups for medical and mental health caregivers who work with this population.

Rhonda Linde, Ph.D.

Rhonda Linde is Chief Psychologist and Coordinator of Mental Health Training and Research at the Fenway Community Health Center in Boston, Massachusetts. She is an assistant attending psychologist at McLean Hospital in Belmont, Massachusetts, and at Harvard Medical School. She is a founding member of the AIDS Action Committee of Massachusetts. Dr. Linde maintains a private psychotherapy practice in which she sees gay men with HIV-related concerns and has lectured widely on issues related to homosexuality and HIV.

Rubén Montano-López, M.A.

Rubén Montano-López is a Ph.D. candidate in clinical psychology at Boston University. He is a certified HIV-AIDS instructor with the American Red Cross and has been a staff psychologist with Alianza Hispana in Roxbury, Massachusetts. He has worked on AIDS-related projects that are particularly relevant to the Latino community and has written on sexual practices and knowledge of transmission of HIV among Latinos.

Walt Odets, Ph.D.

Walt Odets received his training in clinical psychology from the Professional School of Psychology in San Francisco, California, and has done research and writing on HIV-negative gay men. His book *Life in the Shadow: Being HIV Negative in the Age of AIDS* is currently in press. He has presented on the psychological issues related to HIV and has worked as a volunteer for the Shanti Project in San Francisco. He is currently in private practice in Berkeley, California, working with predominantly gay men, many of whom are HIV positive.

Jane K. O'Rourke, L.M.S.W.

Jane O'Rourke holds an M.S. in personnel services and counseling from Miami University and an M.S.W. from Smith College School for Social Work. She interned at Brigham and Women's Hospital in Boston, Massachusetts, where she started her work with gay men diagnosed with HIV and AIDS. She presently works at Maine Medical Center in Portland, Maine, as the clinical social worker of the AIDS Consultation Service. Approximately 90% of the referrals to the service are gay men from Maine. She is on the executive board of the Maine AIDS Alliance, facilitates a support group, and provides pre- and posttest counseling for the AIDS Project.

José A. Parés-Avila, M.A.

José Parés-Avila is a Ph.D. candidate in clinical psychology at Boston University. He is a clinical fellow in psychology at the Robert B. Andrews Unit (an HIV program) at the Massachusetts General Hospital in Boston, Massachusetts. He has worked on a National Institute of Mental Health–funded AIDS research project through Abt Associates in Cambridge, Massachusetts. He is part of the AIDS Action Committee volunteer mental health committee, where he provides support for staff of color. He has been active in the development of programs specifically aimed at Latino gay men to prevent and treat HIV infection.

Claire E. Philip, L.I.S.W.

Claire Philip was practicing psychotherapy in Cleveland Heights, Ohio, until a life-threatening illness forced her to curtail her activities in August 1990. She has worked as a consultant to clinics specializing in chronic illness, and has written about the dilemmas confronting therapists when they are faced with a life-threatening illness.

Rev. Jennifer M. Phillips, D.Min.

Jennifer Phillips received her B.A. from Wellesley College and her M.Div. from the Andover Newton Theological School. She is an Episcopal priest in the Diocese of Massachusetts and is currently rector of the Church of St. John the Evangelist in Boston, Massachusetts, which is a highly diverse inner-city parish with a large outreach program to the gay community and to the poor. The Rev. Dr. Phillips has written widely on the topic of HIV, particularly as it relates to spirituality, the Christian response, pastoral ministry, pastoral counseling, and care for the caregiver. Previously she was the full-time chaplain at the Brigham and Women's Hospital in Boston.

R. Dennis Shelby, Ph.D.

Dennis Shelby is on the faculty at the Institute for Clinical Social Work in Chicago, Illinois, and is in private practice. He has presented widely on HIV-related subjects and is the author of *If a Partner Has AIDS: Guide to Clinical Intervention for Relationships in Crisis*. He is currently researching the experience of gay men who test HIV positive.

Michael Shernoff, C.S.W., A.C.S.W.

Michael Shernoff is founder and codirector of Chelsea Psychotherapy Associates in Manhattan, New York. He has served on the board of directors of the National Lesbian/Gay Health Foundation, is an adjunct lecturer at Hunter College Graduate School of Social Work, and is widely published in the areas of AIDS and mental health services to gay men.

Perry S. Sutherland, A.C.S.W.

Perry Sutherland is a clinical social worker at Community Counseling Center in Portland, Maine, and maintains a small private practice. He received his M.S.W. from the University of Tennessee at Knoxville, with a clinical focus on social work treatment with gay men and lesbians. He has been active vis-à-vis HIV and AIDS and in gay communities since 1985. He was director of the AIDS Project in Portland, was a former member of the Maine AIDS Alliance, and is currently a member of the Maine AIDS Development Plan Coordinating Committee. Over the past 8 years his casework has ranged from 10% to 90% with gay men living with HIV or AIDS.

Bruce J. Thompson, M.S.W., Ph.D.

Bruce Thompson is a social worker who chairs the Social and Health Services Program at Roger Williams College in Rhode Island. He also is an assistant clinical professor in the Department of Community Health, Brown University, and adjunct assistant professor at Smith College School for Social Work. He also has a private psychotherapy practice in which he sees mostly gay men who are HIV infected.

Gil Tunnell, Ph.D.

Gil Tunnell is Director of the Family Studies Unit in the Department of Psychiatry at Beth Israel Medical Center in New York City. He is an adjunct supervisor in family therapy in the Clinical Psychology Training Program at New York University. He formerly chaired the Task Force on AIDS for the New York State Psychological Association, and continues to be extensively involved in the training of health care professionals in areas related to group psychotherapy and HIV. He also has a part-time private psychotherapy practice specializing in gay and lesbian issues, and has written and lectured in these areas.

Preface

Steven A. Cadwell, Ph.D.
Robert A. Burnham, Jr., Ph.D.
Marshall Forstein, M.D.

Acquired immunodeficiency syndrome (AIDS)–related illnesses are the leading cause of death among gay men in the United States. Results from epidemiological studies have indicated that although the rate of new human immunodeficiency virus (HIV) infections continues to increase in other populations (including heterosexuals, women of color and their children, and adolescents), gay men continue to make up more than 50% of newly diagnosed cases of HIV each year. Although research and medical discoveries are producing vast amounts of biological knowledge, less is known about the complex psychological fabric involved in preventing transmission of HIV or coping with the diagnosis of HIV infection and the development of subsequent illness. It is only through an in-depth analysis of individual lives in the context of psychotherapy that we learn how human beings manage their lives in the face of danger, fear, anxiety, loss, and grief.

We are writing to bear witness to how the AIDS epidemic has impacted our professional work. Our purpose is to record the ways in which the epidemic has affected the therapeutic relationship with and the lives of our gay patients. By itself, traditional psychodynamic assessment has a limited capacity to yield understanding of the breadth and power of what gay patients are experiencing. With a view to extending traditional approaches to therapy, the material in this book emphasizes a multidimensional perspective that includes psychodynamic, social, cultural, medical, and political dimensions.

The AIDS epidemic continues to be a central experience in the gay male community and is an unrelenting presence and source of anxiety in gay men's daily lives, regardless of their HIV serological status. HIV, both as a disease and as a symbol of stigma and alienation, affects their friendships, their families, their work, their sexual lives, their dreams, and their beliefs. To better understand the impact of HIV on psychotherapy with gay men, we must look at these men's experience both within a larger social and historical context and more specifically within the tradition of psychotherapy. If you are gay, you will hopefully recognize your own experience here. If you are not gay, you may need to work at trying to fully comprehend the extraordinary experience of a gay man in the age of AIDS. The following exercise may help you understand this experience.

> Imagine for a moment growing up left-handed in a right-handed culture and having the culture tell you not to use your left hand. The majority of the society sees you as sick, sinful, and an outlaw. Whether consciously felt or not, the stigma against your use of your natural left-handedness is emotionally abusive. To fend off the pain of your difference and the loss of opportunities in asserting your natural inclination, you might work to pass as right-handed. A false sense of self would develop. Internal conflict would develop as your true left-handed self would be caught between your needs for integrity and an expression of the self and your need to protect yourself from further social abuse and injury. Even after reclaiming one's left-handedness, there might remain scars as a consequence of passing as right-handed for so long that your sense of cohesion and core value would be shaken.

Of course, this brief exercise falls short of conveying the complex and essential role of sexuality in identity. For gay men, the feeling of being legal, social, cultural, and moral outlaws runs deep and damages early attempts to internalize a positive sense of self. A gay man's work to love himself and then to love another man is a long hard battle with little or no help from society. His attempts to break through to some sense of true self may risk more trauma delivered by the larger homophobic culture. By necessity, he has to find strength by turning inward.

If he is fortunate he will find the support of others like himself, finding solace in his own community of outlaws.

The gay subculture has seized its own power and identity over the past few decades. On Stonewall Street in New York City in 1969, after continued harassment from the police intruding on the privacy of a gay bar, a group of homosexuals fought back against stigma to claim their own integrity as gay men and the modern gay liberation movement took force. Part of the developing, affirmative gay male culture included a celebration of sexuality, often challenging the traditional boundaries and values of the heterosexual society that denied the equality of gay people. Throughout the therapeutic work with gay men there is a profound experience of the existential irony that the emotional freedom sought and sometimes found in sexual activity should be the unwitting vehicle for the biological convenience of viral replication and human destruction. Although some might argue against homosexual behavior on moral or religious grounds, society must come to grips with the issue that the marginalization and rejection of gay people has contributed to the splitting off of affect and relationships from the expression of sexual drive.

The task of replacing the false self with the true self, and of internalizing some positive sense of that self in an antihomosexual society, is an undertaking of ultimate significance for gay men. For those who need help in this, psychotherapy would seem to be a useful resource. But historically, homosexuality has been defined as a mental illness. Instead of a resource for healing, psychotherapy was most often yet another source of oppression. In 1973, the change of nomenclature in DSM-III (American Psychiatric Association 1980) to include homosexuality as treatable only when it was assessed to be ego dystonic cleared the way for a more gay-positive treatment in psychotherapy. Since then, ego-dystonic homosexuality has also been removed from DSM-III-R (American Psychiatric Association 1987).

Although the nomenclature regarding homosexuality has been changed in DSM-III-R, attitudes of mental health clinicians have not kept pace; many clinicians continue to try to treat homosexual patients' sexual orientation or are unsophisticated about the intrapsychic process of coming out in the context of human development. Furthermore, many gay men continue to feel distrust for the profession as they assume that sexual orientation itself will be perceived by the professional as the issue for treatment. The challenge remains for any gay man to feel syntonic and valued in a homophobic society. The more insidious emotional disturbance—society's homophobia—as yet goes largely unassessed and untreated. Homophobia, individual and institutionalized, continues to be socially acceptable, a reservoir of the same prejudice and ignorance that feeds sexism and racism.

In this charged and oppressive atmosphere, the AIDS epidemic festered and grew. In the beginning stages of the epidemic, it was clear that the only resource available for HIV-positive gay men would be therapists who were gay or lesbian and those gay-affirmative therapists who already were committed to providing support and treatment to the gay population. With the initial hope that the epidemic would be short lived, these therapists adapted crisis intervention treatments to cope with the mushrooming devastation of human life. Over the last decade, as the scope of the epidemic became more apparent, therapists tried to keep pace by evolving and developing treatment modalities and therapeutic strategies to meet the ever-expanding needs of infected and noninfected gay men and the people in their lives. The silence and lack of response by society and mental health institutions only served to deepen homosexual individual's sense of being outlawed and invisible in the majority culture.

It is out of this frontier work that we have culled material from therapists who have been immersed in treating gay men with HIV and AIDS. It was not our intent to make this a fully comprehensive book. Much has been written about the epidemiological and medical aspects of HIV, and keeping current with the latest information and treatments is every therapist's responsibility. A great deal has been written about the political and psychosocial aspects of this epidemic. Less attention has been paid to understanding the psychodynamic and behavioral aspects of gay men affected by HIV. If there exists any hope for containing this devastating epidemic, it lies in our capacity to comprehend the complex forces that are involved in how gay men make choices that protect them or put them at risk for infection.

In this volume, it is our intention to examine in depth particular aspects of the psychotherapeutic work with gay men during the unfolding of this epidemic over the past decade. We have invited articles that exemplify an empathic approach to the specific needs of various segments of the gay population. Some of the chapters deal specifically with the issues for gay men who are infected with HIV, whereas others address the needs of gay men regardless of serological status.

The book records the experiences of therapists who have been on the front line. Each of the five sections addresses a different aspect of working with gay patients affected by the AIDS epidemic.

Section I: General Issues

The authors of this first section address those concerns that are more universally experienced across populations and psychotherapeutic modalities. In Chapter 1, Cadwell explores the discrimination faced by gay men who are again stigmatized by their experience of being infected with HIV. The therapist's active acknowledgment of this social marginalization and its personal consequences for the gay man is critical to effective treatment. In Chapter 2, Linde goes on to suggest a model for how the AIDS epidemic, as a social and intrapsychic force, has affected sexual identity development in gay men. Following the emergence of AIDS in our society, the "normative" development for gay men has been inevitably changed. How does a gay man develop healthy attitudes and beliefs about intimacy and love when he must treat every new sexual experience as a potential threat to his life because of HIV?

For members of the gay community, the AIDS epidemic has delivered losses of catastrophic proportions. In Chapter 3, Shelby explores, through a self psychological paradigm, the interaction between personal mourning and the capacity of the gay subculture to process and integrate the meaning of multiple losses extending from the AIDS epidemic. In the context of such devastation, Phillips, in Chapter 4, brings into focus the spiritual dimension of illness, death, and loss in order to help the psychotherapist recognize and facilitate the integration of spirituality within the more traditional context of psychotherapy.

At various stages of HIV-related illnesses, individuals are confronted with how much emotional and physical pain is tolerable, with suicidality sometimes emerging as the only apparent salvation. In Chapter 5, Forstein examines the range of issues confronting therapists working with gay men at any stage of HIV infection. In his discussion he distinguishes suicide as a necessary psychological defense from a "rational" decision to terminate one's life. With the higher rate of suicide among men who are both gay and infected with HIV, the therapist working with gay men will inevitably struggle with understanding and managing patients who are feeling self-destructive.

As HIV affects the functioning of the brain and mind, the impact of cognitive dysfunction on the process of psychotherapy can be at times either profound and obvious or quite subtle and easily overlooked or misinterpreted. In Chapter 6, Beckett and Kassel help the provider integrate the neuropsychiatric sequelae of HIV with psychodynamic concerns that arise in ongoing treatment. Cognitive dysfunction may profoundly affect the process of psychotherapy and often challenges therapists to adjust their treatment style and expectations.

In working with HIV-infected gay males, it is also critical to pay attention to how patients' specific sexual behavior impacts on their physical safety and psychological integrity. Frost, in Chapter 7, provides some guidance on how to incorporate these concerns into treatment. In the context of complicated transferences, initiating a discussion of specific sexual practices often has significant ramifications on the therapy. Finally, in Chapter 8, Forstein examines how a seemingly routine medical test can have complex psychological meanings. HIV-antibody testing presents many issues for the gay man who is assessing his level of risk for HIV, and has implications that may go far beyond the decision to be tested based on a rational approach to risk assessment.

Section II: Treatment Modalities

The AIDS epidemic impacts every gay man's fundamental sense of himself, his social group, his relationship with his family of origin, and his relationship to the man he loves. What is initially and primarily experienced as an assault on the integrity of the self spreads out quickly to involve the individual in every part of human existence: work, play, and love. As psychotherapists, we find that no one modal-

ity of treatment suffices. Individual, group, family, and couples treatment modalities are explored in this section of the book, but by no
means are all the therapies useful for gay men confronting HIV infection covered.

In Chapter 9, Abramowitz and Cohen reveal how the self psychological perspective frames issues of gay men with HIV and identifies
ways of using the individual treatment relationship in intensive psychotherapy.

The power of group therapy is demonstrated in three different
chapters in which three populations of gay men are examined: men
who recently tested HIV positive, gay men who have been living with
HIV, and gay men who are sexually compulsive. In Chapter 10 Brauer
describes how group therapy with gay men who have learned they are
HIV positive can serve as a rite of passage through the rocky, uncharted terrain of integrating difficult news. Peers and leaders work
together to stabilize members and orient them into a more integrated
sense of themselves. In Chapter 11 Tunnell tracks how a supportive
therapy group's development parallels Erikson's stage theory of individual development. He identifies the unique characteristics of AIDS
as an illness (its stigma, the threat of premature death, and a highly
variable course of illness) and the issues related to AIDS patients' homosexuality, and shows how the issues can all be accessed within the
interactive context of the group. If managed effectively, the group
members can do powerful work together on these issues.

In Chapter 12, Baum and Fishman describe how intensive group
therapy can work with gay men who are excessively dependent on sex
to maintain a cohesive sense of self. In group therapy they learn about
their own dynamics and gain control in sexual, interpersonal, and
intrapsychic realms.

HIV also has an impact on the family life of gay men. In Chapter
13 Thompson describes the poignant and complicated family dynamics that can be present when a gay man who is HIV positive or has
AIDS returns home to die. The clinician's assistance in negotiating the
convergence of powerful needs may be critical for the gay man and his
family.

To sustain their relationships, gay couples have had to struggle
against external social oppression and internalized homophobia. In

Chapter 14, Forstein outlines how HIV further stresses their union. He also describes how the therapist can intervene to bolster their strained resources.

Section III:
Specific Treatment Populations

In a book about therapy with gay men, special attention must be given to portions of the gay population with specific treatment issues. We have focused on ethnicity, survival of childhood sexual abuse, substance abuse, the rural environment, and negative HIV status as some of the distinctions that delineate special groups of gay men.

Our inclusion of Chapters 15 and 16 on African American gay men and Latino gay men is by no means exhaustive of the ethnic groups from which gay men come. Although not included specifically in this volume, gay men from Asian, Native American, or Caribbean island cultures have their particular relation with their ethnic culture, with the larger gay culture, and with the nongay society. Being gay and infected or at risk for HIV infection must be understood in terms of how the gay man of color relates to each of these sources of identity. Homosexuality itself may be pathologized within the ethnic group. Resistance in the culture to dealing with homosexuality, bisexuality, and HIV may prevent the gay man from receiving support from his ethnic or racial community. Resistance to dealing with racism may prevent the man of color from receiving support from the gay community. Authors Dowd (Chapter 15) and Parés-Avila and Montano-López (Chapter 16) address the contextual sources of positive and negative identity for African American and Latino gay men. Their clear delineation of the particular needs of these gay men and men who have sex with men points to our need for an increased understanding of the needs of gay men from other ethnic groups.

In Chapter 17, O'Rourke and Sutherland explore HIV-related issues for men living in rural America. There men who have sex with men share a culture that is often homophobic and has limited resources for men who are HIV infected.

Burnham proposes a theoretical framework in Chapter 18 within which to work with gay men who, as survivors of childhood sexual abuse, are dangerously vulnerable to being retraumatized by HIV. For them, HIV can be yet another manifestation of a world that abuses. Tragically caught in the repetition of their early abuse experience, they may fail to protect themselves, or may unconsciously even seek HIV infection as further confirmation of their distorted sense of worthlessness developed earlier. If they are already infected, they may experience the infection as further perpetration of abuse. The work of therapy is to detoxify the trauma and help strengthen the identity of the survivor.

The AIDS epidemic works as a prism through which particular psychological dynamics of gay men can be further fragmented or intensified. To deal with social oppression and subsequent low self-esteem, some gay men use chemical substances excessively, thereby numbing their pain but also damaging themselves physically and emotionally. In so doing, they collude with society's negative opinion of them, extending society's devastatingly negative response as they turn against themselves. In Chapter 19, Cabaj describes how containing this epidemic requires a comprehensive understanding of the relationship between the use of mind-altering substances and the risk behaviors that facilitate HIV transmission.

Another expression of gay men's identification with an aggressor's oppression can be heard in the despair of some seronegative men. Guilty about surviving and unclear about their right to have their needs addressed, seronegative gay men persist in risking unsafe sex in the belief that, because they are gay, they deserve no better than to die. Many other complicated dynamics, elaborated on by Odets in Chapters 20 and 21, can ensnare seronegative gay men. Even if a gay man is able to remain uninfected, he is never unaffected by the epidemic.

Therapists must be vigilant for the particular ways that each gay patient may collude with the larger society's oppression. This vigilance must extend to scrutiny of the therapist's own collusion with the majority culture's rejection of gay men's rights and needs.

Section IV: Impact on the Therapist

As therapists we have learned to take a scientific view of illness, and in so doing we have developed a professional view of experiencing hardship. We have learned to insulate ourselves from physical revulsion, to delimit our identification with our patients' existential suffering, and to strive for a philosophical stance toward the inadequacy of our efforts to help our patients—or so it seemed before AIDS.

AIDS shakes the foundations of these professional coping mechanisms. In Chapter 22, Cadwell describes how the epidemic floods clinicians, who are trained to identify and ameliorate neurotic pain, with wave after wave of their patients' existential anguish as they grapple with the encroaching realities of this debilitating and deforming disease. It is commonplace for mental health practitioners to be caught off guard by the strength of their personal identification with the pain of their HIV-infected patients. Having been trained to analyze positive and negative feelings toward patients by understanding the ways in which the feelings mirror the patients' early relationships and core conflicts, we associate good treatment with methods designed to monitor the ways clinicians identify with patients. However, HIV always confronts the clinician with the interface of neurotic pain and existential anguish. This complicated and dynamic interplay, which necessitates the ongoing renegotiation of the psychotherapeutic contract, can be profoundly confusing to clinicians.

Each of the authors in this section writes from a different perspective about the intricate interweaving of characterological structure, neurotic pain, and the real threat to existence that HIV represents. The following chapters concentrate on three topics of chief concern: in Chapter 22 Cadwell points out helpful versus problematic forms of identification with HIV-infected gay men; in Chapter 23 Fishman illustrates the essential ways in which the psychotherapeutic contract is affected by the disease process; and in Chapter 24 Feingold looks at the development of models of consultation and supervision that help the therapist monitor his or her personal as well as professional experience in the work with gay men with HIV-related concerns.

Section V:
When the Therapist Is HIV Infected

A primary task of the therapist is to enter into the patient's experience and yet not be the patient. The problem for HIV-infected therapists is how not to be in the role of the patient when they are in the role of the therapist. HIV-positive therapists have a significant emotional experience to integrate into their professional life. They must make sense of their own radically changing life. In their therapeutic role, they are challenged to temporarily suspend their focus on their own life in order to attend to their patients' lives. When working with a patient who is also concerned with HIV infection, the relationship between therapist and patient intensifies.

A complex relationship exists between infected therapists and their peers. Colleagues must relate to these therapists as fellow professionals and not be pulled into treating them as patients. The responsibility of noninfected therapists to HIV-infected therapists is to provide a safe haven within which the latter can find purpose and reason to continue to do their work as long as they choose to and are responsibly able to do so. The professional monitoring of peers, difficult under the best of circumstances, is made more difficult by the intense emotional issues engendered by HIV and the potential for a paralyzing identification with the infected therapist.

In this epidemic, we are learning how to take care of each other in new ways. We have had to face our own denial of our vulnerability and the vulnerability of those who have been fighting shoulder to shoulder with us. Over the past decade, having not been prepared to face openly these depths of vulnerability, we have stumbled when our colleagues stumbled. We now must anticipate and be responsible for our inevitable vulnerabilities and potential death. Just as we have learned to contract with our gay HIV patients to be with them through the final stages of their lives, we are learning to contract to be with one another through the hardest times of our careers: facing our colleagues' HIV illnesses.

Gay men and lesbians who are therapists will continue to provide much of the therapy for gay men with HIV. We must continue to develop better ways of addressing our own needs and frailties. The unthinkable must not only be voiced, but planned for: How will I help you address the dilemmas in your practice if you get HIV? and, How will you help me address the dilemmas in my practice if I get HIV?

Inclusion of this section was both urgent and necessarily preliminary. Two of the editors have been part of a peer supervision–support group in which two members were diagnosed with and subsequently died of AIDS-related illnesses. We were with them in their process of coming to terms with their illness and its impact on their careers as therapists. We make no claim to be comprehensive or definitive. In this area, the voices are few. We are enormously grateful to each of our contributors. Their experience and insight contribute to our building an empirical and theoretical base for more complete understanding of this frontier. Philip's wisdom and clarity, evident in Chapter 25, reaches from her own experience with her life-threatening illness to the issues encountered by therapists with HIV. In Chapter 26, Shernoff writes from the position of being a therapist who is HIV infected. In Chapter 27, Hutton describes her experience as both witness and support to a colleague with HIV who struggled with his disclosure of his HIV status to his patients and the closure of his therapy practice. Here, again, we find ourselves adapting and inventing ways to maintain the clarity of our mission and the integrity of our professional and personal lives.

The epilogue offers the personal perspective of the three editors who have brought together the contributors of this volume.

We have chosen chapters that describe critical facets of this complicated work. Different positions are expressed by the different voices of each chapter. We, as editors, do not take one position. We are witnessing, as our authors have witnessed, the always demanding and often painful journey of therapists on the front line who have forged a body of work that is ever changing and developing. Neither static nor definitive, this is a record of brave and valiant exploration of a rich and hazardous new frontier in human experience.

Indeed, we have found that all of our therapeutic work is changed because of our work with gay clients with HIV. It is just this pushing past the bounds of traditional therapy that brings us to new levels of development in mastery of our own professional selves. In addition, and even more profoundly, our personal lives and our inability to deny the existential reality of our own mortality have been changed by this work. We have grown and matured through these relationships: with our patients, with our colleagues, and with ourselves.

We would like to dedicate this book to our colleagues who have labored over this first devastating decade of the epidemic, and to our patients, then and now, who have helped us learn that living and dying are part of the same journey. We are grateful that together we are strengthened, and that makes this work possible. Our hope is that some of their vision and strength will be passed on through this volume.

> And it was in the midst of shouts rolling against the terrace wall in massive waves that waxed in volume and duration, while cataracts of colored fire fell thicker through the darkness, that Dr. Rieux resolved to compile this chronicle, so that he should not be one of those who hold their peace but should bear witness in favor of those plague-stricken people; so that some memorial of the injustice and outrage done them might endure; and to state quite simply what we learn in time of pestilence; that there are more things to admire in men than to despise.
>
> Albert Camus
> *The Plague*

References

American Psychiatric Association: Diagnostic and Statistical Manual of Mental Disorders, 3rd Edition. Washington, DC, American Psychiatric Association, 1980

American Psychiatric Association: Diagnostic and Statistical Manual of Mental Disorders, 3rd Edition, Revised. Washington, DC, American Psychiatric Association, 1987

Section I

General Issues

Chapter 1

Twice Removed:
The Stigma Suffered by
Gay Men With AIDS

Steven A. Cadwell, Ph.D.

B ecause society fears difference, homosexuality, disease, and death, gay men infected with the human immunodeficiency virus (HIV) can be multiply stigmatized. Long before the acquired immunodeficiency syndrome (AIDS) afflicted the gay community, gay men were stigmatized as socially deviant individuals. With the advent of AIDS, they have been further stigmatized as being lethally contagious. Psychosocial theory helps us understand stigmatization as a costly way of managing fear. Thus society contains its terror of difference, sexuality, disease, and death by blaming and isolating people with AIDS (PWAs).

Scapegoating is a predictable process in any group dealing with overwhelming issues. All groups—whether gay or straight—are in a high-risk category for perpetrating stigmatization. Any group could be singled out as a scapegoat. Ultimately, stigmatization injures both the perpetrator and the scapegoated individual or group because it is a dysfunctional and inadequate process for dealing with unchangeable realities, such as difference, sexuality, disease, and death. These are immutable realities despite one's efforts to dissociate from them.

An earlier version of this chapter was first published in *Smith College Studies in Social Work* 61 (3):236–246, June 1991.

The social, political, and cultural context of AIDS in the United States has been fertile ground for scapegoating and stigmatization, of which gay men have been the prime, but not the only, target. When unacknowledged, these social processes threaten to undermine any groups' attempt to deal with the challenges posed by AIDS. By examining in the first part of the chapter how these processes played out in the first decade of the epidemic in the United States, we may be better able to intervene to protect all who are at risk: the perpetrators whose fears go inadequately tended and the individuals who experience the trauma of stigmatization.

In the latter part of this chapter, I explore the impact of stigmatization on PWAs and their support systems, and I present implications for clinical practice and social policy. On the clinical level, understanding the process of stigmatization can deepen our sensitivity to gay PWAs and to the probable manifestation of prejudice in transferential and countertransferential experiences in treatment. On the social level, recognizing the damage stigmatization causes is integral to developing humane and protective policies for PWAs and policies that unify the public in addressing the fears and concerns of all who live in the midst of this epidemic. My premise is that we are all survivors of this epidemic and we all need interventions, both as perpetrators and scapegoats. The dimension of the epidemic I trace here is the social infection of fear and the destructive projection of that fear onto gay men who are infected with HIV.

Historical and Cultural Context

The Norm of Life Expectancy: Fear of Death

In the United States, which has enjoyed decades of general prosperity, human deaths caused by uncontrollable biological factors seem anathema to us. Our propensity to deny death has been underscored by various theorists (Becker 1973; Freud 1917; Lifton 1979). The developments in medical science and the increase in general affluence have doubled life expectancy for most Americans since the turn of the century. This reality of increased longevity coupled with our eager denial of death has created a new social norm that American culture has quickly adopted.

Until the outbreak of AIDS (cancer notwithstanding), the issue of death had been pushed ahead to the "twilight years" for most Americans. Furthermore, we have always attempted to relegate death to formal medical and thanatological institutions, which remove it from integrated experience in our daily lives. The eruption of a disease in our midst that affects large numbers of relatively young individuals has been devastating to this social order. The AIDS epidemic has forced us to confront mortality. In a culture of narcissism (Lasch 1979), this is a narcissistic injury to the entire society. These social circumstances have heightened the psychological terror that illness triggers.

In any group, this fear can unleash destructive impulses. When more constructive means are not available, regressive and paranoid reactions can take over, and the group may seek to exert some control over the situation by extruding the member(s) they see as causing the problem. In the AIDS epidemic, gay men have been just such a target. Homophobic fears (the irrational fear of homosexual thoughts and behaviors) cause society to delineate gay men as a target, but terror and regressive paranoia about illness and death unleash society's destructive impulse to take aim and fire upon gay men, thus further isolating and stigmatizing them.

Fears Fueled by Social Misperception and Uncertainty

The AIDS epidemic underscores the fact that illness is a social state as well as a physical condition (Friedson 1984). Many are still confused about how the virus is transmitted and why various groups are differentially exposed to HIV. This uncertainty and the inability of medical science to develop a vaccine or efficacious treatment for AIDS have left the public feeling exposed and defenseless in the face of a horrible and devastating disease. This exposure has fueled a panic that is virulent and harmful in its own right, a festering state in which preexisting fears further infect the public imagination. Entrenched values and prejudices stemming from socialization and stratification are more likely to become further manifested in this climate of uncertainty.

The media has fed fears that AIDS can be transmitted through nonsexual contact by reporting stories of alleged transmission through food preparation or in child care settings. These reports encourage the public to suspect more people of having the disease than is accurate. Then, as more people are included in this inflated category of being contagious, the public becomes increasingly frightened. People see danger in those who do not actually fit the more scientifically delineated categories of illness but who are only at a higher risk for exposure to the disease. Members of these groups may themselves internalize the public's misperception. The fears and attitudes of the larger public infect a scapegoated individual's self-perception, making it more difficult to keep a balanced sense of his or her own health (Siegel 1986).

One of the most devastating misperceptions in the current AIDS crisis is the inflated health risk attributed to groups that actually have a lower risk of exposure. This distortion has been a constant source of fear for the public. The media's relentless reporting of unscientific beliefs continues to exacerbate the public's fear. As Larry Kessler, executive director of the AIDS Action Committee in Boston, has warned, "What we don't want to do is generate fear. We want to generate a healthy respect for the virus. Fear doesn't accomplish anything" (Bartlett 1988).

Misconception fuels fear, and irrational fears in turn can trigger the negative social processes that function to maintain order at the expense of equality. As fears become inflated in the mass society, escalating panic can lead to the irrational search for scapegoats. Persistent notions of casual HIV transmission, for example, have led to gay restaurant workers being fired from their jobs. Policies such as mandatory testing and the quarantine of people in high-risk categories are two additional examples of scapegoating fed by these same beliefs. Scapegoating can also happen in more subtle ways. In my own clinical practice, a nondisabled PWA who works in the computer industry was "encouraged" to work at home rather than at the main office. By isolating PWAs, society has implicitly identified this group's social deviance as the cause of the epidemic in order to ease its own panic. An in-group–out-group dichotomy, essentially a strategy for social control, is invoked in an effort to master tremendous panic.

The objective reality is that the proportion of individuals within high-risk groups who have AIDS has remained relatively constant in the last several years, with the risk to the general heterosexual public not as high as was once assumed (Boffey 1988). Despite this reality, the public has imposed its own set of beliefs on events; social theory reveals the function of these beliefs. The more the heterosexual population misconstrues its level of risk, the more the disease is described as a *homosexual disease.* In so doing, Americans invoke a process that adds an insidious and brutal form of social trauma to the burden of an incurable illness.

Blaming the Victim

> The stigma, the defect, the fatal difference—though derived in the past from environmental forces—is still located within the victim, inside his skin. . . . It is a brilliant ideology for justifying a perverse form of social action designed to change, not society, as one might expect, but rather society's victim. . . . We must particularly ask, "To whom are social problems a problem?" And usually, if truth were to be told, we would have to admit that we mean they are a problem to those of us who are outside the boundaries of what we have defined as the problem. . . . Now, if this is the quality of our assumptions about social problems, we are led unerringly to certain beliefs about the causes of the problems. We cannot comfortably believe that we are the cause of that which is problematic to us; therefore, we are almost compelled to believe that they—the problematic ones—are the cause. (Ryan 1971, pp. 3–24)

Placing blame is one means by which we turn something incomprehensible and frightening into something explicable and thus potentially controllable and avoidable. In premodern society, disease was explained as the wrath of God or divine intervention. People looked for some evil within afflicted individuals that would account for those individuals' fates. Although we were assumed to have outgrown such a primitive morality, AIDS has pushed us back behind the frontiers of our most sophisticated scientific knowledge, allowing moral judgments once again to be invoked as a way of finding control. Attributing blame outside of one's own social group allows one to believe that the behavior within one's social group is healthy, normal, and secure (Gilman and Nelkin 1988).

As in the case of AIDS, placing blame on another is an attempt to locate risk outside of oneself and within the other. This process is a social construct that reflects beliefs, stereotypes, and political biases of the time (Douglas 1967). A pattern of blaming is pervasive in the popular media's coverage of AIDS in which intravenous drug users, Haitians, Africans, homosexuals, and the promiscuous are among those who have been blamed.

Labeling AIDS as a Gay Plague— Placing AIDS "Outside"

Because AIDS in the United States was first diagnosed among homosexuals, it was initially called *GRID—gay-related immune deficiency—* and has been associated with homosexuality ever since. In contrast, AIDS first appeared in Africa among the heterosexual population and was called the *European disease* or the *slim disease*. Early in the research on the etiology of AIDS in the United States, considerable effort was made to identify the characteristic features of gay life-styles that might be contributing causes to the spread of the disease. The description of gay men as promiscuous or sexually compulsive spawned early stereotypes that all PWAs were promiscuous. Although subsequent research showed that there is great variety in the sexual behavior of PWAs, the initial findings had already captured the public's imagination.

In the United States, the initial labels of AIDS as the *gay plague* and *gay cancer* have persisted over time. Before AIDS, it was the gay liberation movement that brought the invisible minority of gay men into focus in every stratum of society. Once homosexuality became more visible, society, in part fueled by its fear of this clearly present diversity, reacted by mixing its fear of gay men with its fear of AIDS. Fear of AIDS became another expression of fear of gay men. It followed that gay men were blamed for causing AIDS.

As the movement challenged the norms of the old social order by exposing deviance in the midst of every stratum of social and occupational structure, the fear of AIDS became a more strident articulation of the fear of gays. The talk of rooting out the abnormal, deviant homosexual has been replaced by attempts to constrict the groups blamed for causing AIDS. The object of discrimination—gay men—has remained constant.

A major theme in the story of AIDS in the United States is prejudice. In the early stages of inquiry, the media neglected to cover the epidemic with the same widespread attention afforded toxic shock syndrome and Legionnaires' disease. The Reagan administration, anxious to keep a lid on government spending and unsupportive of homosexuals in general, largely ignored the problem. Edward Brandt, the former Assistant Secretary for Health of the U.S. Department of Health and Human Services, initially saw AIDS as a problem for the states to handle, although he later became very involved in the fight against AIDS. The medical establishment also faltered in its commitment to the public. Scientists were routinely advised to stop studying this "homosexual disease" and turn to more legitimate research. Prejudice also existed within the gay community. Some gay businesspeople actively blocked the gay community's ability to rise up unilaterally against the illness at the start (Shilts 1987).

Ultimately, the lesbian and gay community organized the first efforts to raise money for AIDS research and services for PWAs. However, this mobilization may have been counterproductive, serving to further confirm the public's perception that AIDS was a gay disease. The media's coverage of gay groups' activities continues to link AIDS with gay men. If the marked increase in "gay bashing" is an accurate barometer, the public's response to AIDS has been to rigidify its negative attitudes towards gay men and step up its scapegoating of PWAs, ascribing to them total responsibility for their plight. Consequently, PWAs are often denied the generosity, kindness, and support that society at its best can provide to those who are ill (Siegel 1986).

AIDS and Sexual Morality

An understanding of the link between AIDS and morality is crucial to recognizing the social impact of the epidemic. The media has repeatedly underscored the similarity of AIDS and syphilis as sexually transmitted diseases rather than the similarity of AIDS and, for example, hepatitis as viral diseases. Individuals who have AIDS have been treated similar to those who have syphilis—they have been stigmatized as being promiscuous, immoral, and dangerous (Brandt 1988).

Whenever occurrences of a sexually transmitted disease become widespread, the public comes face to face with social conflicts about the meaning, nature, and risks of sexuality. Because many misperceive the cause of AIDS to be sexual behavior (especially lascivious indulgence) rather than a virus, an anxious public is forced to struggle with sexual taboos. Just as the individual psyche engages in certain defenses to process a major disruptive event, society develops mores and norms to create and maintain order when it is challenged by threatening behavior. When an individual or subgroup is perceived as transgressing the norms or breaking taboos, social order is threatened and society reacts to restore order. In the popular consciousness, gay PWAs are judged to have broken an important taboo and transgressed a significant norm: they prefer sexual relations with the same sex and are assumed to be promiscuous in their sexual expression. Homophobia thus further intensifies the rigid rejection of gay PWAs.

Although social theorists converge in their definition of *deviance* as the violation of social morality, they differ in whether they see social morality as absolute or relative. In traditional perspectives, moral rules were seen as absolutes external to individuals. In recent theory, social order is viewed as the outcome of purposeful constructions in which moral meanings are used to create the social context. This more existential perspective views humans as creating their own social order through the establishment of norms and by labeling groups as deviant. By labeling deviancy, the boundaries of group norms are defined (Lemert 1967).

From this existential perspective, one can identify the societal function fulfilled by labeling gay PWAs as *deviant*. First, gay PWAs deviate from the highly valued norm of health. Their precarious health status and probable premature death break the social expectations of wellness and longevity that strongly encourage the denial of death. A gay PWA's illness also threatens the public's inflated belief in medical science's ability to protect us. Second, beyond breaking the death taboo, these individuals' illness provides public acknowledgment that they were sexually active, at the same time as their homosexuality places them outside of the acceptable range of sexuality. Even within the range of homosexual behavior, a gay man's probable engagement in high-risk anal or oral sex stigmatizes him even further. Images of a man being passive and penetrated further threaten the constricted majority view of the proper male sexual role. Thus the social order reasserts itself against the "danger" of gay men's transgressions by labeling them deviant.

Stigma is the mark of social disgrace that sets the deviant individual apart from those who consider themselves normal. The stigmatized member has a "spoiled identity" as a result of others' negative evaluations (Goffman 1963). Rather than facing their fear within themselves, the "normal" people project their fears onto those who are considered "immoral," "bad," "unnatural," and "deadly." The scapegoat carries this bad part away and the herd goes on—at least until its provisional, precarious security is shaken once more. And, despite our hubris, we will be shaken again. We do not have ultimate control over disease or death, an important lesson that the epidemic teaches those who listen.

Impact of Stigmatization

Clinical Manifestations—
The Cycle of Isolation and Shame

Because of the stigmatization they have encountered, PWAs have been left with few of the social supports that can buffer the stress of illness. Often a gay man who has been diagnosed with AIDS experiences multiple jeopardy. He must not only inform others of his diagnosis, but he may also be put in the position of revealing to others for the first time that he is gay. Both admissions may lead to rejection rather than to the support he sorely needs. He can be perceived as multiply deviant by others: as gay, as diseased, and as a transmitter of death. This may be especially difficult to handle if he is also a member of a stigmatized racial or ethnic minority group.

Being isolated and rejected is brutally damaging to a man who has already experienced rejection and stigmatization because he is gay in a homophobic society. Scar tissue may just have formed over that earlier injury when his sense of self is once more assaulted by further rejection over his AIDS status.

Self-Blame and Self-Punishment

Depending on his stamina, the flexibility of his character, and his defensive style, a gay man may successfully manage this new assault on his self-image (and on his healthy narcissism). The danger is that this assault on a more vulnerable gay man may leave him prone to higher risk behavior. He may try to numb his painful shame by abusing alcohol or drugs (e.g., see discussion in Chapter 19). Or he may seek to break his isolation through sex at any cost. Internalizing a sense of being unworthy of a relationship or of love, he may pursue only anonymous serial partners, accepting any sex offered, and not protect himself enough from what may be harmful, injurious sex. Any of these behaviors are dysfunctional means of staving off the conscious experience of shame. To act otherwise could cause the collapse of this man's denial system, leaving him open to feelings of hopelessness, despair, and depression. His whole sense of self could be jeopardized." As illustrated in Case 1, the stigma of AIDS exacerbates a gay man's underlying issues of shame and hunger for acceptance.

Case 1

Mr. A, a 40-year-old gay man with AIDS, had struggled in his life with feelings of shame, failure, inadequacy, and not being loved. Although many of these issues existed before his AIDS diagnosis, he struggled with them in new ways after he became sick. Although he was an AIDS activist, he was wary of becoming the AIDS "poster child." He continued to search for a deeper understanding of his shame. At a point in his illness when he was losing weight and becoming more apparently sick, he had a pivotal dream. He was on a stage speaking and the people from the audience came onto the stage and touched, caressed, and held him. Mr. A wept when he recognized that the dream was a manifestation of his yearning for love, acceptance, and a place to belong.

Increased Suicidality

For a gay man, suicide can seem to be the only way out of this painful stigmatization and shame. The stigma can tear away all of a man's sense of self-worth. His rage at being rejected by others can be turned against himself. By acting suicidally, the gay man identifies with the social attitude that he and society would be better off if he were dead. (See Chapter 5 on suicide.) Case 2 illustrates a patient's struggle with suicidal thoughts as he faces AIDS and his shame.

Case 2

Mr. B, a 36-year-old gay man, had been in treatment for more than 5 years. He had an early history of suicidality triggered by rage at his abusive parents, a rage that he had turned against himself. When he developed AIDS his suicidal thoughts returned. Although he was able to work through the recurrence of his earlier self-punishing thoughts, the AIDS diagnosis was for him another confirmation of his unworthiness, of the fact that he had no right to live. However, once he faced that core shame, he was able to face his life anew and claim his life for himself. He freed himself from the effects of being rejected by his family, a rejection that was duplicated in his experience of being rejected by society for having AIDS.

Stigma Plus Race

For African American and Latino gay men, the social stigma of having AIDS has yet another dimension of intensity. The public response to basketball star Magic Johnson's disclosure of being HIV positive is a relevant case study. The media and public struggled to integrate Johnson as a champion for AIDS. The racial barrier of his being African American was overcome because of his heroic stature as a star athlete. However, he and others scrambled to wipe out any perception that he could be gay. This is an example of the power of both general social homophobia and the intense homophobia within the African American community.

The sources of isolation and stigma for Latinos and African Americans are multiple: sexual orientation, disease, and race. (See Chapters

15 and 16 on special issues affecting these patient groups.) Their subsequent shame may be all the more lethal unless it is worked through. Because of the stigma and subsequent shame of being gay within a culture that vehemently condemns homosexuality, these men are at an even greater risk for further infection because they disavow being gay and thus deny any need to learn about or practice safer sex (Sullivan 1990).

Bisexual men of any ethnic background are in a similar double bind, being crippled by stigmatization for their sexual orientation and disease status. They may revert to covert, anonymous, or paid sexual encounters where safer sex may not be discussed or practiced.

Gay Youths

The stigma gay men with AIDS experience can frighten gay youths who may already be struggling with their homosexual identity and persuade them to keep their sexuality undisclosed. The development of their sexual identity may be stunted, or they may be forced into furtive, higher risk, sexual outlets. At their age, it is normal for them to believe they are "immortal." It takes enormous efforts by responsible adults to help them deal with the frighteningly real specter of AIDS. The reluctance of our society to teach safer sex to any youths, let alone gay youths, has left the latter in a hotbed of unsafe, impulsive, uninformed sexual expression. The San Francisco AIDS Foundation reported that as many as 40% of San Francisco's 20- to 25-year-old gay-identified men may now be infected with HIV (Odets 1991). We can assume that a large portion of these men were exposed in their teenage years. As illustrated in Case 3, a teenager struggles with the dangerous mix of his homosexual desires and his shame in the age of AIDS.

Case 3

Mr. C, an 18-year-old college student who was in therapy for poor self-esteem because of societal and internalized homophobia and family issues, described seeking sex in anonymous places because of his shame. In so doing, he knew he risked his own safety by becoming vulnerable to gay bashing, sexually transmitted diseases, and AIDS. When asked whether he was currently practicing safer sex, Mr. C stated that he knew the parameters of safer sex but stretched his own safety rules after bouts of drinking.

Stigma and the Threat to the Support System

Social stigma can infect and cripple a gay man's support system as well. Family, friends, and even lovers may be unable to withstand the actual and feared rejection of others. Their own inner issues concerning disease, death, and homosexuality may also surface. For the family, the fear of stigmatization can cut them off from being with their son at a time of mutual need.

In a support group I have led for lovers of gay PWAs, members all too often described abandonment by gay friends. It seems that their friends' internalized homophobia and shame were expressed indirectly in their abandonment of friends who had AIDS. This betrayal is devastating and damaging for all involved. By rejecting his friend with AIDS, the gay man may be projecting onto him his own self-hate, which undercuts his own self-esteem. For a gay PWA, the identification with a peer group of gay men has been hard won. To be rejected and stigmatized by one's own peers is a major loss at a time when everything else is in jeopardy. Feelings of internalized homophobia can resurface for the PWA. The gay man can begin to blame himself for the illness. This is but one example of how the destructive process of blame can threaten the cohesion of the gay community; both HIV-positive or HIV-negative subgroups can scapegoat the other.

Clinical Interventions

Individual Therapy

The impact of stigmatization must be addressed in clinical practice with people affected by HIV. The sensitive clinician can effectively treat the isolation, depression, and damaged self-esteem caused by stigmatization. Acknowledging the gay man's experience and enabling him to ventilate his feelings of loss, oppression, and anger are vital steps in healing his injury.

In any clinical work with gay men (especially gay men with AIDS), the therapist must take an empathic, nurturing stance. The goals of therapy are to help the patient identify the real sources of stigma and nurture a capacity in the gay man to be able to be more empathic toward himself. Just as when treating women, African Americans, or any minority population, the therapist must actively acknowledge and validate the real trauma of stigma. Simply assuming that the patient will discover this source of stigma on his own is tantamount to assuming an abused individual can always sort out the source of abuse. Much of the therapist's work will be in identifying and freeing the patient from his own internalized self-hate and identification with the aggressive, stigmatizing "other."

It is important that the therapist acknowledge and interpret the pain, fear, and self-doubt that the patient experiences as separate from the stigma of disease, death, and homophobia. The patient will often need help distinguishing the multiple sources of stigma. The support and holding provided in therapy can be a lifesaving refuge from the harsh stigma outside. Many of these needs are well described in the self psychology model of therapy (see Chapter 9), but any approach to treatment will be enhanced by an awareness of the dynamics of stigma.

Throughout treatment, the therapist must be vigilant in exploring the patient's sexual behavior in a nonshaming way. For example, when a gay man continues to seek unprotected anal sex, the therapist needs to focus on the reasons for his lack of safety. The therapist must understand the patient's stigma- or shame-based motivations for the behavior but not add to his stigma and shame (see Chapter 20).

The impact of stigma may also appear in more subtle forms within transference and countertransference in therapy. Clinicians are not immune to the impact of the stigma against AIDS. Fear of contagion, death, and homosexuality all have been documented in the countertransference responses of clinicians (Cadwell 1993; Dunkel and Hatfield 1986; see also Section IV in this volume, "Impact on the Therapist"). Fear of the contagion of stigmatization is also important to track. A therapist may worry, Will my practice collapse if I am seen as an AIDS therapist? Will I get any other referrals? Awareness of these anxieties and one's capacity to manage them are critical in clinical work with PWAs. Clinicians' own shame and impulses to distance the one stigmatized may be overwhelming at times. They will need to develop their own means of coping. Just as AIDS patients need support and holding, so do their therapists. (See Chapter 22 on treating patients with empathy.)

The transferential issues are significant. A gay PWA has every reason to be cautious about entering therapy with someone who may have prejudices against him. His fears need to be addressed carefully by the clinician. Some of his fears may be expressed directly; others may come out in the process of deepening the therapeutic relationship. One patient dismissed his erotic transference to me by saying that he avoided any sexual fantasy of me because he felt I could never love him because of his illness. Fundamental here is the therapist's recognition of the inherent imbalance of power in the therapeutic relationship. The patient is bound to fear stigmatization and shaming. Being alert to this inevitable dynamic within the relationship is critical. By addressing the manifestations in the process of the treatment, clinicians can work them through, thus ensuring a safe, holding experience for the gay patient.

Couples Therapy and Family Therapy

Any system that is affected by AIDS will be affected by stigma. Clinical interventions with gay couples in which one or both members are HIV positive must allow them to work through their experience of stigmatization. Are they more isolated as a consequence? How does shame play itself out within the relationship? For example, have they stopped having sex? One gay AIDS patient feared that his lover was using his anger over the messiness of their apartment as an excuse for not bringing friends to their home. He thought the real reason was that his lover was ashamed of the patient's sickness.

Families of gay PWAs also must struggle with stigmatization in their communities. This is especially true of families living in less urban settings in which social and religious values may be heavily antigay and AIDS phobic. These families have to struggle alone with their own misconceptions and the social pressure to disavow their attachment to their son. The clinician's capacity to establish a safe, educative relationship in which the family members can explore and work through their homophobic issues is critical. Otherwise, further stigma and isolation will hamper their ability to truly care for their gay son or brother infected with HIV. (See Chapter 13 on AIDS patients returning home to small communities.)

Group Therapy and Support Groups

Support groups are a tremendous resource for gay men struggling with the stigmatization of the AIDS epidemic. The therapist can play a vital role in making patients aware of this resource and helping them over their initial reluctance to join these groups. Addressing a patient's fears about going public and risking stigmatization by the group is important. Once the patient joins the group, the group facilitator has the responsibility for ensuring his fit in the group and helping the group adhere to its task of support. Negotiating a consistent focus on support issues and averting the pull to become engaged in deeper therapy are critical for the safety of a support group.

No matter through what behavior the virus was transmitted, all people infected with HIV struggle with stigmatization. Every member of a support group that I facilitated for HIV-positive patients described how difficult it was to acknowledge their HIV status publicly. They concealed their status because of the fear and prejudice they had seen PWAs experience. They also realized that, by disclosing their status, they would have to contend with their own internalized doubts about guilt, homophobia, and the fear of death. With courage and commitment, they decided to come forth to support one another in this crisis. In this new context, they would not be made lepers. They found strength in establishing their own subgroup. The clinician can build on the power of healing social experience by heightening awareness and access to such organizations.

Group psychotherapy can also be a vital forum for addressing stigmatization and shame. Helping group members identify the social function of stigmatization, examine their own internalized stigma, feel the redirection and support offered in a group, and experience the catharsis of their pain and shame is all part of the healing in group therapy. These activities are an especially powerful antidote to the isolation and shame, and can be an empowering place of belonging. (See Chapter 11 on special issues in group therapy for gay men with AIDS.)

Beyond Therapy: Political Strategies

Just as other stigmatized groups have had to struggle against stigma and shame, gay men and PWAs have organized and gained power to combat stigmatization. Affiliation with the gay rights movement can be affirming for the gay man faced with the disempowering force of social stigma.

The movement by persons with AIDS to claim their own title— *PWAs*—is a self-empowering expression of resistance to social pressure to conform to the constricted roles of compliant "good patients" or "helpless victims." The acronym is reminiscent of *POWs,* and the similarity in the experience of these groups is ominous. Both have engaged in war, and both have felt the shackles of prison. In the case of PWAs, both the war and the prison are here at home.

The activist PWA group called "ACT UP!" is an empowering expression of the will of the group not to be categorized as victims, not to be "spoiled" by stigma. As one PWA relates,

> Not buying into the victim mindset is keeping me alive. To me "victim" implies helplessness and passivity. At this time in my illness, I am not helpless and I am anything but passive in dealing with it. I can look around and I see incredibly courageous men who inspire me with their strength. These men continue to defy the odds and say "No!" to AIDS. They give me hope and strength. (Haney 1988, p. 253)

Stigmatization Sets the Stage for Discrimination

For gay men, the struggle with discrimination is not new. The fact that consenting homosexual acts are still illegal in most states has paved the way for discrimination in housing and employment. AIDS has made gay men even easier targets for discrimination. For example, health and life insurance companies use the HIV-antibody test as a means to screen applicants who might be in risk categories. The prospect of losing fundamental rights is particularly stressful for gay PWAs. Given the background of stigmatization, gay men have every reason to fear mandatory testing. They already have ample evidence of discrimination, the lack of compassionate care, and isolation from the social community.

Implications for Social Policy

Understanding stigmatization and its negative impact on gay PWAs, policymakers must be careful to uncover discriminatory policies and develop more protective policies for PWAs. Health and life insurance, HIV testing, housing rights, family law, employees' rights, immigration, right to free travel, AIDS education, and disability laws are some of the policy areas in which gay PWAs' needs and rights are often violated (Gostin 1990). A glaring example is that the message put forth in some AIDS prevention materials is tempered by a policy of not directly promoting or encouraging homosexual activities. At this late date in the epidemic, educational messages continue to be determined by morality and politics, and not exclusively by public health needs. The government must be compelled to overcome political impediments to funding AIDS education in the gay community. If not, preventable infection will occur.

Another example of discrimination is the futility of the policies that control immigration and travel for persons with AIDS or HIV infection. These policies have clearly affected International AIDS Conference efforts, thereby inhibiting progress in the science of AIDS (Sherer 1990).

AIDS-related discrimination is also found in access to and reimbursement for health care services. An example of limited access is the insufficient number of long-term beds available to care for the AIDS patients (Sherer 1990). An example of insurance discrimination is found in employers who limit or eliminate health care coverage for the disease. In Texas, John McGann learned he had contracted AIDS in 1987. At the time he informed his employer of his status, his employer provided an insurance plan with lifetime medical benefits of up to $1 million. Some months after McGann's disclosure, his employer changed the provisions of the health plan, reducing the benefits to a $5,000 ceiling on AIDS-related costs but not on costs of any other catastrophic illness. McGann, whose $5,000 of coverage ran out in early 1990, died in 1991. In March 1992, the executor of his estate filed an appeal with the Supreme Court and in the autumn of 1992, the U.S. Supreme Court judged the radically reduced benefits *legal*.

Progress has been made in some areas of AIDS-related policy, such as in the workplace. The right of employees with AIDS or HIV infection to remain on the job has been repeatedly upheld by the courts. Persistent efforts to educate legislators, judges, and those in the workplace have had an impact. More advocacy and education are critical to ensure more freedom from discrimination for gay PWAs.

Conclusions

As clinicians we should create a safe place in which the gay PWA can know himself more fully in the face of the oppressive stigmatization of society. Within the safety of therapy, the patient can begin to address and overcome his shame. He can realize the source of the shame—both inside and outside of himself—and become free. This freedom is the essence of successful therapy.

In the larger social context, as clinicians we can identify stigmatization as a dysfunctional and destructive social reaction to the uncontrollable realities of difference, sexuality, disease, and death. We can work to foster better ways of managing irrational fears. Once people face their fears and their mortality, they may be able to embrace diversity with hope, courage, and integrity, and not with hate, fear, anxiety, and despair. They then will be less apt to abuse power and overwhelm others with projection, blame, and victimization.

The societal definition of our collective humanity is being tested by the AIDS crisis and showing new levels of deficiency. As Tony Ferrara, a PWA, said early in the epidemic:

> To those of you not afflicted goes the task of ensuring that our cause
> is not forgotten by the politicians and civic leaders responsible for

allocating funds to carry on the research that feeds our hopes. . . . It is up to you to correct the public's misperception, fostered by often insensitive media representation, that all AIDS patients are ignoble people who are undeserving of attention, let alone the benefits of a worldwide quest to save them from a devastating disease. We are not bad people. We are merely gay, and that is no reason to regard us with disdain. Those of us physically unable to carry on this message look to you for champions. (Ferrara 1984, p. 1287)

Tony Ferrara died from AIDS-related illnesses on 4 June 1984. The pain in his voice still rings clear as raw testimony of the stigma he fought and that gay PWAs continue to fight. Others succumb to the isolation and depression that stigma can cause. The rate of impulsive suicide among PWAs is staggering (see Chapter 5 on suicide). One study showed the rate to be 66 times the rate of suicide in the general population (Marzuk et al. 1988). Case 4 illustrates the fatal combination of stigma, shame, homosexuality, and HIV.

Case 4

Three weeks after testing positive for HIV, Mr. D, who was in his 30s, was referred to me by his sister. He never made contact with me. After he was reported missing for 24 hours, his father called to tell me that he had been found dead. He had hung himself. In subsequent family meetings, we sifted through the family pain and attempted to piece together this man's pain. He could not bear the stigma of AIDS. He also could not bear the admission of his homosexuality. Now his family was left to fight the stigma he could not.

The war against AIDS has many fronts. Clearly, one of the most challenging is the battle against social stigmatization. We must recognize the degree of stigma that our gay AIDS patients experience and work to heal their wounds. On a policy level, we must be ready to both expose stigmatizing policies and develop more protective policies for PWAs.

We have found the enemy, and again it is us: our prejudice and our penchant to create scapegoats to blame. If there is an opportunity for good in the war against AIDS, it is that we can develop healthy relationships that are more humane and capable of embracing differences. We may then truly heal ourselves and our social disease. At our worst, we become perpetrators and create scapegoats out of our cowardice. At our best, we face the truth of our reality—our fears and joys in life and death—with courage.

References

Bartlett E: Scientists condemn findings in AIDS book. The Boston Globe, March 3, 1988, p 77

Becker E: The Denial of Death. New York, Free Press, 1973

Boffey P: Spread of AIDS abating, but deaths will soar. The New York Times, February 14, 1988, p 1

Brandt A: The syphilis epidemic and its relation to AIDS. Science 239:375–380, 1988

Cadwell S: Issues of identification for gay psychotherapists in their treatment of gay clients with HIV spectrum disorder: special vulnerability and its management. Journal of Gay and Lesbian Psychotherapy 2:78–100, 1994

Douglas M: Purity and Danger. London, Penguin, 1967

Dunkel J, Hatfield S: Countertransference issues in working with persons with AIDS. Soc Work 31:114–117, 1986

Ferrara A: My personal experience with AIDS. Am Psychol 30:1285–1287, 1984

Freud S: Mourning and melancholia (1917), in The Standard Edition of the Complete Psychological Works of Sigmund Freud, Vol 4. Translated and edited by Strachey J. London, Hogarth Press, 1950, pp 285–296

Friedson E: The Profession of Medicine. New York, Dodd Mead, 1984

Gilman S, Nelkin D: Placing blame for devastating disease. Paper delivered at the New School Conference on Plague, at the New School for Social Research, New York, January 15, 1988

Goffman E: Stigma: Notes on the Management of Spoiled Identity. Englewood Cliffs, NJ, Prentice-Hall, 1963

Gostin L: The AIDS Litigation Project. JAMA 263:1961–1972, 1990

Haney P: Providing empowerment to the person with AIDS. Soc Work 33:251–253, 1988

Lasch C: The Culture of Narcissism. New York, Norton, 1979

Lemert E: Human Deviance, Social Problems, and Social Control. Englewood Cliffs, NJ, Prentice-Hall, 1967

Lifton R: The Broken Connection. New York, Basic Books, 1979

Marzuk PM, Tierney H, Tardiff K, et al: Increased risk of suicide in persons with AIDS. JAMA 259:1333–1337, 1988

Ryan W: Blaming the Victim. New York, Pantheon, 1971

Sherer R: AIDS policy into the 1990s. JAMA 263:1972–1974, 1990

Shilts R: And the Band Played On. New York, St. Martin's Press, 1987

Siegel K: AIDS: the social dimension. Psychiatric Annals 16:168–172, 1986

Chapter 2

Impact of AIDS on Adult Gay Male Development: Implications for Psychotherapy

Rhonda Linde, Ph.D.

Acquired immunodeficiency syndrome (AIDS) is a devastating disease, not only because it eventually leads to death, but also because it wreaks physical, emotional, social, and financial havoc on an individual's life. It deforms and wastes the body, liquidates one's financial assets, depletes one's social network through fear or attrition, and exposes the infected individual to isolation and rejection. Throughout the course of the disease, independent and productive individuals are forced to become increasingly dependent on others for their care. Even in the earlier, asymptomatic stages of the illness, infected individuals live with the amorphous threat of AIDS hanging over their heads, which influences decisions about every aspect of their lives. Because most of those who are infected with the human immunodeficiency virus (HIV) are between the ages of 20 and 50, they are forced to deal prematurely with developmental issues that normally would occur later in their lives. Those issues will vary depending on the individual's age and the stage of the disease. Psychotherapy can be an effective tool to help the infected individual cope with these converging developmental tasks.

In order to understand the impact of AIDS on the life cycle of a gay male, it is necessary to conceptualize the developmental issues involved. The literature on homosexual development has focused mainly on the "coming out" process of gay identity formation (Cass 1979; Coleman 1981–1982; Hanley-Hackenbruck 1989), a process that can be applied to different chronological ages. The few authors who have addressed age-related developmental issues for gay males have focused on either adolescent (Gonsiorek 1988; Malyon 1981; Zera 1992) or aging (Kimmel 1978) populations. In his book *The Seasons of a Man's Life,* Levinson (1978) presented a model that can be applied to gay male development and the subsequent impact of AIDS on that process. Kimmel (1978) applied his own research on aging gay men to Levinson's model as a way of refuting the myth that older gay men are tragic figures, lonely and depressed. He did not, however, elaborate on his data in a way that was clinically relevant to developmental issues.

Levinson's Model of Male Development

Levinson (1978) presented a chronological spectrum of the developmental issues men face as they go through the life cycle. His work was based on a study conducted from 1968 to 1973 in which 40 men were interviewed. Although Levinson's work reflected the social biases of that era (heterosexuality and traditional gender role values), his concepts remain relevant. Levinson's spectrum covers a process of evolution through several stages of fairly stable developmental *life structures,* which are connected by transitional periods. During each stable period the task is to change the old life structure by making choices about goals and values. Transitional periods allow the individual to "terminate the existing structure and create the possibility for a new one" (Levinson 1978, p. 49) by questioning and reappraising the existing structure and exploring new possibilities for change.

Childhood and Adolescence (Ages 0–17)

Although Levinson (1978) began his discussion with the postadolescent years, it is important to keep in mind that adolescence is a time of "identity versus identity confusion" (Erikson 1950). It is a time to form an initial or provisional sense of self based on one's identification with one's familial and peer role models. Levinson defined *adolescence* as *pre-adult* because life remains centered on family and peer groups and "adult figures are authority figures, helpers, and enemies but not peers" (Levinson 1978, p. 74).

Early Adulthood (Ages 17–40)

Generally in early adulthood, especially from ages 20 to 30, a man is at the peak of his physical and mental abilities. It is a time when he forms a preliminary adult identity by making his first choices about occupation, relationships, residence, and style of living. Although a man of 40 has not lost much in terms of physical and mental abilities, there are cosmetic changes that remind the 40-year-old man of bodily decline that the 20- or 30-year-old man cannot even anticipate.

Early Adult Transition (Ages 17–22)

The main task of a man's early adult transition period is to form a preliminary adult identity and separate from his family of origin by removing "the family from the center of his life" (Levinson 1978, p. 75). This might entail a physical move to a new home, establishing an independent source of income, and giving up the adolescent peer group. With increased distance from the family comes an internal differentiation from parents involving a reduction in emotional dependence on parental support and authority. This is a gradual process. Remaining internally tied to his family in some ways, the young adult male does not want to separate prematurely. This period is a time for the young man to explore his fantasies, experiment with options, and begin to make commitments in a provisional way. Marriage at this point may facilitate this transition.

Entering the Adult World (Ages 22–28)

The task of the next period is for the young adult male to build the first adult life structure around his preliminary choices, while keeping "his options open, avoiding strong commitments" (Levinson 1978, p.

79). He may yet have some major adventures as he continues to shape his life. He must find an appropriate place between the extremes of transient rootlessness and premature commitment without alternatives (Levinson 1978, p. 58).

Age 30 Transition (Ages 28–33)

The task of this period is for a young man to change his initial life structure. Life becomes more serious, more real. This is a time to modify life to include important things still missing from life before it is too late. It is also a time to anticipate the upcoming stable period of greater adult responsibility.

The major tasks of the above two stages (ages 22 to 33)can be summarized as follows:

1. *Forming a dream.* The dream refers to the kind of life the individual wants to lead as an adult. The task involves defining the dream and "finding ways to live it out" (Levinson 1978, p. 91).
2. *Forming a mentor relationship.* Mentors are transitional figures who serve as teachers, sponsors, and guides, and who support the realization of the dream. These mentors are typically slightly older than the individual and serve as parental figures.
3. *Forming an occupation.* This involves not only choosing an occupation but also "acquiring skills, values and credentials" (Levinson 1978, p. 102) and beginning to establish an occupational identity with a corresponding niche in the occupational world.
4. *Forming love relationships, marriage, and family.* The task is to form enduring relationships with both men and women that are based on one's adult identity and needs.

Settling Down (Ages 32–41)

A man's second adult life structure is established around "becoming one's own man" (Levinson 1978, p. 60). It is a time to invest oneself in the major aspect of one's life: "work, family, friendships, leisure, community—whatever is most central" (Levinson 1978, p. 59). It is also a time to realize youthful goals.

Middle Adulthood (Ages 40–60)

The central task of this phase is to come to terms with one's own mortality and assess whether one's life has meaning. By this point in life, it is very hard to be blind to the physical manifestations of the aging process.

Mid-Life Transition (Ages 40–45)

The mid-life transition period presents an individual with the following tasks:

1. *Reappraising the past.* A man in this stage reappraises the life structure of the prior "settling down" period in the light of the awareness of his mortality. He asks himself, What have I done with my life? Where is the dream I had? It is a time of "de-illusionment" (Levinson 1978, p. 192), of seeing whether his life is based on fantasies and whether the old beliefs about himself and the world are true.
2. *Modifying the life structure.* If the course of life is downhill from age 40, then a man must change what he does not like while he still can. Some people dramatically restructure their lives, ending marriages and changing occupations. Others modify existing structures to adjust to the new realities of maturing children and aging parents.
3. *Enhanced individuation.* By this point in life a man is expected to have a strong sense of self and to operate in the world with confidence.

Middle Adulthood (Ages 45–60)

Once in middle adulthood, a man has to negotiate and build a new life structure around the following developmental issues:

1. *Changes in biological and psychological functioning.* There is a gradual diminishing of physical and mental capacity. Biological drives no longer predominate and are better integrated. A man must accept the fact that life changes and mourn for the loss of his youth.

2. *The sequence of the generations.* The task here is "to assume responsibility for new generations of adults, . . . becoming parental in new ways to younger adults" (Levinson 1978, p. 29). A man may have to reverse roles with his parents and become their caretaker. Erikson (1950) called the challenge for this period as one of "generativity versus stagnation." Foreseeing death, the person in middle life can either surrender to stagnation and despair or struggle creatively towards generativity.

3. *Evolving career and enterprises.* The 40s are a time to review the progress of life. Because the middle years are those in which an individual has the most power and the highest level of achievement, changes sought must be made soon for the adjustment of goals and visions to have more meaning and success in reality.

4. *Modifying long-term relationships.* By middle age, the resolution of identity conflicts allows a man to be more intimate. It is a time to step back and assess whether relationships are satisfying.

Late Adulthood (Ages 65–80)

By age 60, a man's bodily decline is evident. He increasingly finds that his peers and family become seriously ill and die. Having fewer responsibilities, he is less interested in societal rewards and more interested in his own inner resources and creativity (Levinson 1978, p. 36). "The developmental task is . . . to sustain his youthfulness in a new form appropriate to late adulthood" (Levinson 1978, p. 35). He must maintain more of an internal sense of youthfulness. Erikson (1950) labeled this period as one of the struggle between "integrity versus despair." As Levinson put it, if during a self-appraisal at this stage a man can find "meaning and value in his life, however imperfect, he can come to terms with death" (Levinson 1978, p. 37).

Late-Late Adulthood (Age 80 and Older)

In late-late adulthood, a man may be preoccupied with bodily needs and personal comforts. His world narrows and he has only a few relationships. "In the end he has only the self and the crucial internal figures it has brought into being. He must come finally to terms with the self, knowing it and loving it reasonably well, and being ready to give it up" (Levinson 1978, p. 39).

Gay Male Development

Although much of what Levinson describes can be applied to the gay male, the difficulties of growing up and being gay in modern society impact the gay male's developmental process. Societal prejudice and the resulting internalized homophobia can impede and delay developmental progress in some areas and foster a more rapid development in others.

In its most basic meaning, *coming out* refers to the process by which a man acknowledges to himself and others that he is homosexual. It represents the first time he recognizes this, the first time he tells someone, and the countless other times he tries to integrate the fact that he is gay into the daily fabric of his life. Most heterosexual people do not question their sexual orientation throughout their lives. They may never have questioned it or, at different developmental stages, may question issues related to it. For example, as a woman approaches menopause she may question her femininity, or as a man enters middle age he may question his masculinity; however, these self-appraisals probably do not entail a reworking of sexual orientation per se. This is not the case with gay men. Different developmental milestones and different situations stimulate second and third periods of questioning or reworking acceptance of gay men's sexual orientation. Each time a gay man is confronted with gay-related prejudice or discrimination, at some level there is the thought, If I weren't gay this wouldn't be happening, or, Straight people don't have to go through this. It would be easier if I were straight. In addition, whereas the world has rituals to mark and celebrate developmental milestones for heterosexual individuals (e.g., marriages, engagements, births, bar mitzvahs), it has none for gay individuals, thus leaving these individuals feeling excluded and unacknowledged. These issues are reexperienced as the biological clock ticks for gay men. For example, the issue of having children raises questions about what it would be like to bring them up in a straight home versus a gay home, and what society's reaction to gay parenting would be. People rework these issues over and over again, striving to find a comfortable place in their gay identity as new situations present themselves. Although occasional self-examination and soul-searching are good and foster growth and change, constant reexamination and reaffirmation of something so basic to the core of one's being are counterproductive.

Adolescence

Malyon (1981) eloquently described the additional roadblocks that gay adolescents must face during this very trying developmental time. Adolescent identity formation relies on extensive experimentation. Teenagers try out different behaviors and personae on a trial-and-error basis, searching for themselves. Both separation from family of origin and the establishment of new primary love relationships require intense social involvement with others. Due to the "antipathy associated with homosexuality, many critical social experiences are not available to homosexual adolescents. For example, their most charged sexual desires are seen as perverted, and their deepest feelings of psychological attachment are regarded as unacceptable" (Malyon 1981, p. 326). There are few activities or institutions available to gay youth, leaving them isolated from gay peers, alienated from heterosexual peers, and not yet part of the adult gay community. Gay adolescents are left with the perplexing dilemma in which they must

> Complete the developmental process in a hostile and psychologically impoverished heterosexual social environment or must decide to seek peer support and social opportunities in the homosexual community. Neither alternative is very satisfactory. The decision to remain in the heterosexual community nearly always results in estrangement and confusion. A move into the homosexual community precipitates a separation from parents, and requires premature assumption of adult responsibilities and social roles. (Malyon 1981, p. 328)

It is quite difficult for heterosexual teens to make it through adolescence unscathed and ready to form healthy love relationships.

Straight male adolescents have to struggle with forming an identity based on the accepted norms of what it means to be a man. Gay youths face the additional roadblocks of external and internalized homophobia as they attempt to come out as homosexual individuals and form healthy peer and love relationships. Straight male adolescents have their fathers and other straight male role models with whom to identify. Gay adolescents must fend for themselves without respected gay male figures to serve as examples. They must overcome considerable societal hatred and self-hatred simply to label themselves as "gay." They must face the real possibility of rejection by their families and peers if they openly disclose their sexual orientation. These are some of the reasons why many people delay the coming out process, isolate themselves from the culture in which they grew up, or lead double lives. In any of these ways, the coming out process may disrupt and delay the developmental milestones Levinson described.

Early Adulthood (Ages 17–40)

Gay men may or may not proceed through early adulthood along Levinson's timetables. Some gay men are so distressed by their homosexuality that they either automatically repress it or consciously decide to suppress it. These men may marry young in an attempt to deal with their feelings. Although on the surface they may appear to follow Levinson's model, their lives could fall apart as they enter middle age and experience their children leaving home. Other gay men may find the world so hostile that it is easier for them never to leave home. They may avoid the issue of adult object choices and never alter old familial ties. Gay men in these two groups have great difficulty forming positive, integrated identities. For some, this may inhibit the ability to think of themselves positively in other arenas, compromising, for example, efforts to find careers that are gratifying. For others, unexpressed libidinal energies may be invested in work to the exclusion of social and intimate relationships.

For many gay men, coming out delays some of the tasks of late adolescence into early adulthood. They may have to delay sexual experimentation until leaving home. The development of peer relationships may be delayed because of feeling "different" during adolescence. Adolescent socialization and dating, which form the basis for later, more mature relationships, frequently occur during early adulthood or even later for gay men. There are many reasons why a segment of the gay male community appears not to develop many lasting primary love relationships. Without early examples of gay male intimacy and male coupling, there is no early model comparable with what heterosexual men internalize as their ideal. It is only much later in the gay man's development that he may cognitively and then affectively create such an internalized ideal. In addition, there is no societal support for gay relationships, resulting in few models for committed relationships. There are no societal institutions or rituals such as marriage for fostering lasting relationships. On the contrary, society labels homosexual coupling as wrong and promotes the stereotype of gay men as promiscuous and sexually abusive of young boys. Further, it is more acceptable for men in this society to play the field sexually. Whereas women are socialized to be "attachers" and emotional, men are expected to be individually oriented and nonemotional. Gay male couples, then, are subject to the effects of this socialization.

Because of this projected male sex role, the sexual revolution of the 1960s, and the lack of nonsexual gay male institutions available prior to the last decade, a gay male ethos initially developed in which sex was split from intimacy. For some men this was a perfectly acceptable way of life, and they experienced no desire to settle down with one person. Other men established long-term relationships that eventually became quasi-platonic and nonmonogamous. Another segment of the gay male community appeared to follow Levinson's model of establishing long-term monogamous relationships. Some men did this early and others later. Those who did settle down later were simply in step with the increasingly common heterosexual practice of waiting until the late 30s to make a lasting commitment.

Middle Adulthood (Ages 40–60)

For some gay men, developmental issues during middle adulthood are identical to those for heterosexual men. It is a time to reexamine and assess the value of both career and relationships. For example, a gay man may buy a house with his significant other, plan for retirement, make out a will, and take other legal steps to institutionalize his relationship.

For gay men who have built much of their self-esteem on being physically attractive, middle age presents a crisis of identity and social interaction. They may feel increasingly rejected and abandoned for their lack of physical attractiveness. The task for these men is to redefine their own self-worth. They may also have to learn new ways of relating to other men that are not based primarily on an ideal of youthful sexual attractiveness.

Late Adulthood (Age 60 and Older)

The gay man in this phase of life may have to revisit some of the conflicts he confronted in adolescence as he once again becomes dependent on a society that sees him as unacceptable. Because there usually are no community services for elder gay individuals, they must retire to straight retirement homes and communities where homophobic stigma may again isolate and inhibit them. When the appropriate developmental task is to integrate one's self with one's life, the elder gay male is once again thrust into a dependent position within a hostile environment, often retreating to the safety of invisibility (Kimmel 1978).

Impact of AIDS on Gay Male Adult Development and Related Therapy Issues

Positive Impact

Even given the horror and destruction of AIDS, there are several ways in which dealing with this disease actually spurs some gay men along with their developmental tasks. First, the threat of AIDS often incites a gay man to reevaluate his life. This self-examination may lead to personal growth if the developmental crises are successfully negotiated. Often people do not take the time to assess whether their lives are fulfilling. The specter of AIDS affords some gay men the opportunity to make productive changes. It gives them the chance to focus on the overall quality of life.

Second, the realities of AIDS have led gay men to begin using traditional instruments for protecting their possessions and partners (e.g., wills, powers of attorney, and life insurance policies). This process of preparing for their death, whether from AIDS or another cause, in turn facilitates their developmental progress by allowing them to acknowledge the serious threat of the disease, as well as their responsibility toward their partner, and also marks certain developmental milestones for them. Using these also adds further stability and legitimacy to gay relationships.

Third, AIDS has caused many gay men to reexamine the role of sex in their relationships and has encouraged some to integrate sex with more intimacy. It has also forced the gay community to develop nonsexual institutions, such as service organizations and activity-centered clubs, as alternatives to sexually oriented bars and bathhouses. This gives gay men the chance to experience more of their total selves in a safe, nonsexual, gay environment.

Negative Impact

For the most part, AIDS has completely disrupted the gay male life cycle. It has forced gay men to deal with developmental issues that do not normally confront others in a similar age bracket. In some cases it fosters regression and in others a leap to subsequent developmental phases.

The overriding general issue is prematurely facing death and loss. Although probably no one is ever ready to die, people in Levinson's last stage of development are more apt to be ready than someone at age 30. People need time and the experience of living to be able to accept death. In Levinson's model, one has not typically thought of death as it relates to the self before the age of 40, unless one has experienced a near-death trauma or the death of loved ones. A 40-year-old man still has many years ahead. Because the majority of the gay men who have AIDS are between the ages of 20 and 50, they have much psychological aging to do to be ready to accept illness and death. One needs to have achieved the stage of becoming a senior member of society during middle age to be able to reflect on professional accomplishments and relationships. The gradual, yet perceptible decline of physical capabilities and appearance gives individuals the opportunity over the course of time to accept change and aging in a way that is not sudden and traumatic. Before reaching this stage, one still thinks in terms of what could be rather than what is or what has passed. It is more difficult to let go psychologically of something one still has not achieved or is still searching for than something one has already accomplished.

In the next section I examine some of these issues and give examples of how they are manifested in the course of therapy.

Illness and Development

The age of the individual and his stage of HIV illness determine the quality and magnitude of the conflict between his chronological age and the developmental issues he faces. A gay man who is HIV positive and either physically asymptomatic or not severely symptomatic has decisions to make about how to proceed with his life. Does he go on with business as usual or does he automatically act as if he were 65 years old and ready to retire? Does he date and look for a long-term partner? When does he tell a dating partner that he is positive? Does he continue his demanding graduate program or does he take his savings and travel to Europe in order to fulfill a lifelong dream? Does he put the issue of being HIV positive on the back burner of denial or does he focus on it in anticipation of its consequences? Certainly, the age of the individual and where he is in accomplishing his dream greatly influence how he answers these questions.

In my clinical practice, I have found that these dilemmas present me with difficult decisions about therapeutic strategy. I am caught between continuing with the long-term issues on which I have been working with the patient, and switching to more focused, supportive work concerning grief and acceptance of death. It is not easy to know when the albatross of HIV seropositivity is the principal, overriding reality, and when a patient is using it as a way of resisting moving on with life. In the next section I outline the different clinical issues that apply to the various stages of HIV infection, and in the following section discuss how they can be manifested at different developmental stages. I also present several case examples that illustrate these issues.

Clinical Issues at Different Stages of HIV Awareness

Status Unknown: Deciding Whether to Get Tested

The decision to be tested or not to be tested is one that challenges a person's defensive structure and coping skills. It begins with the need to assess realistically one's risk status and behavior, a process inevitably affected by psychological defenses and beliefs. An individual who relies heavily on denial as a defense mechanism may allow this denial to cloud his assessment of prior behavior and lead him to think he is not at risk and therefore not in need of being tested. On the other hand, an individual who feels very guilty about his homosexual behavior may overestimate his risk and interpret a negative HIV test result as an indication of his "goodness," or a positive result as punishment for his acts. For most people, except for those in acute denial, this is a period of extreme anxiety. Those who have an intellectualized defensive structure may feel better knowing the result of the test, even if it is positive. Others who feel endangered by the possibility of a positive result may prefer not to know so that they can hold on to some ray of hope that they are HIV negative. The job of the therapist is to assess the patient's defensive structure and accordingly help him more realistically assess the pros and cons of testing, as well as to anticipate his reaction to hearing the results. (See also Chapter 8 on testing.)

Finding Out Test Results

Discovering that one is HIV negative may be a double-edged sword. On one level there may be relief and, for most people, a feeling that they have a new lease on life. The therapeutic challenge here is to help the individual maintain safer sexual behaviors. The other side of the sword involves dealing with the mixed blessings of surviving in a community that has been devastated by AIDS. On a basic level, the work involves helping the patient navigate through a series of deaths of friends and lovers. There is perpetual grief as layer after layer of the patient's supportive social network crumbles. For some people, being a survivor also means having *survivor guilt* (i.e., feeling guilty for being HIV negative when so many loved ones are HIV positive [Fishman and Linde 1983]). The therapeutic task is to help the patient understand all of the underlying issues contributing to the guilt and to manage the feelings in a safe way. These patients are vulnerable to depression and may unconsciously seek to join their HIV-positive friends either by sabotaging their own success in life or by putting themselves at risk for infection. (See Chapter 21 on survivor guilt.)

Discovering that one is HIV positive may cause extreme panic. Some individuals take the news to mean that their death is imminent. Others become acutely suicidal as they have not anticipated or prepared for this possibility. The task in therapy is to help the individual slow down and adjust to the reality of his medical situation. Usually, if the patient is physically asymptomatic and tests positive, he has time to adjust to his diagnosis before acute illness sets in.

Adjusting to Being Positive and Physically Asymptomatic

Those who get tested soon after infection may experience a long period of health before symptoms appear. If their T cell counts remain high, there may be no actual intrusion of HIV into their daily lives. The task is to help them decide how to live their lives with the knowledge that somewhere down the road they will become somatically symptomatic. They will have to decide how to approach decisions about career, relationships, sex, and recreational time. Some men, once having set these general parameters, are able to put HIV on a back burner and not preoccupy themselves with it on a daily basis. Others, however, always live in the shadow of HIV even though they are physically asymptomatic. They may become mired in the uncertainty of the disease's progression and unable to find a comfortable way to live with the infection.

When T Cell Count Drops to 500

Although still physically asymptomatic, an individual who is HIV infected may be required to deal more actively with his condition when
his T cell count drops to 500. This is the point at which most medical
providers believe that some preventive action must be taken. A decision must be made about taking antiviral medication. This event can
be a major assault on denial. Patients who need to maintain their denial may decide not to begin antiviral treatment. In contrast, those
who decide to begin treatment will be reminded of their infection
every time they take their next pill. They may also have to deal with
disturbing side effects. Sometimes hard decisions have to be made
whether or not to continue treatment in the face of severe side effects.
At other times, the side effects of medication mimic immunosuppressive symptomatology and must be coped with as such.

When T Cell Count Drops Below
500 and Some Symptoms Occur

An individual is much more susceptible to opportunistic infections,
especially Pneumocystis carinii pneumonia (PCP), when his T cell
count drops below 500. Prophylaxis for various opportunistic infections is usually initiated at this point. The patient's anxiety often increases as he realizes he is more vulnerable to opportunistic infections
and that his T cell decline has not been checked. Obviously, the appearance of a symptom raises anxiety; the severity of that anxiety depends on the nature of the symptom, whether it interferes with
functioning and enjoyment, and the symbolic meaning it has to the
individual with regard to prognosis.

First Diagnosis With Kaposi's
Sarcoma or PCP or First Hospitalization

For most patients, being diagnosed as having Kaposi's sarcoma or PCP
signifies they have AIDS. Although a patient's first bout with one of
these illnesses may be mild and he may quickly resume his prior level
of functioning, he usually also experiences a profound shift in his

emotional state. Even though the patient has been living with the knowledge that he is infected with HIV, he had not yet been diagnosed as having AIDS. Now he must adjust to the notion that he does, in fact, have AIDS, and he must integrate this into his identity.

The first hospitalization generally has the same impact as, and in many cases may coincide with, the first diagnosis of AIDS. It brings the added reality of the constraints of hospitalization: feeling out of control, feeling helpless, and being dependent. Furthermore, being hospitalized can frighten one with thoughts of terminal illness, the process of dying, and death.

End-Stage Illness

The final stages of AIDS may precipitate physical deterioration so profound that extreme weakness or paralysis confines a person to bed, sometimes without muscle, bladder, or bowel control. Mental deterioration may be as mild as forgetfulness or as severe as dementia. The major psychological issues involved at this stage of the disease are adjusting to increasing dependence on others and approaching death. Often the primary task in therapy is to help the patient adjust to relying on others. His anger and frustration must be addressed. It also means helping the patient tie up loose ends, both concretely (e.g., wills and living wills) and emotionally (e.g., reviewing his life and coming to peace with what has been done and what will be left undone).

Interaction of Stage of HIV Infection
With Patient's Developmental Stage

There is an interaction between a patient's stage of HIV infection and his developmental phase: the developmental phase affects the perception of and ability to cope with each stage of HIV illness, and the stage of illness greatly impacts the course of personal development.

HIV infection forces young and middle-aged adults either into a regression to preadolescent dependence on their family or into a fast-forward movement into late-late adulthood in which preoccupation with bodily functions and personal comfort prevail. In either case, these men are forced into situations that are developmentally inappro- priate, without having time to help ease the transition.

Fear of Becoming HIV Infected at Any Developmental Stage

Regardless of the gay male's developmental stage, the specter of HIV infection may delay his coming out. He may either be frightened of becoming infected and feel inhibited in being sexual, or incorporate societal prejudice against gay males and AIDS and experience an over- whelming surge of internalized self-hatred.

The fear of AIDS may keep some adolescents and men from com- ing out of the closet for a long period of time or forever, which in turn can delay their personal development. If one is fearful of becoming or is infected with HIV because of gay sexual activity, internalized homo- phobia may resurface, which makes it much more difficult to form a positive gay identity. If a gay male who has not previously disclosed his sexual orientation plans on being tested or has symptoms of HIV infection, he may be forced to come out to health and social service providers before he is developmentally ready to do so (Fishman and Linde 1983). If individuals who are ill need the support of their fam- ilies, they may have to face the double whammy of coming out to families as both gay and HIV positive at the same time. They may not be psychologically ready to do this, but may be forced to do so by the severity of their illness.

The fear of AIDS forces people already out of the closet to rework coming out issues. The thought, If I didn't have homosexual sex, I wouldn't be at risk for AIDS, intrudes. Individuals who grew up in religious households are especially vulnerable to reexperiencing a surge of guilt at being gay and at being sexual in the face of AIDS. The fear and guilt may be so extreme that they send more vulnerable males back into the closet.

The fear of AIDS may interfere with forming relationships as well. Individuals who are HIV negative may be so scared of becoming in- fected that they avoid all sexual contact. Individuals who are HIV pos- itive may also avoid contact out of fear of infecting others or out of fear of rejection. HIV complicates already intricate human relationships by making sex a life-and-death matter.

HIV Infection and Early Adulthood Developmental Issues

Men in early adulthood must travel the farthest developmentally in dealing with HIV-related illness. Young adults often have no hint of the experience of mortality. They are fearless, believing that illness and death have nothing to do with them. For them, sex, adventure, and experimentation carry no risk, and HIV infection is a remote possibility at worst. This age-appropriate denial can be a major roadblock to efforts to educate young adults about HIV and to help their personal risk. This denial is a liability in negotiating the phases of HIV testing and adjustment to a potentially positive result. Young adults may see no real reason to be tested because they feel they could never, under any circumstances, be infected. If they are HIV positive, they may never process this fact while remaining asymptomatic. In conjunction with this denial they may continue to practice unsafe sexual behavior or avoid seeking medical care. For young adults, denial may continue even after initial symptoms develop because they persist in denying mortality. However, when major debilitating symptoms occur, the young adult's denial may be shattered all at once, and he may be hit with an emotional punch he never anticipated. He may then be flooded with overwhelming fear and panic. He has not had the life experience to assist him in coping with loss and anticipating death. It will be extremely difficult to come to terms with an approaching death when the youth feels so cheated out of life.

In turn, learning one is HIV positive can also affect one's early adult developmental issues. Early adulthood is the time when a person begins to construct a more stable identity via career choice and responsibility in relationships. A premature death warrant can bring development in these areas to a standstill. The fact of being infected with HIV can stifle the gay man's motivation to go out into the world and develop a life. Later stages of illness dramatically stall development and easily foster regression if the young adult has to return to his family of origin for care. Also at this age, a young gay man may derive much of his self-esteem from his physical appearance. HIV infection can dramatically alter this and precipitate an identity crisis. Case 1 illustrates how learning one is HIV positive can stall early adult development.

Case 1

Mr. A, a 31-year-old recreation director for a cruise ship, was referred to me after he experienced panic attacks for the first time while traveling in rough seas during a storm. He had worked on cruise ships since he graduated from college. He told me that he was HIV positive and suspected he had been so since he was at least 24 years old. At that age, even though he had not been tested for presence of the HIV antibody, his platelet count dropped significantly and he underwent removal of his spleen to correct the problem. He reported that he had had no other symptoms of HIV illness since that time.

In exploring the panic attacks, it became clear that there were two precipitating events: 1) immediately preceding his first panic attack he had gone to see his doctor for a regular checkup, where he had learned his T cell count had dropped dramatically to under 500; 2) he was about to turn 30 years old. After further exploration I told him how I understood what had happened: precipitating events had combined to break through his denial about his own mortality, and he was experiencing a loss of control over what up to that point had been a very orderly and controlled life. I explained that turning 30 is a major developmental milestone; it makes one think about getting older and makes one review whether life is unfolding as expected. Because he had been physically asymptomatic since the removal of his spleen, Mr. A was able to deny his HIV infection until he discovered that his T cell count was dangerously low. Finally, the rough seas he had experienced on the cruise brought his unconscious fears about his well-being to the surface. I commented that things in his life had become rough and stormy, and he felt out of control.

The immediate crisis was not Mr. A's only problem. His original awareness of being HIV positive had come when he was 24 years old. What became clear was that he had put his life on hold at that time. He had always expected that he would go to sea only until he was 30 and then change careers. Meanwhile, he had never had a primary love relationship as he had decided not to bother getting involved with anyone. Because he was HIV positive, he felt that no relationship could be a long-term one. He also did not want to burden anyone with his illness. He had had only short involvements that were not very intense.

Mr. A's father was simple, hardworking, and autocratic. His mother, who kept the children at home with her, allowing them to go only to school, may have been psychotically depressed. No family member had ever had personal interests or aspirations. Even if Mr. A had not been HIV positive, I suspect he would have had difficulties in the areas of career and relationships. He had never developed an occupational dream, and had chosen to work on a cruise ship because his older brother had been able to leave home and escape an oppressive mother doing this type of work. He had no idea what motivated him or where his interests or skills really lay. He responded to his parents' attempts to control him by playing the role of the good boy. He had never challenged them or experienced an adolescent rebellion. He had gone away to college and came out of the closet fairly easily once away from his parents.

Early in therapy, Mr. A decided to take a leave of absence from his job and use therapy to figure out what he wanted to do. I debated whether his therapy should focus on long-term developmental issues—career development and the impediments and characterological roadblocks to forming relationships—or on more immediate issues. Mr. A estimated that he had been HIV positive for at least 7 years and that he probably had 2 more healthy years and then 2 years of decline before he died. He did not want to switch to a career that would take any more than 1 year of schooling. He appeared paralyzed over what to do. Although he wanted to do something personally meaningful, he was reluctant to do the long-term work required. I wondered if he had the time to do long-term characterological work. Was it realistic to think he might have only 4 more years left? What was I to work on with him? Awareness of HIV infection at an early age had blocked his development in the areas of work and love. Although it was likely that he would have experienced difficulty in these two areas without HIV infection, he might also have had greater motivation and experienced more hope for a successful resolution of these developmental challenges had he not been infected. He might have attempted the work earlier. Now he was using HIV as an excuse for not addressing his developmental difficulties.

Interaction of HIV Stage and Middle Age Developmental Issues

A middle-aged man may be better equipped to deal with some of the developmental consequences of HIV infection than his younger counterpart. He has already begun to think about getting older, his changing attributes and declining physical capacity, and his own mortality. He may have had a parent become ill and die. Illness and death may already have been a significant part of his life. He probably has experienced some disappointments and accepted these as part of life. He may already have realized significant portions of his dream in the areas of career and relationships. These experiences may better prepare him to accept the constriction of illness. He may, in fact, sail more smoothly through the initial and middle phases of HIV illness.

On the other hand, the middle-aged man is at the height of his independence. He is years away from having lived with his family of origin and years away from retirement. He is at the peak of his power in the workplace, and an authority and mentor to the younger generation. It will be hard for such a man to accept having to rely on others for his care during the later stages of HIV illness. A man who is president of his company will find it particularly humiliating and frustrating to have to wear diapers and be fed his meals. A man who is a respected sage may not easily accept memory loss and confusion. A working person will not be pleased at having to rely on welfare and social service agencies for the first time in his life.

When an individual with AIDS has to return to his family of origin for care, the potential for regression is great. It is very hard to avoid returning to old patterns of interaction learned in childhood, which may be quite dysfunctional for the independent adult. Parents may infantilize their son and prevent him from doing what little he still can do for himself. Likewise, elderly parents also face a return to a phase of development they thought they had left many decades before. They may have been looking forward to a time of retirement that involved traveling and little family responsibility. They may be infirm themselves. It can be quite a strain for all parties involved. It is even more complicated if the parents either did not know of their son's homosexuality or disapproved of it. It is hard for the person with AIDS to achieve some sort of peace before death in such an environment. On the other hand, if the family can rise to the occasion, it can be a very repairing experience. Old wounds can be healed as everyone has a second chance to express acceptance, caring, and love. (See Chapter 13 on returning home to die.)

HIV infection may present a middle-aged gay couple with issues that are commonly experienced later in life. The necessity for one partner to become his lover's caretaker places an inevitable burden on the relationship. It shifts the balance of power and often has negative consequences. The man's lover may feel guilty for wanting any time to himself, or he may displace anger at the disease and at his own helplessness onto his dependent partner. If the lover is also infected, he has to deal simultaneously with the fear of his own illness. If the lover is HIV negative, he has to deal with survivor guilt. The illness forces the relationship from its appropriate chronological context and causes the couple to confront some of the challenges they would not normally face until later years. These couples, like elderly couples, may no longer have friends to help. Their entire network of friends may either have died or be in the throes of the illness themselves. Lovers who care for partners with AIDS face the same sense of isolation and overwhelming burden as the husband or wife with a sick spouse. They must turn to social agencies for help. (See Chapter 14 on couples therapy.)

A gay man in his late 30s or early 40s may have made an earlier commitment to a career and already have achieved success. He may have been through a series of earlier serious relationships and finally found the person to whom he wants to make a lifelong commitment. Once he discovers that he is HIV positive, how does the couple plan for their lives together? Do they proceed with the age-appropriate tasks of buying a house, involving children in their lives, or continuing their successful careers? In fact, people cope in varying ways. For example, one of my patients who was HIV positive and whose lover was very ill was determined to finish law school and take the bar examination. His lover died a couple of months later, and he himself got sick and died about 1 year later. Another patient who was fairly healthy decided to give up his successful business and move to Provincetown, a coastal gay resort. He chose quality of life as a priority.

Cases 2 and 3 illustrate two different ways in which HIV can alter development in middle age.

Case 2

Mr. B was HIV negative but his partner of 10 years had been HIV positive for 5 years. Although the lover was asymptomatic, he had a T cell count of less than 500. The lover had started treatment with zidovudine (AZT) the previous year. Both had very responsible jobs and made a decent living. Over the years they had become closer and had come to a point in their relationship where they wanted to "nest" more by buying a house together. At the time they lived together in a small apartment in the city. They began looking and found their dream house in the country. They debated whether they should buy this house. Financially, it would be difficult and require that all Mr. B's salary go toward the house expenses. His lover's salary would cover the couple's additional living expenses. His lover did not have life insurance and could not get it because he was HIV positive. I explored the pros and cons of buying the house with Mr. B in therapy. He feared that his lover's health would deteriorate soon after purchasing the house. They would then have the burden of an expensive house, only with less income and possibly no way to sell the house quickly in the current sluggish real estate market. On the other hand, his lover could be fine for many more years. Even if he was well for only a short while, they wanted the chance to share what little time they had left together in the way that would have the most meaning and pleasure for them. They wanted a piece of the American dream just like any other committed couple. My main concern as a therapist was that I wanted my patient to be able to look at all the issues and not deny the grimmest possibilities, but at the same time be able to hold on to the excitement and pleasure of enhancing the couple's life together. He was not avoiding issues of loss; as a matter of fact, the thought of buying his first house had revived issues of grief over the death of his parents. This was someone dealing with age-appropriate issues but with the cloud of death hanging over him. He had to evaluate the suitability of this first home not just as a starter house but also as a retirement home with its potential of conversion for wheelchair use and easy accessibility.

Case 3

Mr. C was a very successful businessman. Although he was physically symptomatic for about 1 year, this did not impede his normal life in any consistent way. Suddenly he began to sleep a great deal and lose the energy to leave the house. Although I had offered to make home visits many times before while he recuperated from operations, he had refused, being a very proud, formal man. However, when his energy deteriorated, he asked me to visit him at home. He was barely able to get up to answer the door. The most distressing thing for him was that he began to nod off during our talks. Although this was embarrassing, we discussed how he wanted to handle this. He asked me to repeat his name so that he would awaken. We had no choice but to table our ongoing work and focus on his acute situation. He also began to have periods of incoherence. This was very difficult for him because mental acuity was required in his line of work. His medical providers could not identify the cause of his changes in mental status. Ultimately, we had very little time to adjust to these changes because his health deteriorated quickly and he died within a matter of 2 months. We barely had time to say good-bye.

Interaction of HIV Stage and Late Adulthood Developmental Issues

Developmentally, the older gay man may have the most syntonic experience with HIV illness. Although physical deterioration, greater dependence on others, and mortality are part of his normal phase adaptation, there are aspects that are not. A man in his late 50s and early 60s who has worked hard and is looking forward to retirement may feel particularly disenfranchised by AIDS. He is angry that his enjoyment of retirement has been stolen. He may be better at accepting the notion of mortality, but he may not be ready for it to happen at that very moment.

The older gay man grew up and disclosed his sexual orientation in a very different world. When he was young, being gay was less accepted, and he was more influenced by the pervasive societal prejudice. The older gay man may not have had as much freedom to be openly gay. He may resent that HIV infection has further inhibited his ability to express his homosexuality and may be bitter and jealous of the freedom of younger gay men. Older gay men often feel invisible, both in the straight world and in the gay world. Segments of the gay culture value youth and may not reach out to aging men. There may not be many organizations or supports directed toward the interests of aging gay men. This may lead to isolation and may be particularly difficult for the older man infected with HIV. He may feel especially wounded by the additional stigma that HIV infection brings, and he may not be able to reach out for the supports that are available to him.

Summary

Human emotional development is linked inextricably with physical development. Early stages of both types of development are defined by the infant's inability to survive physically or cope emotionally with the demands of life on his own. Both processes move slowly from a state of dependence on others for care and nurturing to a time of prolonged independence. Gradually this independence gives way to the need to rely on others once again as the body begins the decent into the infirmities of old age. In the course of normal development, one would have several decades to deal with age-related physical deterioration and adjust psychologically as one goes along. However, after having developed AIDS, a person may have only several months or years to live. It is quite a psychological challenge for people with HIV infection to deal with a lifetime of developmental issues in a compressed period of time. Their physical condition and their emotional stage of development become disconnected and increasingly out of synchrony. Gay men who are infected with HIV face the additional work of having to deal with the impact of societal and internalized homophobia on their personal development.

Psychotherapy can be a useful tool in helping people cope with the emotional ramifications of HIV infection, but the therapist is not immune to the dilemmas that HIV presents either. It is a challenge for therapists who work with HIV-infected patients to help them deal with the coming of winter when they have just begun to treasure the warm seasons.

References

Cass V: Homosexual identity formation: a theoretical model. J Homosex 4:219–235, 1979

Coleman E: Development stages of the coming out process. J Homosex 7:31–43, 1981–1982

Erikson EH: Childhood and Society. New York, Norton, 1950

Fishman J, Linde R: Informed consent: making appropriate choices about AIDS from an informed perspective. Gay Community News 10:8–9, 1983

Gonsiorek J: Mental health issues of gay and lesbian adolescents. Journal of Adolescent Health 9:114–122, 1988

Hanley-Hackenbruck P: Psychotherapy and the "coming out" process. Journal of Gay and Lesbian Psychotherapy 1:21–39, 1989

Kimmel D: Adult development and aging: a gay perspective. Journal of Social Issues 34:113–130, 1978

Levinson DJ: The Seasons of a Man's Life. New York, Ballantine Books, 1978

Malyon AK: The homosexual adolescent: developmental issues and social bias. Child Welfare 60:321–330, 1981

Zera D: Coming of age in a heterosexist world: the development of gay and lesbian adolescents. Adolescence 27:849–854, 1992

Chapter 3

Mourning Within A Culture of Mourning

R. Dennis Shelby, Ph.D.

The experience of loss has become an integral aspect of the lives of the several generations of gay men who have directly encountered the acquired immunodeficiency syndrome (AIDS) epidemic. If one's only exposure to AIDS is through the mainstream media, it is easy to lose sight of the fact that AIDS does not occur in a vacuum. We all live in and are sustained by a matrix of relationships. Hence the death of one man to AIDS also means the death of a son, a partner, a brother, a friend, a colleague, and perhaps a hero.

The Difference Between Grief and Mourning

In approaching the topics of grief and mourning, a clarification of terms is in order. In this chapter, *grief* refers to the affective experience that accompanies a loss, whereas *mourning* refers to the process of integrating the meaning of the loss. Grief refers to affect states, mourning to the process of self-reorganization following the loss of someone central to a person's life. Mourning involves three distinct dimensions: 1) the affective state—or grief, 2) an initial withdrawal from relationships, and 3) a process whereby affects gradually become less intense, overwhelming, and volatile, and the individual reengages with his world and the people in it. Numerous theorists from Freud onward have discussed relationships, their loss, and the mourning of the loss in the structuralization of the mind. As Bowlby (1980) pointed out,

> Authors regardless of theoretical framework agree that the process of healthy mourning involves to varying degrees the withdrawal of investment in the lost person and that [it] may prepare the way for making a relationship with a new one. How we conceive of their making this change, however, depends on how we conceptualize affectional bonds. (p. 25)

Thus in order to discuss mourning, we must understand the very nature of relationships, the theoretical framework we use to understand them, and the consequent implications of their loss.

Understanding Mourning Within a Self Psychology Paradigm

In a previous work (Shelby 1992), I outlined the development of analytic theories on mourning and the problematic aspects of those theories when they are applied to the mourning process of gay men. The central issue is that of psychic structure. The theories state that in order to mourn one must have the capacity to resolve ambivalence, a capacity that is theoretically reached with the Oedipal level of development. In traditional drive theory and subsequent object relations theories based on drive theory, homosexual men are viewed as not having achieved the Oedipal level; hence they are unable to resolve their ambivalence toward the lost individual and are theoretically unable to mourn. Another aspect of these theories that is troublesome is that the role of other people in the mourner's life and the cultural rituals that accompany a death are simply relegated to the realm of reinforcing the reality that the deceased was indeed dead.

I have proposed that, for clinicians who strive to work with gay men and lesbian women from a depth psychological perspective, the framework of self psychology is the most logical fit (Shelby RD: "Oliver Button Was a Sissy: Clinical Theory, Homosexuality and the Problem of Gender." Unpublished paper, 1991; Shelby 1992). The self psychology model, with its emphasis on the coherence of the self rather than on drive or object relations development, avoids the theoretical pitfalls one invariably encounters with the other two paradigms when trying to understand the phenomenon of homosexuality.

As Kohut (1977) stated, "[There] is no mature love in which the love object is not also a selfobject, or to put this depth formulation into a psychosocial context, there is no love relationship without mutual self-esteem enhancing, mirroring and idealization" (p. 141). In a self psychology model, the loss is viewed as the loss of a selfobject relationship, which brings about an imbalance in self-esteem (Palombo 1981, 1982; see also Chapter 9 for a more thorough theoretical overview of self psychology). In many cases, the imbalance in self-esteem is more accurately described as a massive disorganization of the self and a shattering of self-esteem. Relationships vary in the degree to which individuals rely on one another for specific selfobject functions; hence the degree to which the loss of a particular relationship psychologically impacts on a mourner will vary in accordance with the meaning of that relationship.

Shane and Shane (1990) extended formulations of mourning theory within a self psychology framework. Although they focused on children, they argued that it is not the degree of psychic structure that enables the child to mourn, but rather it is the presence and the ability of the surviving parent to tolerate, mirror, sustain, and share the range of the child's affects regarding the lost parent that helps the child to mourn. In other words, the surviving parent must provide essentially a "compensatory self structure . . . to repair the weakened aspects of the self, but facilitate continued or renewed development" (p. 119). Even though Shane and Shane indicated that the presence of an "optimal selfobject environment [is] more readily available to the adult," they did not elaborate on the nature of the role of the selfobject matrix (or environment) in adult mourning.

Mourning and the Selfobject Matrix

In my study (Shelby 1992) of the impact of AIDS on established gay male relationships, the integral role other people play in facilitating adult mourning was clearly demonstrated. The ability of others to tolerate and be in tune with the mourning partner's affect states was a highly meaningful experience, and often resulted in the partner's having a greater coherence to and an increased ability to reengage with the world of the living. Granted, this is also where many men encounter difficulty. Problems can arise with the deceased partner's family; some families may even challenge the will, creating a great deal of anger and anxious uncertainty just when the surviving partner greatly needs support and reassurance. At a time when men long to feel comforted by their family of origin, the families of some surviving partners may not acknowledge the depth or the validity of the relationship. However, with the exception of men who had sustained parent loss in childhood, surviving partners tend to find people who can acknowledge and validate the depth of their grief.

To help bridge the cultural and intrapsychic aspects of mourning in the face of AIDS, the following formulation on the nature of selfobjects may be enlightening:

> Selfobjects are not experiences. They are not distinct and separate beings. These two ideas insist on the boundary between individuals and demand that we maintain what is internal in opposition to what is external. Selfobjects are the others that allow one to achieve and maintain an individual integrity. They are what makes us what we are, our very composition. But the individual is not reduced to these selfobjects, since there is an "owness" inhering in the individual that goes beyond and is logically distinct from, these relations. They are joined together to form the self. Therefore we never become free of our selfobjects, nor should we, because they are our constituents. (Goldberg 1990)

Our selfobject matrix is part of the fabric of our lives. I make a clear distinction between the *selfobject matrix* and *supportive relationships*. The former implies the integral nature of our selfobjects in the very sustenance of the self, whereas the latter implies relationships that support defensive aspects more in line with formulations that rely on a clear distinction between self and other. Thus with every death of a partner, friend, or family member from an AIDS-related illness, one aspect of the self is lost and, on a broader level, part of the gay culture is lost. The warp and weft of life gradually slips or is ripped away, leaving the gay community to try to make sense of the enormity of its experience, whether it be on the most personal level, as with the death of a partner, or the more existential level with a sense of losing its culture. For the gay man mourning the loss of his partner, often the most painful and confusing aspect is the desire to be comforted by the very person who is gone. This highlights another crucial distinction between the selfobject matrix and supportive relationships: the mourning partner is not yearning or searching for a lost figure, object, or any representation thereof; rather, he is experiencing the absence of his particular, unique experience of that individual, the dialogue between the selfobject dimension and the dimension of shared experience that comprises an intimate relationship.

Palombo (1990) pointed out that all meaning is embedded in culture. Hence there is some overlap between private or intrapsychic meanings and the meanings that have evolved within the larger culture. In the 1970s, the gay culture dramatically exploded onto the scene. Suddenly there were gay communities (some called them *ghettos*), gay health clinics, gay social service agencies, gay newspapers, gay therapists, gay doctors, gay resorts, gay politicians, gay bars, and gay celebrations of memorable magnitude. These structures were put in place by the gay community to tend to its needs. Gay men carved out their own territory in a larger cultural matrix that tended to ignore or minimize, if not scorn, their needs and validity as human beings. One way of viewing the gay liberation movement is as a process of establishing new cultural meanings vis-à-vis the phenomenon of homosexuality.

In the 1980s the gay community developed agencies to care for its ill when no one else would. Also during this decade, gay men had to learn to mourn their dead. Many of the people who had contributed to the evolution of gay culture were now dying. The culture that evolved in the 1970s suddenly seemed to be in danger of slipping away. One could argue that developing rituals for mourning and honoring the dead represents the ongoing evolution of a culture. Unfortunately, the massive loss of lives came rather early and suddenly in the gay movement. Considering this, the gay community has done reasonably well in honoring its dead and validating the enormity of its loss. From a clinical standpoint, mourning is ultimately an individual issue. However, the potential exists for the accumulation of grief within a culture to be so great that the community members neglect the needs of people who have lost central relationships. They may pull back from the grief of others rather than acknowledge and sustain them, or they may attempt to minimize the impact of their own losses for fear that they will be swallowed up in intense sadness and despair.

Far from crumbling as a result of the massive loss of lives to AIDS, many of the gay cultural institutions appear to be stronger than ever. From a social welfare standpoint, one can argue that the ability of a minority group to create and sustain institutions that tend to the group's needs within a cultural context is a sign of the group's cohesiveness. The rapid creation, maintenance, and expansion of institutions whose role is to tend to the needs of people living with human immunodeficiency virus (HIV) has been unprecedented in the history of social welfare in the United States. A more ardent seriousness about being gay is also evident in our culture. AIDS and the effects of loss are ultimately humanizing. As men mourn the loss of a partner or friend, their narcissistic defenses lose some of their power. Gay men often become less afraid and less tolerant of homophobic bigotry. Loss reminds us that we are indeed human, because loss is one of the most basic experiences of being human. Many straight people are taking increasingly ardent stands against bigotry and HIV discrimination as well. Here again, in the face of the loss of a gay friend or relative to AIDS-related illnesses, the "straights" are not missing and mourning the "gay"—they are missing the human being.

Epidemiological research into the effects of loss in the gay community (Martin 1988; Martin et al. 1989; Neugebauer et al. 1992) has indicated that depressive symptoms, depressive disorders, and demoralization are not dominant, nor is their frequency increasing dramatically. As Neugebauer et al. (1992) postulated, "Changes in normative expectations regarding AIDS deaths and mobilizations against AIDS within the gay community may account for the lack of depressive symptoms and depressive disorder" (p. 1374). Although the results of psychometric testing completed over the course of 1 day may yield general indications, these data do not account for the reparative and shifting processes of life and mourning. As clinicians, we are well aware that a person may be considerably depressed during a certain day, week, or month, but not during another. Our patients will most likely be those for whom depressive symptoms do predominate and persist, eventually eroding the quality of their lives.

From the clinical perspective, the issue is the nature of the mourning process for a particular individual and what factors tend to facilitate or impede the process. If we take the basic Kohutian stance that people strive for coherence in their lives, then the question becomes, How do people regain and maintain their coherence in response to loss or massive losses?

A Reformulation of the Mourning Process

In a previous work (Shelby 1992), I proposed the following reformulation of mourning: the process of mourning is one of reorganizing affects and constructing a new or modified *narrative*—an account of the loss that can then be integrated into the self-organization. The person that has become accustomed to an intimate, ongoing dialogue based on the bedrock of shared experience with another must now integrate the experience of being alone. Initially the self of the mourner is in a highly disorganized, vulnerable, and deficient state. Affects are intense and volatile and self-esteem is diminished and unstable; consequently, the person withdraws from an environment that feels very unsafe and unfamiliar. The work of mourning involves the gradual reorganization of the affect states and their integration into the overall experience of the self. As affective states become less intense, a narrative can be formed. The mourner makes meaning out of his loss and the narrative gradually supplants shifting affect states. The loss becomes viewed as a complicated and painful event in the context of a larger life experience. As this occurs, the self regains its coherence, self-esteem becomes more stable, and the person reengages with the world, often establishing new relationships.

The central figures in the mourning process are not so much the mourner and the deceased individual, but rather the mourner, the deceased individual, and the selfobject matrix. This process has personal and public dimensions. Initially the mourner's self is in a deficient state. The mourner often treasures the belongings of the deceased, other symbols of their life together, and their loss. The interaction with these symbols, visits to the gravesite, and other rituals, as well as ongoing conversations with the deceased person help complete the reconfiguration of the deficient self in a personal way by providing the mourner with the essence of his shared experience with the deceased person. In so doing, the mourner's affects are soothed and modulated.

By responding to the mourner's affect states and the real meaning of the loss, the surviving people in the mourner's matrix assist in soothing and organizing the mourner's affect and help him complete the reconfiguration of the self in a public way. Public encounters serve to orient the self towards the world of the living and rekindle the hope that the self can become enriched through participating in experiences with the living, rather than finding meaning and solace in attempts to recreate the experiences shared with the deceased person.

Through the personal and public soothing and modulating of affect, the construction of a new or modified self-narrative is formed and gradually integrated. The mourner is able to become increasingly engaged with his world, the self regains its coherence, and self-esteem becomes more stable. Thus mourning involves varying degrees of withdrawal from the world of the living and personal and public attempts to validate, modulate, and soothe the grief associated with the loss. Then, as the self regains its coherence, a greater degree of engagement with the world of the living becomes possible.

In my study (Shelby 1992), two different kinds of public encounters stood out as being highly meaningful for surviving gay partners. The first was the "special person." The special person was usually a sibling, most often a sister, of the ill partner. In the absence of a sibling, the mother of the ill partner tended to take on this role. The mourning partner often formed a strong bond with the special person during the partner's illness, a bond that was solidified during the acute phase of illness and death and that continued well into the mourning process. During the times when the surviving partner missed the deceased partner more intensely, such as on holidays or anniversaries, he often turned to the special person to share his grief. Given the centrality of their relationship, the pace of the mourning process for the special person was often in tune with that of the surviving partner, and they were able to share their mutual grief and loss. By so doing, the surviving partner helped to facilitate the mourning of the special person. Often after such encounters, men found themselves feeling more alive, spontaneous, and more able to participate in holiday celebrations and to feel they were a part of the world of the living.

The other highly significant area of public experience has been the AIDS quilt. Gay men tend to be a creative lot, and have often found ways to meet their needs despite their status in society. For years, despite adverse societal pressures, they have established families, created social networks, established communities, and greatly expanded their culture. The AIDS quilt is an outgrowth of their need to create structures for themselves in a society that does not readily acknowledge their participation, let alone provide any structures for them (e.g., the lack of recognition of same-sex marriages).

For the individual mourner, the quilt is a chance to create: to conceive, design, and construct a panel that conveys the essence of the person who has died and the meaning of the relationship with them. Some panels are made privately; others are collective efforts of close friends. The creation of individual panels affirms the centrality of the loss and modulates affect. Placing thousands of the panels together creates a powerful symbol of the enormity of private and cultural loss. The quilt creates its own, giant holding environment that mirrors, sustains, and encourages the experience and expression of grief. The individual mourner first encounters the enormity of the quilt as a validation of the enormity of his loss. He must search for the panel of his partner, friend, or friends as he wanders through the symbols of the losses of others—just as he may search and yearn for the lost experience of the relationship. Finally he finds the panel. He created it, sent it on, and may have seen it go all over the country, but once again he finds it. The memories flood, the tears well up, the sadness and pain return. Gradually the mourner's intense affects subside. It is time to move on, time to go on living.

Many people report feeling cleansed after a visit to the AIDS quilt, often feeling that the visit was an affirmation that "yes, something horrible did happen. The pain and sorrow are real." The enormity of the quilt also affirms just how hard it is to understand, to make sense of the epidemic and its individual and collective impacts. Some men will find themselves dancing later in the evening, wondering why they now feel so connected and joyful. Again, as the sadness and pain are acknowledged and tended to, men are able to feel more a part of their world. The quilt serves to express, soothe, and organize grief. It helps people mourn.

The healing power of rituals, whether they be personal, cultural, or religious, is not in the rituals themselves, but in the personal meanings people arrive at through participation in them. The ritual provides a context for the experience, expression, and modulation of affects related to the loss or losses. As affects are modulated, new meanings regarding the loss often emerge.

Living With AIDS, Loss, and Mourning

The AIDS epidemic is an ongoing, dynamic entity. Some men have died, some are dying, some are taking antiviral medications and holding their own, some are contemplating which medical approach to take, some are asymptomatic, and some are struggling with whether they should be tested or not. The game rules keep changing as well. Initially, gay men were advised not to be tested. At the time there was no treatment for the illness and the test results might have been held against an individual. Then zidovudine (AZT) was made available for "compassionate use," then for those with a T cell count below 200, then for those whose count was below 500. Now gay men are encouraged, if not pressured, to be tested. Should they try combination therapy? Pneumocystis carinii pneumonia (PCP) prophylaxis? Which drug should be tried and when should it be started?

In a current study, I am looking at how gay men manage the psychological impact of living with AIDS. Just how do men manage to keep a sense of coherence in their lives when the rules for managing such a deadly illness keep changing while they keep on living? Again, their relationships with others play a central role. As HIV-positive men join groups and establish relationships with other HIV-positive men, they often find that their terror, isolation, and confusion diminish. Men also form friendships that strongly reflect the sentiment "we are in this together." A great deal of comfort, reassurance, and hope can come through these relationships.

Many times gay men identify one or several other seropositive men in a group as their mentors. The mentors tend to be physically well and appear to be managing the psychological impact of seropositivity in such away that they maintain a hopeful, if not enthusiastic view of life. The idealization of the mentor helps the new group member find his own strength and courage. However, the progressive nature of the disease becomes highly problematic for many men. If the mentor-friend becomes ill and dies, isolation, terror, and despair often return to the survivor. The game rules change once again. The initial comforting thought of, If he can make it, so can I, suddenly becomes, If he dies, so will I. The warp and weft of life continues to unravel. Men are faced with mourning the loss of not only their friend but also the comfort, reassurance, and hope they had experienced as a result of the relationship.

The Mourning Experience of Seropositive Surviving Partners

In my study of the impact of AIDS on established gay relationships (Shelby 1992), I found an important difference between the mourning process of surviving partners who were seropositive and those who were seronegative. Essentially, the mourning process of a seropositive surviving partner is often more protracted and complicated than that for a seronegative partner. The mourning experience of the former overlaps with their basic experience of being seropositive. Furthermore, powerful dynamics sometimes evolve. Often one observes a continued idealization of the deceased partner and an identification with his illness and death. This can lead to considerable withdrawal, diminished self-esteem, and in some cases a major depressive disorder. The same virus that killed the survivor's partner is inside the survivor. It may come to represent a powerful and deadly tie to the deceased partner that cannot be loosed. Although his medical status may be quite stable, the self of the seropositive partner may become increasingly organized around impending death, which dramatically erodes the quality of his life.

Although seropositive surviving partners may receive optimal help in facilitating their mourning from their existing selfobject matrix, the responses of those who comprise this matrix tend to be in the understandable and recognizable realm of loss and grief. In contrast, the complicated mourning often seen in seropositive survivors is a direct outgrowth of the epidemic. As clinicians, we must be able to recognize and identify the difficulties faced by these men, and tailor our interventions based on an understanding of their more complicated mourning process.

I worked with Mr. A, who is discussed in the following case example, in individual and group treatment for 61/2 years. As a seropositive surviving partner, he was often certain that he too would be dead within a few months. However, he continued going strong. Over the years, Mr. A maintained his efforts to manage the impact of his partner's death and his own seropositivity in order to remain engaged with his world.

The following interventions evolved over the 6 years of Mr. A's treatment: 1) using the therapeutic relationship to facilitate his mourning; 2) attempting to engage with a wider selfobject matrix; and 3) reworking the meaning of his partner's death. I also noted that there was a massive loss of mental coherence when symptoms emerged.

Using the Treatment Relationship to Facilitate Mourning

Case Example

I initially saw Mr. A and his partner as a couple because of difficulties they were having managing the impact of the partner's diagnosis of AIDS. AIDS was still fairly new to Chicago then. The anxiety, uncertainty, and terror associated with the disease were heightened by the disease's newness and were greatly impeding the couple's ability to talk to each other about the disease and their many fears. Mr. A was relieved and excited to have the forum of couples therapy to work through some of these issues. His partner was somewhat suspicious and reluctant. Gradually, a dialogue between us opened up, and the two men were able to sort out several miscommunications that had resulted in hurt and anger. It was unfortunate that after the second session Mr. A's partner developed a second attack of PCP and died several weeks later.

Mr. A spent the next month at his parents' home in a neighboring state. He called me during his first day back at his office. His voice trembled, he began to cry, and he told me he did not understand what was happening to him and that he was afraid he was "losing it." We made an appointment for later that evening. In my office, he was repeatedly overwhelmed. He related that while at his parent's home he had felt shaky but not to the degree he was currently experiencing. After returning to his home and work, he began to feel intense waves of sadness and anxiety. He missed his partner deeply and was terrified of facing life without him. Mr. A had never lost a person so central in his life, he had no idea of what mourning was like, and he was afraid that he was indeed losing his mind. I pointed out that I did not think he was losing his mind, but that in a way his mourning had been put on hold while he was at his parents' home and now that he was back in his own environment where reminders of his partner's absence were more evident, the mourning process was beginning.

Mr. A quickly formed an intense attachment to me. In the early months of our work together, the treatment relationship was used to modulate, contain, and organize his often intense and shifting affect states. He experienced his sessions as a place where his feelings could be tolerated and understood, where he could feel and be less afraid of being overwhelmed. I affirmed the centrality of his loss, pain, sadness, and confusion as he attempted to function in a world that "no longer made sense." Mr. A began keeping a journal to record his experiences and a series of letters to his partner. He would often bring his writings to his sessions. Although they expressed his longing for his partner, the letters also were a reconstruction of their life together, including the emergence of his partner's illness and their life in the face of AIDS. Although the daily act of writing became a ritual that served to modulate affect, the journal was also part of Mr. A's attempt to make sense of what had happened.

Mr. A kept in close contact with his partner's family. There were many phone calls in which they shared their mutual grief. Mr. A's parents had known of his relationship and had been very supportive during his partner's illness, death, and funeral. However, they appeared to be in a quandary about why their son was so grief stricken.

Mr. A related his growing anger over feeling discounted by them in his sessions. During a phone call his father implied that it was "time to get over it." Mr. A angrily replied, "How would you feel if Mother dropped dead?" His father apologized, and Mr. A was delighted that he had succeeded in getting his father to understand him. This was also the beginning of a wider dialogue with his parents regarding his homosexuality, a topic that had not really been discussed in the family.

As time progressed, Mr. A's affects gradually became more stable and predictable. Approximately 6 months after his partner's death, the families and Mr. A gathered to disperse his partner's ashes. The chosen site was a family vacation home in a remote woodland that had been a favorite place of his partner since childhood. Mr. A dispersed a portion of the ashes in each of his partner's favorite places on the property. As he did so, he carefully photographed each place. On his return, he brought the photographs to the session. He related that I had been such a central part of his mourning that he wanted me to somehow participate in the dispersal of the ashes.

Shortly after this, Mr. A became increasingly preoccupied with his own antibody status. He had tested positive for HIV during his partner's first episode of PCP, but had put his own antibody status in the back of his mind while he tended to his partner and was preoccupied with the early phases of mourning. However, the impact of being HIV positive was beginning to surface. He began to feel increasingly damaged, ill, and doomed. Being seropositive began to feel like a monkey on his back that would not go away. Very gradually, Mr. A's preoccupation with his antibody status declined, he moved to a new apartment more suitable for one person, gave away many of his partner's belongings, and subscribed to several publications in order to keep abreast of developments in the treatment of HIV infection.

Emergence of Symptoms and the Ability to Hope

For many years, surviving partners of those who have died from AIDS-related illnesses live in fear of their own illness. The emergence of symptoms or the need to begin taking AZT is often experienced as the beginning of the end. The clinical question is, What is the terror related to? From my work with these men, it has become clear to me that it has to do with the illness and loss of their partner. It is related to the experience of having relationships and sustaining connections ripped away from them. Further, with the emergence of their own symptoms, they experience a fragmentation of their lives and often become profoundly withdrawn in an attempt to manage their fears. It is as if they are reexperiencing their first realization that their partner is dead and they are alone. This sense of aloneness and isolation is at the core of the intensity of their reaction; in the self-organization, they are unable to recall present and past experiences of benign and helpful people. It is often helpful if the therapeutic alliance is solid enough to point out to the patient that AIDS did destroy the relationship with his partner, but that the patient still has a number of relationships that will be there for him.

Mr. A had been in twice-weekly treatment for 3 years when he became symptomatic. The treatment had evolved into addressing preexisting self-esteem issues as well as his experience of mourning and the complications secondary to his being seropositive. Mr. A's T cell count dropped considerably. Just as he had achieved a degree of equilibrium regarding the decline in his laboratory values, he developed a severe and extremely painful case of shingles. He canceled several sessions, often just before they were to begin, saying he was not feeling up to leaving his home. After the third cancellation, I gently insisted that he come in. He had spent the last 10 days holed up in his apartment, groggy on pain medication and attempting to keep at bay the terror he felt. He related that he feared if he sat across from me, he would experience the terror full force. (Although his physician had explained that the shingles were not necessarily HIV related, Mr. A experienced them as the "beginning of the end.")

In the course of the session, Mr. A did experience intense affect, mingled with considerable relief. He related that he felt intense terror and kept being flooded by images of his partner on his death bed. He alternately felt acutely alone, isolated, terrified, and enraged. In the session, he repeatedly experienced these states and affects. He experienced himself as in the process of dying. The events that he had feared for so long were now happening. He too was dying just like his partner, and it had come too soon, much too soon. At the end of the hour, with some surprise, he reported, "You are still here, and I am still here. There were times when I felt you slipping away, but we are both still around."

After this experience with me, Mr. A attended sessions regularly, but a pronounced withdrawal was evident for several weeks. In part this was related to the narcissistic withdrawal often experienced by people during illness. The other crucial aspect was his preoccupation with the death of his partner and his own death. He was avoiding contact with his family because he experienced their concern and anxiety as overstimulating as he felt they were a confirmation that he was indeed seriously ill and dying. I quietly but firmly pursued him during this period. Gradually, the terror, withdrawal, and preoccupation with his partner eased as we were able to establish more firmly the symbolic connection of his symptoms to the ripping away of his relationship with his partner. He was once again able to take considerable comfort in his family relationships.

Eventually, Mr. A compared the experience of his partner calling to him to that of Captain Ahab (from *Moby Dick*) who, when entangled in the harpoon lines, beckoned to Ishmael. I, on the other hand, was calling him back. There was also a transference connection: his wish that, within the context of the idealizing transference with me, which he experienced as very sustaining, if he did everything right, he would not get sick. Thus the emergence of symptoms also represented a transference disappointment. This same sequence was experienced several months later in a much milder and less protracted form when Mr. A's T cell count declined to the point where his physician recommended he begin taking AZT.

The Tie That Binds—Separating One's Illness From A Partner's Death

Mr. A's experience offers a number of potential insights into the experience of surviving partners as they face their own illness. In making initial explorations for this chapter, I encountered numerous professionals who related similar experiences with surviving partners who became ill. The clinicians were struck by the degree of withdrawal, often rapid decline, and lack of enthusiasm for treatment that they observed in surviving partners. Several of the symptomatic survivors I encountered in the course of the study tended to have varying degrees of apathy, an "as if" quality about them. They were only partly present, as if they were going about the motions of living. Several were actively saying and doing all the "right things" in their own treatment and in their outlook for the future, but were actually highly disengaged. Essentially, their personal dialogue was very different from their public dialogue.

Mr. A's experience offers insights into the dynamics that contribute to this at times dramatic process of turning inward, if not gradually shutting down the self and its involvement with the world of the living. Because surviving partners tend to identify their infection with their partners' deaths, their intense and often complicated affect secondary to their own infection makes it extremely difficult to form a narrative in which their potential illness and death are separate from the illness and death of their partner. Illness and death represent an ongoing shared experience. In the wake of the trauma of illness, the self organizes along these lines, and the survivor views his current experience as an extension of his experience with his partner. If the survivor is already significantly ill when his partner dies, or symptoms emerge early in the mourning experience, this process may be difficult to modulate or reverse.

This part of the mourning experience shades into the nature of the capacity to hope and of hope itself. Hope ultimately represents past experiences of having had sustaining people available and the subsequent integration of these experiences into the self-organization. At a time of trauma, overstimulation, or anxiety, a relationship has calmed or soothed and helped to restore coherence. Hence hope is ultimately related to the idealized parental imago, the self-structure that develops out of the idealizing selfobject relationship a child has with his parents. In a patient who has severe deficits in this area, ultimately due to selfobject failure or severe disappointments, one often sees an inability to hope, let alone trust, that people can be useful in helping him manage anxiety or trauma.

The surviving seropositive partner has already experienced several severe, often acutely traumatizing disappointments. He may have hoped that he would be seronegative, hoped that he could sustain his partner until a cure was found, and hoped that he would not become ill himself. The emergence of symptoms ultimately represents another disappointed hope. Repeated disappointments, the assault on the self that AIDS represents, and the overall erosive effect of a protracted emersion in the experience of HIV-related problems tax even the most resilient self.

When the patient is not severely traumatized and is able to make use of the distinction, it is often useful to point out the difference between hope and contingent hope or wishes. The hope of being negative, of sustaining his partner until a cure is found, and of not becoming symptomatic himself is ultimately more related to wishes or *contingent hope*—the belief that results are contingent on doing things right, on being a "good person." It is often helpful to point out to the patient that, although his wish to remain symptom-free has been dashed, and his wish to not lose his partner to death was also dashed, and that relationship was ripped away, his hope comes from the experience of others being there for him. The therapist is still available, as are other sustaining connections. However, in the face of the terror of becoming ill, the patient may not readily be able to call upon them. The therapist's task is to work with the patient in such a way that he can feel calmed, reassured, and, once again, begin to call on his past experiences and the people who are able to be with him.

Moving From Isolation to Engagement

Throughout Mr. A's experience of mourning, he maintained a high degree of withdrawal from the larger social networks available to him. His experience of mourning and being in therapy resulted in a considerable reworking of his experience in his family. Just as a dialogue regarding his long-standing experience of "feeling weird and different" was opened up in the treatment relationship, a broader dialogue was begun with his family, and he began to experience himself as an actively involved member of his family. A central problem with the family concerned both parents' difficulty in helping Mr. A feel comfortable outside the family. The transitions from home to grade school to college appeared to have been traumatic for all. The lack of encouragement and support left Mr. A feeling abandoned and frightened as he ventured out on his own.

Mr. A had made several attempts to attend the meetings of a large seropositive support-educational organization. However, he frequently became anxious and overstimulated, especially if anyone attempted to strike up a conversation. Often he would make plans to attend but would then fall asleep and miss the meetings. He was at once chagrined and relieved by this behavior. In the transference relationship, he would both ask me for help and then dare me to do anything about it. Lengthy discussion of this dynamic did not result in enabling Mr. A to attend the meetings. I then suggested that he might want to join the group for seropositive men that I was forming. He was anxious but interested. I took a neutral stance. He eventually decided not to join, but would periodically ask about the group. Several months later an opening was available in the group and I related this to him. He again was anxious but interested. This time I casually remarked that, "I just might insist that you join." Mr. A laughed, and the next week announced that he wanted to give the group a try.

During the first several sessions with the group, Mr. A experienced considerable anxiety around revealing that he was a surviving partner, and interpreted several group members' responses as attacking and overstimulating. However, he was also surprised that there was another surviving partner in the group. For several weeks his individual sessions (which followed the group sessions by several days) were spent in helping him organize his experience of the group and understand the acute vulnerability he felt in the group. Very quickly his anxiety diminished and he became an active member of the group.

Facilitating Engagement

Five years after the death of his partner and 20 months following his withdrawal from his family and the larger social networks available to him, Mr. A was enthusiastically engaged with his family and with a large support-social organization for seropositive men, was an active member in the group led by myself, and had begun to attend social events for a group of gay men and lesbian women who shared his vocational interests. In a group session in which the members were talking about their experience of isolation, he remarked, "Looking back, being so isolated was like being dead."

The combination of past trauma and the ongoing self-esteem difficulties inherent in HIV infection may prevent gay men from engaging with potentially helpful relationships. Although the selfobject matrix may offer considerable reassurance and sustenance and a sense of belonging, we as clinicians often need to help our patients engage with other people. It is not unusual for homosexual children to have considerable difficulties in peer relationships. The temperament of the homosexual child is often radically different from that of heterosexual children; hence the peer group may mock and deride them and label them as an outcast, a "sissy." Memories of these earlier experiences often reemerge as men attempt to join groups for HIV-infected people. If people are able to engage, what they soon find (to their relief) is that membership is contingent on being different or having a "problem," and that difference is not grounds for exclusion. Thus a reworking of earlier experiences of rejection may occur as men address self-esteem issues inherent in being HIV positive.

Power of the Matrix to Facilitate New Meaning

By his sixth year of treatment, Mr. A had become an integral member of the group and developed a friendship with another group member. In the course of the group, the partner of another member died. Mr. A repeatedly reached out to the grief-stricken member, conveying his understanding of the depth of his loss. His friend also enlisted his help in leading a smaller group for men who needed extra help and support while they were joining a large support-educational organization for seropositive men. During a session following one of these groups, Mr. A related that a very shaken, anxious, and overwhelmed young man had come to the group and that he had spent a great deal of time with him, listening, reassuring, and answering his many questions. Mr. A reflected on his own sense of amazement and accomplishment that he had helped someone deal with being HIV positive, an issue that he himself had felt so helpless about. I pointed out that he had also helped a group member mourn, another experience that had initially left him feeling helpless.

Several weeks later, his friend asked Mr. A to accompany him to the hospital to visit a friend on the AIDS unit. Mr. A was anxious at first but went along and spent several hours visiting with the patients. The session following his visit proved to be productive and intense. Initially, Mr. A related his sense of mastery at having gone to the hospital where his own partner had died 6 years earlier. Since the visit, he had felt very spontaneous, happy, and engaged. How different this was from the time when his partner had been hospitalized! There was no AIDS unit then. There had been a great sense of anxious mystery. This time on the unit, things felt more normalized. Gay men were visiting with each other. There was a sense of belonging. Gradually, as his associations with the patients on the unit deepened during his many visits, Mr. A became more sad and somewhat frightened. He related how in the past he had become very shaky and overwhelmed if he even looked at or went near the hospital. Now instead, he had walked in, visited other men, and walked out. His assumption was that the next time he entered the hospital would be during his first AIDS-related illness. He would be acutely ill, on a stretcher, gasping for breath, going to meet the same fate as his partner.

I sensed there was more to his feelings, something still deeper and urged him to continue. He went on to relate a solemn vow he had made the night his partner died: that never again would he be happy, that happiness would no longer be a part of his life. I reflected on the penitential quality of the vow, like a monk depriving himself of worldly pleasures, locked away in his cell, flagellating himself for his sins. Mr. A began to cry, "I killed him didn't I! I am the one who gave it to him. Why should I have what he can't?" Mr. A was both horrified and amazed. As he spoke these words, he began to realize the extent to which his life had become organized around his partner's death and the responsibility he felt for it. Eventually he asked, "My God, what have I been doing to myself all of these years?"

Healing Potential of the Matrix

We must be very careful in our assumptions regarding a culture of mourning. Though many of the people within an individual's selfobject matrix may be in mourning themselves, they can still facilitate the process for each other. In responding to the grief of another group member, Mr. A was also acknowledging and reworking his own grief. Mr. A's friend visited the hospital as a member of a committee whose task it was to look after ill members of the large social-educational group to which he belonged. He had done this because of his own fear of and inexperience with death. He had felt that by being around ill and dying people, he would feel less anxious as his illness progressed. In inviting Mr. A along, he had no idea of the impact it would have, or how it would help Mr. A bring into focus deeply rooted and influential meaning structures regarding his partner's death and his own illness.

Mr. A's realizations in treatment are an illustration of my earlier assertion that, in seropositive surviving partners, one often sees a powerful combination of continued idealization of and identification of their infection with the partner's illness and death. Illusive, but highly influential meaning structures can evolve that become central organizers of the surviving partner's experience of self. Though in the course of treatment we had touched on these issues many times, it was not until through interaction with his selfobject matrix that Mr. A was able to bring his vow and its impact so directly into his conscious experience.

Continued Growth and Engagement

In the 10 months following his hospital visit, a great deal happened in Mr. A's life. On a visit to his parents, he came across his high school yearbooks. As he read the inscriptions, he saw evidence that others viewed him more differently than he had assumed. He was clearly well liked, in some cases idealized; was considered funny, brilliant, and outgoing; and was voted "most likely to succeed." "Who was this person?" he asked. Again he was amazed and shaken. The disparity between others' experience of him and his remembered experience of himself was considerable. Two distinct but highly interrelated lines of association followed. The first related to his questioning of whether he had "made himself over" in the wake of his partner's death (i.e., vis-à-vis his assumed responsibility, his vow, and his own seropositivity). Had the severe damage to his self-esteem resulted in his remaking his own history? The second line of questioning was related to his emerging sexuality. Back in high school, his homosexuality had been a deep, dark secret that no one knew about—certainly not the people writing in his yearbook. What would they have written if they had known about it? He realized that these two areas of meaning had converged. His partner's death and his own infection had concretized his secret evolving sexual orientation and his sense of being weird and different, if not evil.

Over the next few months, Mr. A reestablished contact with several old high school buddies who were also gay. To his delight he was warmly received. As his T cell count approached 200, Mr. A began to consider retirement. He had ample financial resources through disability policies. He found that, during a 1-week vacation when he stayed in the city, he was able to keep busy and entertain himself. I interpreted this along the lines that he did not have to become ill and die as his partner did, but rather he could take charge of the situation and determine how he wanted to approach his life in the face of his illness. He also obtained dideoxycytosine (DDC) and began combination drug therapy. He was surprised that he had approached the new regimen with a sense of calm, radically different from the great turmoil he felt when he began AZT treatment. Again, I pointed out that he was viewing himself in a radically different light as he had realized the extent to which he had organized his illness around his partner's death.

Mr. A's friend who had engaged him in the larger group and invited him to the hospital was diagnosed as having AIDS and became acutely ill for several weeks. Mr. A found himself very engaged with his friend, and reported that the whole experience of his friend's diagnosis and illness was a calming, rather than a wrenching, experience. He found himself feeling considerably less frightened of illness and death.

Mr. A's brother visited him for several days. Although he found himself having a great deal of fun and enjoying the visit immensely, Mr. A also found himself engaged with his brother in long conversations about death and dying and trying to make sense of these experiences. His brother, a professional firefighter, faced death every day. He had had numerous "close calls" and experienced the death of colleagues and people he had hoped to save. Again, Mr. A found the conversations calming, and was delighted at the depth to which he and his brother could understand each other.

Mr. A also stopped smoking. He reported that he had realized the connection between smoking and his partner. During his illness, his partner was simply unable to smoke. His partner had wanted Mr. A to stop as well but he was unable to do so. The smoking periodically became a source of conflict. Mr. A felt ashamed that he was unable to stop for his partner's sake. He realized how this experience had prevented him from stopping smoking following his partner's death: if he was unable to stop for his partner, how could he stop solely for himself?

Concurrently, Mr. A found his memories of his partner changing. They focused on his partner not as ill and dying, but rather as well and living. Mr. A was consistently better able to access memories of their many travel adventures and shared interests. As Mr. A reported, he was more able to smile when he thought of his partner, as opposed to being filled with empty longing and a sense of dread.

Mourning, HIV Infection, and Meaning

Saari (1988, 1991) described the self as a *meaning system*. Mr. A's journey illustrates just how interrelated the areas of meaning can become. Long-standing self-esteem issues may become mingled with the narcissistic injury of loss and HIV infection. Consequently, the sense of being damaged and different may come to dominate the person's experience of self. The more Mr. A was able to view his partner's death as separate from his own infection, the more his ability to cherish his partner and their dialogue was enhanced. As his self-esteem became more stable, Mr. A was able to engage more intensely in a number of relationships that were helpful and sustaining and that facilitated further growth.

Although Mr. A still faces HIV infection and probable severe illness, his *experience* of his infection has changed radically over the years. This is an important distinction to make. As clinicians we are working with our patients' experience of their infection and illness. Theorists from Freud onward have pointed out that people often view events in radically different ways. Our task as clinicians is to help our patients understand the meaning that they bring to HIV infection and to realize that their experience of others during the course of HIV infection may enhance or modulate the degree of distress they feel.

Clinical work with people living with HIV infection often involves helping them engage with the wide range of selfobject relationships that are available. As self-esteem problems are addressed and men become more engaged, they are exposed to relationships that enhance their sense of belonging. The strengthening of family ties can offer a great deal of reassurance and comfort. Engaging with others who are HIV infected can offer the experience of being a part of a group working to mourn and manage the psychological impact of HIV infection. Loss is often a central aspect of HIV infection and AIDS—not just the loss of people, but also the loss of a sense of future, dreams, and goals. As men engage with others facing the same losses, their grief is validated and the depth of their loss is affirmed.

Summary

Loss and the need to mourn a loss have become central aspects of the AIDS epidemic. In my practice, the majority of new patients have lost a friend or partner to AIDS. Grieving for those who have died involves a complicated and painful set of affects. Mourning is the complicated process of soothing these affects and integrating the meaning of the loss into one's life.

The potential exists for the collective, cultural grief to impede individual mourning, and for the gay community to become dominated by sadness, withdrawal, and a lack of hope. The potential also exists for the culture to facilitate mourning as rituals and structures evolve, and as gay institutions provide opportunities to help others. The AIDS quilt and memorial day observances for people lost to the epidemic serve to organize and help the gay community express affect and integrate the experience and meaning of loss.

Ultimately, grief and mourning are individual processes. As clinicians we will be asked to facilitate the mourning of our patients. Although this involves the use of the therapeutic relationship to contain and organize affects, it also involves enabling the patient to take advantage of the relationships available to him. Partaking in a larger cultural expression of grief, such as is represented by the AIDS quilt, is often a powerfully healing experience. Being with others facing similar losses affirms that one is a part of, rather than apart from. By tending to the individual's pain from loss, the clinician often enhances the patient's ability to take part in these larger, powerful, healing rituals. As professionals in the community, we need to encourage and support cultural rituals and structures that provide for the collective experience of grief.

As clinicians on the front line of the epidemic, we are a part of the larger culture of mourning emerging in the wake of so many deaths. We have experienced and will continue to experience the deaths of our patients, friends, and perhaps our partners. Grief can be profound or it can be insidious, quietly eroding our joy and hope and gradually causing us to withdraw from sustaining relationships and activities. The challenge to us is to tolerate our own grief; to face, soothe, and modulate it so that our sadness does not interfere with our capacity to tolerate and sustain the grief of our patients. Given our unique position in the epidemic, there may be limits to our capacity to integrate so many losses. Ultimately, we need to find ways of compensating for the sustained effects of loss. Just as we must say good-bye to our patients, and far too often friends and partners, we must also move on to participate in the continual unfolding of human experience.

References

Bowlby J: Attachment and Loss, Vol 3: Loss, Sadness and Depression. New York, Basic Books, 1980

Goldberg A: The Prisonhouse of Psychoanalysis. Hillsdale, NJ, Analytic Press, 1990

Kohut H: The Restoration of the Self. New York, International Universities Press, 1977

Martin J: Psychological consequences of AIDS-related bereavement among gay men. J Consult Clin Psychol 56:856–862, 1988

Martin J, Dean L, Garcia M, et al: The impact of AIDS on a gay community: changes on sexual behavior, substance use, and mental health. Am J Community Psychol 17:269–293, 1989

Neugebauer R, Rabkin J, Williams J, et al: Bereavement reactions among homosexual men experiencing multiple losses in the AIDS epidemic. Am J Psychiatry 149:10, 1992

Palombo J: Parent loss and childhood bereavement: some theoretical considerations. Clinical Social Work Journal 9:3–33, 1981

Palombo J: The psychology of the self and the termination of treatment. Clinical Social Work Journal 10:46–62, 1982

Palombo J: Bridging the chasm between developmental theory and clinical theory, II: the bridge, in The Annual of Psychoanalysis, Vol 18. Edited by Goldberg A. Hillsdale, NJ, Analytic Press, 1990

Saari C: Clinical Social Work Treatment. New York, Gardner Press, 1988

Saari C: The Creation of Meaning in Clinical Social Work. New York, Guilford, 1991

Shane M, Shane E: Object loss and selfobject loss: a consideration of self psychology's contribution to understanding mourning and the failure to mourn, in The Annual of Psychoanalysis, Vol 18. Edited by Goldberg A. Hillsdale, NJ, Analytic Press, 1990

Shelby RD: If a Partner Has AIDS: Guide to Clinical Intervention For Relationships in Crisis. Binghamton, NY, Haworth, 1992

Chapter 4

The Psychotherapist as Spiritual Helper

Rev. Jennifer M. Phillips, D.Min.

Historically, the relationship between psychotherapy and religion has been like that of two sisters who, despite much mutual suspicion and scorn, remained connected by familial bonds that cannot be argued away. Psychotherapists have dismissed religious beliefs as infantile projections, self-deception, or worse. Religious practitioners have regarded psychotherapy as an arrogant attempt at self-healing without regard for the divine source of all healing and the role of sin. Yet both disciplines remain committed to the process of healing, the goals of healthy work and right relationships, and the condition of genuine inner peace and self-awareness. Ideally, both further these ends. Realistically, both sometimes fall short.

The North American Nursing Diagnosis Association has recognized *spiritual distress* as a diagnosis, defining it as a disruption in the life principle that pervades a person's entire being and integrates and transcends biopsychosocial nature. Spiritual distress may be catalyzed by challenges to an individual's belief system, through estrangement from one's roots in a community of faith or spiritual culture, through abrupt confrontation with mortality, or through moral decision making that crosses previous ethical boundaries. Although some patients may express spiritual distress in explicitly religious language (I don't know what I believe anymore! Maybe God has abandoned me!), many may use more diffuse language to raise questions of meaning, purpose, causality, and destiny (Why should I go on? This isn't what I expected of my life. I feel like the universe is against me.). Religious questions may be about God, heaven, or right and wrong as defined in particular sacred scriptures or traditions. They may also appear as reflections about an eternal dimension to life, a sense of being part of a reality that transcends oneself and the concrete world, or an awareness of purpose larger than one can fully understand and appreciate.

In a culture and age in which many find it easy to talk about sexuality, spirituality sometimes remains a taboo subject. Although we think of spirituality as being private, it is in fact a shared dimension of humanness, enhanced by the supportive presence of others (Phillips 1989b). And even if some psychotherapists are profoundly uncomfortable with the idea, they are in an ideal role to be spiritual helpers to patients in distress. Espousal of a personal religious belief system is not necessary in order to help, but a willingness to suspend one's own adamant disbelief and to avoid reducing all religious questions to psychodynamic language is necessary; if these conditions cannot be met, the therapist would do well to refer such questions to a member of the clergy or other suitable religious caregiver.

A gay man who has been diagnosed as infected with the human immunodeficiency virus (HIV) is likely to be facing at least two sources of spiritual distress. First, if HIV infection is diagnosed as a result of obvious clinical symptoms, members of the patient's community of faith, his family, friends, or acquaintances may confront him over issues of sexual orientation, sexual practice, or intravenous drug use. In most religious traditions and in the prevailing secular culture with its Judeo-Christian residue, homosexuality is still regarded as an illness, a moral deficiency, or both. The publicly gay man may have already either left or been ostracized from a religious community because of his sexual orientation. In the best of circumstances, he may have had to rethink his relationship with the cosmos or God and renegotiate his status, whether formal or informal, as a member of a community of faith. Second, HIV infection itself can be a spiritual stressor, raising questions of unworthiness, uncleanliness, sinfulness, punishment, fear, and destiny before and after death. The questions may be raised by the patient himself or may be pressed by those around him. They will almost certainly arise in psychotherapy in some form. To help, the psychotherapist need only be willing to ask gentle and open-ended questions that allow the patient to explore his own spiritual resources, and to listen for the sacred in ordinary conversation.

The material in this chapter derives from my 10 years of hospital chaplaincy during the period in which HIV infection first began to be diagnosed and treated in the eastern United States, 5 years as an inner-city Episcopal parish priest to a congregation touched early and deeply by the acquired immunodeficiency syndrome (AIDS), and an overlapping 8 years as a community AIDS educator, chairperson of several HIV-related organizations and task forces, and a pastoral care and counseling resource person for the AIDS Action Committee in Boston. The chapter is organized around the central issues of spiritual distress and healing that are likely to arise in some form for most patients.

Why Is This Happening to Me?

This question may come to the psychotherapist's ears in many ways, either as a question or as a set of assumptions comprising an answer of sorts. The tone may be bewildered, wondering, angry, bitter, sad, or resigned, as exemplified in the following excerpts:

◆   As the 27-year-old son of a second-generation Irish immigrant family, raised in and long fallen away from the Roman Catholic Church, and to whom God, the punitive Great Father, was seen as unexpectedly harsh and exacting, stated:

>   I know I haven't been everything my Ma and Pa brought me up to be, and I don't hold with everything the Catholic Church puts out, but I guess I've gone right on believing in God. What kind of God would do something like this to anybody, no matter what they had done?

◆   As a Roman Catholic gay man in his 40s, who was a member of a congregation of gay Catholics, stated:

I guess my luck ran out. I probably got infected 8 or 9 years ago when I was doing the bathhouse scene. How could any of us have known back then what AIDS would turn out to be. Someplace in the Bible it talks about rain falling on the just and the unjust alike. I guess AIDS is like that. I don't think God made it happen. My own choices sure helped. It's just one of those things that happens if you're in the wrong place at the wrong time. I believe he'll give me the strength to fight it.

◆ As a 28-year-old man who was Buddhist by affiliation, although he had grown up vaguely Protestant on the West Coast, stated:

My teacher said to bear in mind that everything is always changing and passing away, and that to pretend that you can stop it, that you can keep things the way they were is to be trapped in illusion. Still, I wish to hell this hadn't happened to me! But I'm trying to keep meditating and to just take things as they come . . . you know, with openness and calmness.

The question of, Why HIV? may find concrete, rational answers for some patients: "Because I slept with a guy who had it; I did risky things, so why not me?" For others, the answers are sought on the cosmic scale as they wonder, Is there a deity in charge of things who caused this, someone I can blame? Ideas about and images of God for those patients claiming some belief in a deity are constructed out of the complex web of family nurturing or its absence; subsequent experience in the world and in important relationships; cultural material (e.g., film, literature, television); and faith traditions encountered throughout life. They may be comforting, challenging, or threatening; functional or dysfunctional; and may reflect the beliefs of a particular faith tradition accurately or idiosyncratically. Within any one faith tradition there may be diverse and even conflicting ideas about who God is and how the divine and the human interact. For example, within the Judeo-Christian tradition there are those believers who focus on a stern and judging God who "separates the sheep from the goats" and consigns some to everlasting fire, and who tests people's mettle through suffering and adversity. Others, also building their understanding on sacred scriptures, emphasize that God is all-loving and all-forgiving and does not willingly afflict the children of earth.

It is seldom helpful for a spiritual advisor to try to talk a patient out of his ideas about God. It is helpful to listen hard for those ideas that seem superficial and pat, and those that are deeply rooted, and to reflect back the difference between the two. It may also be helpful to ask the innocent question, Do all Christians (or Buddhists, neopagans, Jews, Baptists, and so on) believe as you do? The question offers a larger context for the reexamination of closely held beliefs.

Freud and his followers were by no means wholly incorrect in maintaining that images of God are often projections of early childhood needs and experiences—the feared or wished-for or ambivalent father (or mother) of infancy writ large (see Rizzuto 1979). If the capricious and punishing God closely resembles the abusive father of the patient's own life, the therapist may rightly offer that observation to the patient in the process of examining those first family relationships. It is helpful to recognize that when a patient heals to the point of no longer allowing the abusive, neglectful, or unreliable parent to exercise power over his present life, that the parentlike image of God may also be debunked from his throne. Relief may be accompanied by spiritual panic over not having a viable image of God to replace the old image. At this juncture it would be congruent with the teachings of any religious tradition to remark that, if God exists, surely God is not defined or limited by our ideas about God, nor is God identical to our parents. The question can then be posed fruitfully, What do you think that God must be like in order to be God? The therapist may also find food for understanding by asking the patient to draw or describe how God looks to him, or to draw or describe a scenario in which God and the patient meet face to face.

For the patient whose earliest familial experience was one of neglect and abandonment, God is more likely to be envisioned as harsh and judgmental rather than as abandoning. As with parents, it is often less devastating to experience an angry and unkind authority than to believe that one has, and somehow deserves, none at all. If during therapy the patient's understanding of God crumbles, then great sensitivity is needed to discern whether or not he needs to construct a life free of all religious ideas for the present, as religion may have become synonymous with abuse. Alternatively, the patient may need encouragement to explore his spirituality anew because he continues to yearn for or experience a numinous dimension to his life.

What Can I Trust?

Change and unpredictability are the hallmarks of living with HIV infection. Indeed, they characterize all life. The awareness of HIV infection magnifies these variables dramatically as spiritual stressors. As a 30-year-old history teacher who was asymptomatic but aware of his HIV infection described the disease, it is "a sword of Damocles just hanging over me by a thread. . . . I never know when it's going to come down, maybe kill me right then, maybe just lop off an arm or a leg or scratch me some; and nobody else knows it's there—this nagging fear."

As HIV-positive patients become more knowledgeable about their infection and begin to cope with the symptoms, they are likely to become increasingly vigilant. Attempts to take control of their health through diet, prophylactic treatment, changes in life-style, alternative therapies, and meditation or positive thinking may offer the hope of delaying the onset of symptoms, but at some level these patients are likely to realize that despite "doing everything right," sometimes disability and death strike. In terms of their spiritual life, the whole universe may begin to feel like a dangerous and hostile place. God may be seen as the sadistic or indifferent gamester who plays dice for one's life. The rapidity of change may feel overwhelming, either because it is an inexorable process of loss and decline or because it is an unpredictable succession of hopes dashed and restored.

The best remedy for the spiritual distress resulting from the roller-coaster ride of unpredictable illness may be redefining one's own role in a less passive way. The patient may not be the driver, but he does not need to be the helpless child just hanging on for dear life either. Case 1 illustrates the beginning of just such a transition from passivity to empowerment.

Case 1

Mr. A was a very shy 30-year-old Indian man who described himself as being brought up Hindu but not much involved in it since college.

He had had a closeted relationship with a lover who had died from an AIDS-related illness 2 years previously. At the time I met him and had the following conversation with him, he had been hospitalized twice with Pneumocystis carinii pneumonia (PCP) and had lost massive amounts of weight:

Mr. A: I'm really fed up with being sick. You know, my landlord is making trouble again because my rent is late. I haven't felt well enough to finish the drawings for my two clients, and they're calling every day. Makes me want to hide! You know?

Priest: Sounds like a lot of pressure on you when you're feeling sick.

Mr. A: I ask myself why I have to go through all this, what for? And just to end up like [my deceased lover] anyway. It's too much. But then it's not like I have much choice, is it?

Priest: You're reminding me of Arjuna. You know about Arjuna?

Mr. A: Yeah. In the *Mahabharata*. I saw it on television, and I remember some of it from when I was a boy.

Priest: Arjuna is standing with Krishna on the eve of the battle and saying, "I'd really rather not do this. A lot of good people are going to get killed and there'll be general devastation and I'm going to suffer a lot of losses and maybe die myself." And Krishna says. . . . Do you remember?

Mr. A: Krishna says something about, "Well, you're a warrior and it's your *dharma* to do the work that is given to you and do it nobly, so quit complaining," or something like that, right?

Priest: Uh huh. Does that fit for you?

Mr. A: I haven't thought of AIDS as my work before, or my destiny; and I sure haven't thought of myself in this state as any kind of a warrior. [He laughed.] Huh! Well, it sure does feel like a bloody battle some days.

It was in the work of Viktor Frankl (1959), an author who survived the Nazi death camps to write of his experiences, that I first heard the truth that when all of life is out of control and full of suffering, one retains a single arena of freedom and power: the right to choose one's attitude. Much of therapy has to do with reminding patients of this choice and helping them form selves with the power to choose. In the great epic *Mahabharata,* Arjuna chooses to fulfill his destiny by fighting the battle against injustice and God, in the person of Krishna, drives his chariot. Mr. A returned to this image again and

again in the two subsequent hospitalizations before his death. Despite
increasing weakness, he was able to see himself as a responsible agent
in the drama of his own life.

What Am I Worth?

HIV infection inevitably raises questions of guilt, shame, and self-
esteem. For many gay patients, these are old and familiar arenas of
struggle.

Guilt is the negative self-appraisal arising in response to the question, What have I done that I should not have done or what have I
failed to do that I should have done? For those patients active in 12-
step recovery programs, this question is prompted by the successful
completion of the step in which one takes an honest moral inventory
of one's life and actions. Therapists are well aware that guilt may be
functional or dysfunctional. It may lead the patient to make restitution
or amends for commissions and omissions of the past, and to institute
changes in present and future conduct in order to achieve greater con-
gruence between espoused and lived values, or it may reflect an inflated sense of personal power and responsibility with little basis in
reality. The therapeutic task of drawing the distinction between reality-based guilt and illusion-based guilt and bringing both to resolution
is helpful to the spiritual task of amending life and seeking and receiving forgiveness from self, others, and God.

Every religious tradition offers an avenue of repentance and forgiveness, although each does so in its own particular language.
Change of life in the direction of good is always possible, no matter
what has gone before. The Christian tradition posits this truth by saying that God is all-merciful and will forgive any and all sins where
there is repentance; the only unforgivable sin is blasphemy against the
Holy Spirit, which is variously defined in the tradition, but which to
this author means denial that there is a spirit with power or the will
to forgive. For a patient trained in a sacramental religious tradition,
even when confession has taken place in the therapeutic context and
some degree of self-forgiveness has occurred, a ritual enactment of the
process of confession and absolution may be helpful and even neces-

sary. Although in the Roman Catholic or Anglo-catholic tradition any priest can offer absolution in the Sacrament of Reconciliation of a Penitent, the therapist might suggest that the patient choose a confessor or church carefully in order to maximize the likelihood of receiving compassionate and helpful counsel during confession. A multiservice AIDS organization should be able to provide suitable referrals to HIV-sensitive and gay-affirmative clergy.

Whereas guilt focuses on action and inaction, *shame* focuses on being and the thorough realization that "I am not the person I should be." From a therapeutic standpoint, the primary goal is to promote self-acceptance; a secondary goal may be to change oneself in a realistic manner in the direction of one's ideals.

Various religious traditions offer slightly different frameworks for understanding shame. In most Protestant and Catholic traditions of Christianity, shame is seen as the common lot of all humanity because, according to the formative myth of Genesis, it derived from when Adam and Eve, tempted by the Serpent, ate the fruit forbidden them by God. In some Christian communities, continual acknowledgment of one's personal fallen condition is stressed. In others, the emphasis is on the belief that all humans as sinners, or as some subset of humanity that has a particular relationship to Jesus Christ, have been saved from sin, redeemed by God's grace, and brought into the promise of eternal life. Jewish tradition shares the same myth, but tends to stress the common lot of all humanity descended from Adam, and the importance of continual efforts to do righteous deeds as prescribed for the Covenant People in the Torah. The history of the collective call, falling away from God, and being recalled, repenting, and returning to a right relationship with God offers the context in which an individual's life can be conducted. Buddhism offers an emphasis on compassion as a sign of the enlightened life; when one slips from the path of compassion and becomes aware of the lapse, one offers compassion to oneself and simply tries again to live compassionately.

In some religious traditions, change of the self and behavior may be valued as a higher priority than self-acceptance. Even within Christianity, some denominations stress one's worthiness to stand before God, whereas others declare, "We are not worthy so much as to gather up the crumbs beneath God's table!" A patient's spiritual response to feelings of shame may have much to do with the religious understanding with which he was raised. The therapist as spiritual helper may find it more efficacious to explore the remedies for shame within the framework of the patient's religious beliefs than to try to change his beliefs or debunk them entirely.

For the patient with an unworthiness-based religious understanding, the therapeutic work of coming to self-acceptance may lead to the insight, If I can forgive and accept myself, then surely God can forgive and accept me too. For the patient with a worthiness-based religious framework, acknowledging that God loves and forgives endlessly may provide firm ground for the therapeutic task of self-acceptance.

Questions that may help the patient explore spiritual healing from shame might include the following:

◆ Do you believe there are limits on God's ability to forgive? If so, why?
◆ Do you believe your own sins or faults are unique? (Spiritual directors in the Christian tradition have long been alert for the peculiar "spiritual pride" evinced by those who believe they are the chief of sinners!)
◆ Do you believe that God can hate what God has created?
◆ What might be necessary for God to forgive you or love you? Does God expect the impossible from you?
◆ When God looks at you with the eyes of compassion, what do you think God sees?
◆ What is good or lovable about you?

As a spiritual concern, self-esteem has twin facets: What is my worth in my own eyes? and What is my value in the eyes of God or in the great scheme of things? For the gay patient who is HIV positive, feelings of self-loathing, uncleanliness, and unworthiness may stem from beliefs about his sexuality as well as about his disease. If the patient belongs to or has come from a religious community that regards sexuality itself as suspect and homosexuality as particularly sinful and aberrant, his ability to make peace with his sexuality in a spiritual context may be best helped by a believer of his own tradition who represents a more tolerant point of view. At times only a member of the clergy has sufficient religious authority to interject an alternative interpretation of religious tradition, as illustrated in Case 2:

Case 2

Mr. B, an Anglo-catholic Episcopalian in the last stages of AIDS, was concerned about issues related to the reaction of his religious community and his funeral planning. When I visited him as his parish priest, we had the following conversation:

Priest: Have you had a chance to think about your funeral planning since we last talked?

Mr. B: I know you said that Episcopalians are supposed to have their bodies brought into church for the funeral, but I'm still wondering if it would be better to be cremated right away and have a memorial service later.

Priest: What makes quick cremation seem better to you?

Mr. B: Well . . . I don't know. . . . I mean, people in the parish know I have AIDS. Maybe they wouldn't be very comfortable having my body right there, especially with an open coffin and visiting hours and stuff. It seems kind of creepy anyway.

Priest: It is a different idea than lots of us grew up with, but bringing the body back to church means coming home for the last time to your community, the people who have loved you, the place where you were welcomed and came looking for God. And you know they welcome you now, alive, and knowing you have AIDS.

Mr. B: My body has these ugly sores, and I'm so skinny.

Priest: Yes. And we love you in it. Your body is precious to God and to the community; it's the same flesh that God took in Jesus when he came into the world. No part of you—your body, your sexuality, your illness—is unacceptable to God. You can still be cremated afterwards if you choose. There are quite a few people in the parish who haven't seen you in a long time and might feel the need to see your body to say good-bye. Your baptismal covenant means that you, including your body, don't just belong to yourself anymore but to your community and to God.

Mr. B: Then it would really be all right for me to be there, even like this. I'm glad. Will you explain all this to my Mom and Dad? I'd like them to understand too.

This pastoral response came out of an Anglo-catholic Episcopalian understanding, but the issues raised by the patient may be generalizable to patients of many faiths. The handling of and response to the body during life and after death expresses in a profound way the acceptance of the bodily (and sexual) self by the self and others. Thus in the therapeutic context, although a therapist may make it a rule to never or seldom touch her or his patients, respectful and appropriate touching of a patient who is HIV infected may signify that love is stronger than any fear of contagion or distaste of the body and its ills.

As a spiritual task, the discovery or construction of a self never occurs in isolation; the spiritual self is by definition a self in relation to others and to the Holy One, however the latter is understood. For the Christian, that truth is expressed by the baptismal covenant; for a Jew, by God's covenant with the people of Israel, of which each Jew is a part; for a Hindu, because each person is related to Atman, the Divine Self. The self that is found to be of value to the self and to the world is a self embedded in the human community and with a sense of transcendent value that is not solely dependent on affirmation by others.

What Does My Life Mean?

Closely related to the issue of self-esteem and value is the question of meaning. The experience of suffering gives the task of unraveling meaning a great urgency. The question of meaning moves a step beyond Why am I suffering? to What difference does my suffering make? What is it for? How do I understand it and make sense of it for myself? The determination of meaning is highly conditioned by religious as well as ethnic culture. It is also highly personal. An individual may entirely reject a meaning commonly accepted in his or her culture. For example, in Irish Roman Catholic culture, the endurance of suffering is often seen as a test in which one shows one's true mettle and devotion. In other strands of Catholicism I have heard suffering variously interpreted as bearing a share of the whole world's suffering on behalf of some weaker person who could not bear it, as a kind of offering to God, as spiritual purification, or as mortification (suppressing the physical being in order to advance the spiritual being). From people of a variety of backgrounds I have heard the thought that God never gives one more suffering than he or she can cope with uttered as an acceptance of a personal challenge to bear up. For others, suffering is indeed unbearable, although just being able to interpret the meaning of suffering may make the difference between experiencing it as bearable or unbearable. Case 3 illustrates alternative ways of interpreting suffering within one family.

Case 3

Mr. C came into my office one morning furious with his aunt who had stopped by the apartment he shared with his partner to drop off a cake. Mr. C's partner was experiencing excruciating pain in his feet from Kaposi's sarcoma (KS) and had been effectively chair- and bed-bound for several weeks.

Priest: What's happened [Mr. C]? You look really angry.
Mr. C: I am really pissed! It's my aunt butting in again. Do you know what she said to [my partner]?
Priest: What did she say?
Mr. C: She took a look at his feet and the pain he's in and she said, "Now you know what it's like to walk the way of the Cross like Jesus." What bullshit! Is that supposed to make him feel better?
Priest: Do you think she intended to make him feel better?
Mr. C: I guess so. She told me she'd been saying novenas for him.
Priest: How do you think [your partner] heard her?
Mr. C: Oh, he just smiled and said he was doing his best.
Priest: But it certainly didn't seem to make you feel better.
Mr. C: That's for sure. Like his pain was some sort of wonderful gift he should be glad for!
Priest: Have you and [your partner] talked about what going through all this means to each of you?
Mr. C: You know him! He just says it's making him a more patient person, making him appreciate the good things more.
Priest: And for you?
Mr. C: Sometimes I think it doesn't mean a damn thing. But in a way he's right. It's made me realize how much I love him and how grateful I am to have him in my life.

Mr. C experienced his aunt's attribution of meaning to his partner's suffering as a violation; indeed, interpreting someone else's suffering in any but the most tentative way is likely to be felt as an intrusion. Yet for Mr. C's aunt, interpreting her own suffering as the way of the Cross likely brings great comfort.

Issues of meaning may be caught up in a patient's impressions about the fairness or unfairness of God, fate, life, or the universe. Does the patient feel that he has been singled out for misery? That there is a particular lesson to learn? Some expiation to make for deeds or choices of the past? Is his suffering a random event or part of a cosmic plan? When the question of fairness arises, the spiritual helper must inquire what the patient's expectations have been. Was he raised to believe that what you reap, you sow; that a good life would be rewarded with happiness and freedom from pain? Is he outraged that some explicit or implicit set of cosmic rules has been violated by his misfortune? Does the patient believe that God's sense of justice and fairness should be identical with his own? All of these may be useful questions for the spiritual work of unraveling meaning, along with the primary question, What does your experience mean to you? I do not believe that suffering has intrinsic meaning; rather, I believe that the courage of the human spirit seeks to weave meaning out of the mystery of suffering rather than be defined by it.

What Will Happen to Me?

This question may arise out of wondering speculation, curiosity, fear, or dread. Its focus may be on a short-term, long-term, or eternal scale of time. It may be a rhetorical question expressing anxiety about the unknown future, or a concrete question eliciting a specific answer (e.g., What will happen to me if I am not well enough to take care of myself when I get out of the hospital?). If the question is a spiritual one, the patient's answer will stem in large part from the responses he has formulated to the previous questions, and on whether the universe is for him a trustworthy or dangerous place to inhabit. The most clarifying responses may be questions themselves, such as, What do you expect? What do you hope for? or, What do you fear?

At the onset of severe symptoms or with the advance of symptoms, patients commonly ask, "What will happen to me when I die?" meaning, What will my dying be like? and, What will happen to me after I die? (Phillips 1989a). The first of the latter questions may indicate very clear expectations in the mind of the patient. Most gay men with HIV infection to whom I have been a spiritual helper have seen friends, lovers, and colleagues die from AIDS-related illnesses, and many have a dread of dying in the same manner. A gay patient whose lover died of PCP in choking respiratory distress may be terrified of the same fate when he has his first bout of pneumonia. A man who has cared for a friend who became demented and infantile may harbor a fear of following in his footsteps. To these specific fears, the therapist, like other caregivers, may only be able to reassure the patient to the point of saying, "Each person's situation is different and yours may be quite unlike his," and then remind the patient about the supports that are available to help him cope with whatever happens, as in Case 4.

Case 4

Mr. D's health had been in a gradual decline from AIDS for about 2 years. He had been making concrete preparations for his death at the time of the following conversation. His former lover had died of PCP, and he had lost more than two dozen friends to AIDS-related illnesses.

Mr. D: What will it be like when I die?
Priest: What would you like to have happen?
Mr. D: I'd like to just go to sleep and not wake up. But I don't want to be alone.
Priest: Who would you want to have with you?
Mr. D: Oh, my mother and sister, you, and my friend.
Priest: Well, when the time comes, we'll try very hard to make that happen.
Mr. D: In your work you've seen a lot of people die. What is it like?
Priest: Everyone leaves the world in their own way, and usually it kind of fits the person that they have been in their life. Some people fight hard, some let go peacefully. In my experience, with good doctors like yours, patients are generally not too un-

comfortable. But it's often kind of like being born, or giving birth, a process that sometimes has hard labor attached and one that sometimes just happens on its own. And I believe that there are arms to catch you when you pass out of this world just as there were arms to catch you when you slipped into it.

Mr. D: And do you believe in heaven?

Priest: Yes. Do you?

Mr. D: I'm not sure. What do you think it would be like?

Priest: Well, there are all sorts of different images in our tradition: pearly gates and streets of gold, a city on a hill, green meadows. I don't know for sure. But I know that God loves us, and so heaven will be a place where we know and feel love fully, with nothing in the way—just face to face with God. And I believe the people we have loved who have died will be there and we will finally love and understand one another fully.

Mr. D: I like that. You know, when my friend died, he was in a kind of dreamy state and he was talking to his grandfather who had died when he was a kid, just like he was there in the room. Do you think the grandfather had come to meet him?

Priest: Just before my grandmother died she told me she had a visit from her brother who had been dead for decades. Yes, I think that's very possible.

For the therapist as spiritual helper, conversations about the afterlife may be more or less uncomfortable depending on the therapist's own beliefs. At times the response, "I don't know, what do you think?" may be the most authentic one. When the patient is well and in the midst of life, preoccupation with death and heaven may be a distraction from the important issues of the present, but as HIV-related illnesses produce symptoms, thinking and talking about one's fate after death is as important a part of preparation for dying as making a will.

The only way to become comfortable with such explorations with patients is to explore one's own beliefs about afterlife and God, and one's own feelings of fear, grief, or aversion in connection with one's own mortality. In the ancient Christian tradition, meditating on one's dying (often very concretely: What will the deathbed scene be? The funeral? The burial? What's the soul's-eye view of the dying moments? What do other people say and do?) was felt to be an essential part of every believer's spiritual discipline throughout life. "Thou oughtest in every deed and thought so to order thyself as if thou wert to die today," wrote the medieval author of *The Imitation of Christ* (Kempis 1882, p. 64), a devotional classic. Such thoughts were not seen as morbid, but as evincing a proper humility in the face of personal human finitude, and as being a strengthening and clarifying process.

One of the therapist's tasks as a spiritual helper for the patient facing death may be to relinquish his or her own image of "the good death," and acknowledge that the patient will die in his own way. For example, one patient swore that he was going to fight AIDS and win. He was adamant about not wanting to leave the new and wonderful relationship he had found, and during the night that he died he kept crying out, "No! No! I'm not going to go! I don't want to die." His nurses, physician, and friends shared afterward that they felt they had failed him because they could not help him to come to a peaceful acceptance of his death, and because they could not help him hold death back. It seemed to me that this patient's anguished dying held great integrity, for he had left the world just as he had chosen to live in it: as a fighter passionately connected to the world and the people he loved.

Who Am I Now? . . . And Now?

With physically healthy patients, a central goal of therapy may often be to produce a stable and peaceful sense of self. AIDS-related illnesses may complicate this process of learning and growing by effecting personality and role changes (Phillips 1988), cognitive debilitation, and physiological changes that are injurious to the patient's sense of self. Whereas a physically healthy patient might feel closer to normal every day and week as therapy progresses, AIDS dementia and physical illness may produce a situation in which the patient never knows who he will be when he wakes up the next morning. Both global and progressive losses and sudden and unpredicted changes can produce a profound sense of dislocation from all that is dear, predictable, and reassuring. The following examples illustrate some of the physical disfigurements AIDS-related illnesses can cause:

◆ A 26-year-old hospitalized patient had uncontrolled KS lesions that were attacking his organs and that had turned his whole face into a mass of weeping, purple and red, raw sores. He looked as though he had been badly burned. He said to me, "I'm afraid to look in the mirror when I wake up in the morning. I don't know the man I'm seeing."

◆ A 36-year-old patient saw his weight drop to 92 pounds, walked hunched over like an elderly man, and had hair that was as thin and patchy as a cancer patient on chemotherapy. One day he took a dog-eared photograph out of his bureau and showed it to me. In it a sturdy 6-foot bearded man posed for friends on a Provincetown beach. Only something about the brown eyes struck me as familiar. "That's a great picture of you!" I said. "Thank God you recognized me!" he answered; "I showed it to two of my nurses and they asked who it was."

◆ A young chef in his mid-30s who had been admitted to the hospital with toxoplasmosis lost normal functioning so quickly that he could no longer read or write, and when friends came to visit he had only a dim sense that they were familiar and that he ought to know them. As I sat by his bed, he turned his head back and forth from one side to the other, repeating his name over and over again. "I'll never forget your name, and neither will God," I said to him. Clearly, he was desperately afraid he would lose his own name and with it, himself.

The book of the prophet Isaiah depicts God as saying to God's people, "I will not forget you. Behold, I have graven you on the palms of my hands." Perhaps only by serving as a companion to someone in the process of losing himself, or facing that loss personally through injury, illness, or psychosis, can the poignancy of that promise be fully understood.

In religious traditions as diverse as Judaism and Shintoism, as well as in several of the faiths of the indigenous peoples of the Americas and Australia, remembering the dead is understood as a sacred task. The patient losing himself through AIDS-related illness has an urgent need to know that he is being *re-membered* (i.e., put back into membership with himself, God, and the human community) even before he dies.

As his or her patient's memory fades, the spiritual helper might ask, What do you want me to remember most about you? How do you hope people will tell the story of your life and who you have been? and offer the assurance that this legacy is treasured and will be preserved. There is much mourning for both the patient and the therapist to do, as who the patient once was is inexorably changed and diminished. At times, the patient may be mercifully unaware of the changes, especially as he moves into the more advanced stages of illness. In such cases, it may be the patient's loved ones who most deeply experience the loss of who that individual once was.

Not all patients face such total assaults on the self, but perhaps a majority who progress to debilitating illness must cope with some degree of regression. Parents in particular may travel a parallel path with the very regressed patient, becoming the parents they used to be to the infant or small child their son now resembles. Because regressive behavior often comes and goes, and because the patient is an adult, even if acting childishly, conflict between parents and adult children is common. In the spiritual life, the same dynamics are often at work. The patient may revert to an understanding of faith or religious practice from childhood. Sometimes this can bring great comfort. Nursery bedtime prayers may be soothing and helpful. At other times, the patient may be embarrassed by such childish needs and thoughts, and need some reassurance that, yes, he is still recognized as an adult and such thoughts and feelings are normal for a seriously ill patient. Although when well the patient may have worked out an adult-to-adult relationship with God in which he cherished his own sense of responsibility and freedom, when seriously ill and regressed, he may revert to seeing God as a "superparent" whom he can blame or complain to or invoke for rescue.

The therapist will receive some of these God projections just as he or she receives many others. By his or her own constancy and care, the therapist will best reflect the love and reliability of God to the patient.

Has God Abandoned Me?

Whenever despair and desperation come to the patient in the whole of his life, they will come to him in his spiritual life also. Although the belief that God has abandoned him may mirror the patient's experience of being abandoned by significant others, either in the past or the present, there is no absolute correlation. At times, for a person of deep faith, God is the only one who proves reliable. For others, God seems the first to go. A gay identity, with or without being infected with HIV, may be seen as the cause, result, or major symptom of God's withdrawal of love. At times, God seems absent because God has not been looked for.

The patient's spiritual task in the apparent absence of God is to contain his anxiety, and wait and seek God in patience, trusting that God wills to be found. This is far easier to say than to do when one is frightened and lonely. When the patient poses the question, Why does God seem to have abandoned me? it may be an invitation to the therapist and other important people to move closer and hold the patient tighter. It may be a sign of depression and the need for therapeutic intervention.

In the Christian monastic tradition, the experience of feeling isolated and out of touch with God, even in prayer, is one type of "desert experience" known at some time to every journeyer on the spiritual road. At this stage, classic spiritual guides recommend perseverance in the practice of prayer, even if it feels empty or without meaning; consultation with a spiritual director; and patience—in other words, remain willing to wait for God. Christian scripture depicts even a dying Jesus feeling abandoned by God. In Jewish scripture many of the psalms and writings of the prophets are cries to God from a position of abandonment, either personal or of the whole community. For those feeling abandoned in contemporary times, praying these ancient prayers can offer a powerful means of expressing their anguish. Patients with nontheistic belief systems may verbalize their own isolation or the failure of their devotional practices to bring solace without personalizing the source of the abandonment.

Anxiety-producing feelings of divine abandonment or isolation are often accompanied by a clenching of the whole being against the fear and hurt. A spiritual helper may do well to suggest trying to open the heart enough to allow for the possibility of discovering that one is not so alone. Questions such as, How are you looking or listening for God? or, How would you know if God had come back? or, Why do you think that God might have abandoned you? may be useful avenues of exploration.

What Will Be Left to Me?

The losses associated with HIV infection are massive and continual. Although some fortunate patients gain something from their diagnosis (sometimes a new support system or group of friends through AIDS service organizations), many more feel like everything they have is slipping away. And indeed the process of dying does involve the ultimate loss of everything that belongs in this world. Each new loss involves a reactivation of the grieving process. Although grief may be continual, particularly for patients who become ill early after learning they are HIV positive or who are cast out by those they love, it need not be all-pervasive. One of the earliest and most aggravating losses is the loss of the feeling of being in charge of one's life.

Every new loss in life is connected to all previous losses. For this reason, grieving is like casting out a net into a pond expecting to catch only a fish. Instead, along with the fish comes an old boot, some driftwood, maybe a flat tire, a bunch of rotting weed, or a rusty refrigerator. All the old sadnesses reemerge and combine to make the load backbreakingly heavy. Each piece of the past must be examined and removed from the net, one by one; each loss must be acknowledged and mourned again. As the therapist sits with the patient through this mourning, she or he will be hauling in her or his own net of memories and feelings and also grieving, though privately. The patient is losing his life. The therapist is losing the patient. There is considerable comfort in grieving in harmony with another human being.

Discovering a gay sexual orientation and coming out as a gay man may bring a whole separate catalog of losses for some patients. A man may have to relinquish dreams of himself as married with children. He may have to cope with societal and family disapproval of himself and any partner he chooses. He may lose a job or the possibility of certain kinds of employment or the freedom to express his affection publicly without fear of violence. His housing options may be threatened. His connection with a religious community may be lost or drastically changed.

In Case 5, Mr. E gives an account of his life story, chronicling a history of losses of which his diagnosis with HIV was just the latest and greatest blow:

Case 5

Mr. E: I never knew my dad. I guess my mom didn't know him much either. [He laughed mirthlessly.] We moved around a lot. For a while we lived with my grandmother, but then she died, and because she was only renting, we had to leave. I ran away when I was 13. Mom could hardly take care of herself. What did she need with a kid? I never thought about being gay . . . I mean as a description of me. I met a guy in Central Park—an older guy, well-dressed, who talked nice. Well, he took me home and had sex with me and bought me stuff. I lived with him for a couple of years. But he used to drink some and get pretty mean. One day he just up and told me to get out. I liked being with an older guy, helping him and everything, so I started looking out for guys like that. Some of them thought I was pretty hot stuff. Dressed me up and showed me off to their friends and stuff. But none of them lasted long.

You're a minister, right? A priest's some kind of minister?

Priest: That's right.

Mr. E: My mom was a Catholic. Taught me to believe in God and took me for my first Holy Communion and everything. I guess I liked it at the time, I don't really remember. All that stuff went down the tubes when I left home. Now I've got HIV. Why should I be surprised? It's just like my whole life. At least it won't go on much longer.

Mr. E was one of those lucky men who, through the tragedy of HIV infection, finally made some lasting human connections that stayed with him until his death. He moved off the streets and into sheltered housing, made friends with his fellow residents, had the first birthday party he'd had in 16 years thrown for him, and became involved in a whole range of activities through an AIDS center. He also found people to cry with him as he mourned the pain of his life. He was able to say during his last month that the 2 years since having been diagnosed as HIV positive were the best years of his life. What a humbling mystery that so little could seem like so much!

In doing the spiritual work of mourning and accepting some degree of loss of control with equanimity, the patient may have to go
through the process of also grieving the dashed expectation that God
would be his rescuer. Perhaps he has prayed urgently for a cure. Perhaps he has secretly believed that God would turn his diagnosis into
some sort of medical mistake, or keep him from ever developing
symptoms. Perhaps he has tried to strike a bargain with God that if he
prays hard enough, or stops having gay sex, or repairs his relationship
with a parent, or gives up drugs or alcohol, that God will keep him
healthy. Disappointment of such hopes may bring anger and feelings
of betrayal as well as of sorrow that the all-powerful one has not in-
tervened on his behalf.

In any individual's faith life, ideas of God or a particular religious
world view falls apart at intervals, making way for a reconstructed and
generally more mature and expansive sense of God and the universe.
The losses of HIV infection coming thick and fast may cause cataclysmic and repeated crumbling of the spiritual architecture. The therapist
may be helpful by acknowledging this process as normal and a part of
spiritual growth during which room is made for something new. Useful questions for exploration might include the following:

- Have there been other times in your life when everything you be-
  lieved or felt about God fell apart? What happened afterward?
- Could it be that God might be different than you had thought?
  How do you think God feels about your illness?
- Could there be other kinds of healing for you besides being cured
  from HIV?
- It feels very sad (angry, scary, and so on) when you don't get res-
  cued from this illness, doesn't it?

The sorrow that pervades the gay community is often pushed
down under the pressure of rallying resources to help the latest wave
of afflicted men and under a kind of enforced good cheer and frenzy
of activity. Even religious communities can be negatively affected by
an avoidance of grieving. It is not enough simply to bury the dead and
pray for the sick. The communal processes of loss require ongoing
rituals and expressions of mourning. The Jewish congregations ac-

complish this well through the practice of saying a daily Kaddish for a deceased loved one with other mourners for a year. The Greek Orthodox make *Kolivah,* a spiced wheat mixture that is cooked by mourners and brought into church on the 40-day and first-year anniversaries of a death. After prayers for the dead, it is eaten by the worshipers as a way of incorporating the memory of the deceased into the body of the living community.

If a community beset by continual loss does not find ways to mourn corporately, the energy to love and care for one another, invest in new relationships, and work effectively dissipates. Currents of anger and bitterness move beneath the surface. Members drop away and conflicts increase. Depression becomes pervasive and in time the community begins to become fractured.

As therapists work with increasing numbers of patients with HIV infection, their professional organizations and collegial networks also will need new ways to mourn together and remember the dead. It is not enough to work through loss in private therapy or with supervision. Rather, grief work needs to be shared in order to acknowledge that a larger social fabric is being torn and that all lives are changed as a result.

Who Will Love Me?

The public sharing of a diagnosis of HIV infection, like the sharing of gay sexual orientation with others, brings with it the voiced or unvoiced question, Will you still love me? To be realistic, at times the answer is a painful no, both from family members or friends, and from a religious community. Such a rejection may be accompanied by the worse blow: "And what's more, God doesn't love you like that either!" It is as unhelpful for a patient to remain a part of a community of faith that responds in such a fashion as it would be for one who has experienced domestic abuse to stay with the abuser and continue to be assaulted. Neutrality from the therapist may be less helpful to the spiritual recovery of a person battered by his community of faith than the strong affirmation of his lovableness and the identification of the community as abusive.

The exploration of a patient's need to remain in an abusive relationship will be a familiar task to most therapists. It is as appropriate when the abuser is a congregation or member of the clergy as when it is another person or group. But just as the patient needs nonabusive relationships (including his relationship with his therapist) to heal from family abuse, he will need a nonabusive and kind spiritual relationship and community to heal on a spiritual level.

When the diagnosis of HIV is made for a person who does not know how his religious community or adviser might respond, he would do well to find a few allies who, upon hearing about his infection, will continue to stand by him before he makes his diagnosis more widely known. He may do well to check out the reaction of the pastor of a congregation before telling the whole group, as the congregation members are likely to follow their pastor's lead. Case 6 illustrates this cautious approach to disclosure.

Case 6

Mr. F decided to come out in both ways—to disclose his being gay and his being HIV positive—to his Alcoholics Anonymous group before doing so in his Methodist church. "Once my sponsor had hugged me and said he loved me, and a whole bunch of the folks had gathered round to pat me on the back and wish me well, I felt brave enough to try telling the pastor of our church," he confided. The pastor turned out to be fairly kind, but advised this man to keep his diagnosis quiet because he didn't know if the parish was ready to deal with either his homosexuality or seropositivity. Mr. F decided that wasn't good enough for him and chose to find another church where he was sure of his acceptance as an HIV-infected gay man.

Important questions to explore with a patient seeking a spiritual community or pondering a change of community might be as follows:

◆ Does your spirit get fed and nourished in the (new or old) community?
◆ Do you know that you are loved for yourself or do you have to conceal parts of yourself? If the latter, at what cost to you?
◆ Do you feel like there are at least some people there you can trust and count on?

◆ Do you feel that the congregation and clergy are willing and able to learn and change, and to talk openly about HIV and homosexuality?

◆ Can you bring a lover there without either of you being badly treated or having to pretend you are not together?

◆ And very importantly, Do you find and feel God's presence there?

If the answers to these questions are negative, the patient needs to find a new community of faith. A therapist would do well to have a file of welcoming communities and religious leaders, just as he or she would keep a file of other helping professionals for referral. Gay-affirming and AIDS-sensitive congregational leaders frequently know of other trustworthy colleagues of different denominations and faiths and can help with a particular referral.

How Shall I Find God's Presence?

This final question is one of religious practice, which may be the area in which the therapist feels the least expert. Even if the therapist chooses to refer a patient for instruction in his life of faith, there are some useful guidelines he or she may supply.

Religious practice frequently changes with illness. Sometimes the patient has neglected his spiritual life, or never developed one at all, and the onset of illness prompts him to inquire in this direction afresh. Suddenly the meaning of life and death and the existence of God are not abstractions but urgent personal matters. In rare cases, a patient may abandon a longtime spiritual practice following a personal disaster, like the diagnosis of HIV.

Illness may disrupt habits of prayer and worship. Perhaps a patient can no longer attend church or synagogue. Perhaps he is in too much pain or is too immobile to sit for accustomed meditation. Perhaps medications disrupt his abilities to concentrate, think clearly, and remember. Maybe nausea and vomiting make it impossible for him to receive Communion. Maybe a central nervous system disease makes it impossible for him to read or speak. Maybe he is stuck in the hospital without the aids that helped him pray at home: the woods to walk in, the favorite prayer bench or rosary, the devotional books, the icons or candles, or simply his familiar and private home surroundings. Any of these may constitute a loss to be mourned.

The best advice I have ever heard about the practice of prayer is this: Don't try to pray as you can't; pray as you can. No matter what the religious tradition, if it has a practice of prayer or meditation, there will also be an understanding that when illness strikes, the best practice of prayer one can manage will be good enough. In the Christian tradition, even the intention to pray and the desire to pray are recognized as beginning forms of prayer.

Earlier in this chapter I suggested that for the very regressed or the very sick patient the method of prayer learned as a very small child may be helpful again. Or possibly illness may prompt a patient to broaden his repertoire of prayer ways. There are dozens of methods of praying. Most religious traditions use only a few. Among the most common are repeated written prayers, intercessions (prayers for other people and concerns), petitions (asking for things), thanksgivings, spontaneous verbal prayer (aloud or silent, in one's own words), chants and sacred songs, and the use of prayer beads. Various forms of centering prayer, contemplative prayer, and meditation may require some instruction from a practitioner. There are also prayers of the body, like Zen or Tibetan walking meditation or sacred dance. One may pray through writing letters to God, poems, a journal, and so on. Sacred scriptures may be read and used as the subject or inspiration for meditation, with the suppliant possibly focusing on each word for a period of time, or using his imagination to recreate a scene and enter into it. A *mantra*—a word or sound that occupies the active mind, leaving the rest of the mind open to the divine and free of distractions—may be used. Instrumental or vocal music listened to or performed may be a method of praying. A single word or thought aimed at God in the middle of activities can constitute a prayer. Doing ordinary activities in a God-mindful manner can be a form of prayer. And there are others. In various ethnic traditions, religious practices vary greatly. In some, practice is focused when the community gathers and prayer occurs there. In others, private devotions or household group devotions are the norm. Some have few requirements of prayer, per se, and instead center on living in a certain manner and observing particular customs of diet, dress, or interaction.

The question, How shall I find God's presence? may contain a further question: How can I find an anchor for my hope? Just as some patients fear the pain of going through the grieving process, others fear that they are going to lose the ability to hold on to hope and become hopeless.

In my experience, losing hope is an illusory fear. Those who seek to protect a patient from losing hope are often defending against the patient's and their own grief and fear. Human beings are remarkably skillful at finding ways to invest their hope. At the time of diagnosis, the first hope may be that the diagnosis is wrong, or that illness will never come. Later, when reality presses in, the patient may hope instead for recovery from a particular illness. He may hope for healing in relationships or for new relationships. If he becomes more seriously ill, hope may find a nearer and more finite goal, like having a pain-free day or hour, being able to walk or sit up or eat, or having a visit from a particular loved one. When the illness progresses to the life-threatening stage, the world shrinks to the size of a single room, or part of a room, or just the patient's bed, and the patient may hope for his next pain shot, or to see his lover's face, or to go to sleep and wake in heaven, or even simply for death to come. Changing hope is not loss of hope.

As with grief, the patient's shifts in hope will likely be accompanied by changes in the ground of hope for the therapist too. He or she may look forward to smaller increments of progress in therapy or to just maintaining ground; to the patient being well enough to show up; to seeing him one last time; to wishing that he be pain-free and at peace from a distance; and finally, to hoping that after death he is in the embrace of a kindly God or universe and at rest. (For an extended discussion of the caregiver's hope, see Phillips 1991.)

Conclusions

The therapist need not be a spiritual expert nor even a believer in order to help a patient with his journey of faith. Questions about religion are not too personal to ask in the therapeutic context; indeed, they are very important when working with patients around issues of sexuality, homosexuality, and HIV infection. As I have advised nurses and physicians, so I also suggest to mental health providers:

> [Such questions] communicate an honest concern for the person and family. If a patient should be distressed by being asked even a simple question about religious preference, he . . . is communicating something that is helpful . . . to know. "That seems to be a distressing question," is a comment that may elicit information about what the patient has experienced at the hands of a religious community or person, ways in which he . . . feels estranged from religious roots, or feels let down or betrayed by God. Like other pains, spiritual pains heal better with discovery and care than concealment. (Phillips 1989a, pp. 229–237)

It is an immense privilege to be a witness and companion to another individual on his or her spiritual journey. One grows in one's own spirituality in the process. A lively and kindly curiosity about matters of the spirit is the most important credential for any spiritual helper, along with a willingness to look honestly at one's own beliefs in or antipathy to religion. As with most aspects of therapy, patients seldom need to have answers provided for them by their therapist; they need to be validated in the asking of their questions, and helped along by the questions of a fellow human being who has their interests at heart.

References

Frankl VE: Man's Search for Meaning. Beacon Press, Boston, MA, 1959

Kempis T: The Imitation of Christ. London, JC Nimmo & Bain, 1882

Phillips JM: AIDS and ARC: pastoral issues in the hospital setting. Journal of Religion and Health 27:119–128, 1988

Phillips JM: Spirituality and AIDS: some transcultural perspectives, in HIV/AIDS Patient Care. Boston, MA, Massachusetts Hospital Association, 1989a, pp 229–237

Phillips JM: Nurturing the spirit, in Comfort in Caring: Nursing the Person With HIV Infection. Edited by Meisenhelder JB, LaCharite C. Boston, MA, Scott, Foresman, 1989b, pp 199–211

Phillips JM: Sustaining hope and care in the face of AIDS, in HIV Positive: Perspectives on Counseling. Edited by Tallmer M, Calson C, Lampke RF, et al. Philadelphia, PA, Charles Press, 1991, pp 124–136

Rizzuto A: The Birth of the Living God. Chicago, IL, University of Chicago Press, 1979

Chapter 5

Suicidality and HIV in Gay Men

Marshall Forstein, M.D.

R ank (1945) wrote, "Most men reject the gift of life to avoid the debt of death" (p. 251). What is it, then, that makes some men, when confronted by the fear or reality of being infected with the human immunodeficiency virus (HIV), contemplate or embrace what is to them the gift of death in order to avoid the unbearable pain of their life?

Suicidality is a common and often terrifying aspect of psychotherapy with gay men who are at risk for or known to be infected with HIV. One might go so far as to assume that if the question of suicide has not appeared in the course of psychotherapy with someone facing HIV infection, the therapist and patient are in collusion to avoid a core existential issue. Although some data have been gathered concerning the rates of suicidality in people infected with HIV (see section on research data below), the issue ultimately is a unique, existential one with which the patient himself and the significant people in his life, including his therapist, must grapple.

After defining some critical terminology and reviewing the few data published regarding suicidality in HIV-infected gay men, I discuss this issue from a psychotherapeutic standpoint. Although there are complicated moral, ethical, legal, and strategic questions involved, some of which I address in this chapter, most of my focus is on the existential and emotional issues that are inextricably related to suicidality in this patient population.

Defining Suicidality in HIV-Positive Gay Men

Suicidality in gay men with HIV-related concerns must be distinguished from suicidal ideation that results from characterologically determined vulnerabilities. HIV-related suicidality may be present in 1) gay men who are concerned about their antibody status based on their estimation of risk; 2) those who are diagnosed with an HIV-related illness, throughout the spectrum of infection; 3) those in the terminal phase of the acquired immunodeficiency syndrome (AIDS); or 4) those experiencing grief related to the loss of others to AIDS.

Suicidality includes *ideation* (i.e., thoughts of suicide, self-destruction, or annihilation), *suicide attempts* (i.e., acting on the ideation), and *completed suicide*. Suicidality may be evaluated according to both the degree of suicidal intent and the lethality of the method considered or used for the suicide. True suicidality must be distinguished from a cry for help, an accident that was intended to incur a feeling of risk but not death, or self-mutilating behavior that is known to the patient to be nonlethal. True suicidality exists when the patient intends to die and believes (however inaccurately) that the method being considered will be successful.

Self-mutilating behavior must be distinguished from suicidal behavior and ideation; the former generally predates HIV infection and is an attempt to find a way to periodically release the pain rather than to die. People with characterological propensities for self-abusive or mutilating behaviors may be at higher risk for suicide sooner after being diagnosed HIV positive because of their more tenuous sense of self and greater impulsivity. The diagnosis of HIV seropositivity may exacerbate acting out feelings of self-loathing and unworthiness.

Passive suicidal ideation differs from *active suicidal ideation*, and perhaps should not be termed suicidality. The psychological meaning of wishing that life would take its natural course more quickly may be significantly different from that of questioning how to hasten that natural process, whether by doing or not doing something.

Rational Suicide

Clinicians often hear patients about to be tested for HIV antibodies predicting that they will take their life if they find out they are positive, usually with the justification that they could not live with the diagnosis. Some speak about the decision to take their life only when a particular event happens or a change occurs in their health status, such as they become cognitively impaired, incontinent, or blind, or lose the ability to live alone. These parameters are often set forth by patients before the fact, and are intended to help frame their response to their illness.

How are we to understand the very purpose of the contemplation, planning, and finally execution of the suicidal behavior itself? How do we begin to make psychodynamic sense out of one's wish to assault one's self? Is it possible for self-annihilation to make sense? It is apparent from clinical experience that some individuals confronting an unwanted assault on the integrity of their self (e.g., such as that from a progressive debilitating illness) do think about dying in order to make sense out of life

The psychodynamic meaning of a patient's projected suicidality is the immediate clinical issue to address, rather than what will actually happen to the patient in the future. The right to end one's life, like the right to refuse treatment, becomes a philosophical issue discussed as *rational suicide*. Thus the question remains, as framed by existential philosophers, What is the purpose and value of contemplating self-annihilation? Socrates reportedly was asked by a student, "Why do we philosophize?" He replied, "We philosophize in order to learn how to die, so that we might learn how to live."

Rational suicide, sometimes referred to as *self-deliverance,* is usually discussed as an option freely chosen by the patient. Siegal's definition of rational suicide has been summarized as having three essential characteristics (see Goldblum and Moulton 1989):

1. That the patient has an accurate and realistic assessment of his particular situation
2. That there exists no diagnosable, treatable psychological illness or emotional distress that impairs the patient's decision
3. That a majority of uninvolved observers from the patient's own community or social group would understand and affirm the motivation for such a decision

I would add a caveat that a substance abuse disorder or acute intoxication precludes the rationality as described above.

Rational suicide is more easily thought about as a reasonable decision to terminate one's pain and discomfort for which there is no physical or psychological relief. The right to terminate treatment, even in the face of hastening one's own death, has been upheld as legal as well as ethical, and has brought about a revolution in thinking about living wills. But the step from refusing potentially life-sustaining treatment to self-administering an agent that brings about death is still a complex psychological and social issue. For example, unless one takes the position that actively taking one's own life is never rational, the debate seems clearer when the individual is at the point of irreversible *physical or cognitive (neurological) deterioration.* Less clear is whether suicide would be acceptable when a patient's *psychological pain* is irreversible and at an unbearable level, as determined by the patient himself. Are there malignant and irreversible psychological states that are not amenable to treatment and of such existential or spiritual magnitude that the value of life is rationally determined to be less than the value of death?

Another question that needs to be addressed is, What time interval should pass between the point of wanting to die and the objective, expectable point of death in order that the decision to terminate one's life is judged as rational and not irrational? Does imminent death, say within weeks rather than months or years, change our acceptance of the rational nature of a decision to terminate life? Does a gay man who has lost his job, housing, and countless friends to AIDS; who is clearly in the throes of unremitting grief; and who is himself facing what he believes to be an unbearable life for months or even years choose suicide rationally or irrationally? Is the decision of another individual to choose suicide ever rational to those who do not contemplate such an act for themselves?

Complicating the picture even more are those psychiatric disorders that render the patient incapable of rationally choosing suicide. Because depression, anxiety states, and substance abuse disorders are common in gay men infected with HIV, the burden of proof appears to be on therapists and physicians to rule out a treatable organic or reactive illness throughout the spectrum of HIV infection that might account for the patient's despair and wish to die. On the other hand, the patient's sentiments may appear rational to his community of peers, themselves experiencing the metapsychological impact of the epidemic on an already stigmatized and outlawed group (Forstein 1992a).

To me, in order for a suicide to be considered a rational suicide, every available treatment known to be possibly effective in treating anxiety and depression should be tried before the patient can be assumed to be free of a psychiatric illness or the emotional distress that would impair the mental process leading to the decision to terminate one's life. It may be easier to rule out a psychiatric disorder as a complicating factor than it is to understand the spiritual issues that may factor into the decision to terminate one's existence. Empathy that permits the clinician to understand and even support the individual who rationally decides to die must not lead to overidentification with the patient's reasoning to the extent that the therapist misses a treatable disorder (see Chapter 22). Case 1 illustrates how empathy for a terminally ill person's sense of hopelessness and resignation might preclude appropriate diagnosis and treatment.

Case 1

Mr. A was a 41-year-old gay man who had end-stage cytomegalovirus retinitis, for which he was being aggressively but not successfully treated. Having lost vision in one eye, being threatened with imminent blindness, and having survived to a birthday that he had not anticipated reaching since being diagnosed as HIV positive, he became acutely suicidal. At the time, Mr. A was living at home with his parents, who were quite supportive and emotionally available to him. He had discussed the option of suicide with them, finding that they could understand his wish to end his life while his mental processes were still intact but that they could not help him with that process. Mr. A understood their position and assured them that he would not ask them to participate; still he sought assurances from them that they would not hate him for "taking the easy way out."

One night, without telling his therapist or his group, he ingested five secobarbital sodium (Seconal) pills and six lorazepam (Ativan) pills, placed a plastic bag over his head, and lay down to sleep at midnight, expecting that his father would find him dead in the morning. His attempt was unsuccessful. Following this, Mr. A's family called his primary care physician, who decided to monitor Mr. A's vital signs at home through the use of visiting nurses. In this way, the family was intent on honoring the discussions they had had with their son regarding the issue of self-determination and rational suicide.

After 2 days, Mr. A was brought to the health center where he met with his therapist and a psychiatrist. Unusually meticulous in his profession and personal life, Mr. A had actually been sloppy about his suicide attempt, having not ingested enough pills to ensure his death. Mr. A was able to acknowledge that his ambivalence about dying was the reason. Seen in this light, Mr. A's suicide attempt had to be interpreted as a plea for help in containing his terror and rage at his disease and at dying. A long-avowed agnostic, Mr. A found himself in the spiritual chains of his early Catholic upbringing, not at all clear about what he really felt and believed about ending his life rather than seeing it through to the end. He was relieved to be finally discussing his doubts about rational suicide with the psychiatrist, who was new to the treatment team, rather than simply receiving permission to die, as he had from his parents and caregivers, who had colluded to avoid facing the issue of dying. In their efforts to be empathic and understanding, the family, physician, and therapist had confused their own anxiety about dying with that of the patient.

A short course of a psychostimulant was prescribed for Mr. A after discerning that he was depressed to a degree beyond despair and grief. He rapidly responded to the antidepressant effects of the psychostimulant and proceeded to engage in a powerful and painful struggle to make sense out of his living and dying and to face the real choices he had to make. The outcome was that he proceeded to work in therapy and with his family on dealing with the ongoing ravages of the illness. Mr. A died several months later, having determined for himself that life was worth living to its natural end.

Incidence of Suicidality Among HIV-Positive Gay Men

Research Data

Available research data provide a confusing picture of the extent of HIV-related suicidality. Early reports from New York (Marzuk et al.

1988) and Lackland Air Force Medical Center (Rundell et al. 1989) showed that patients who were infected with HIV had a risk for suicide 35 to 40 times that of HIV-negative individuals. More recent studies (Holland and Tross 1985; O'Dowd and McKegney 1990; O'Dowd et al. 1989) showed lower rates, not dissimilar to those found in non–HIV-infected populations. Research has also shown that differences exist between populations infected with HIV; suicidality and emotional distress are less among people with an AIDS diagnosis than among asymptomatic and symptomatic HIV-positive patients who anxiously await an AIDS diagnosis, which would seem to make the future clearer (McKegney and O'Dowd 1992).

Clinical and anecdotal reports confirm that suicide is a potential consequence of HIV infection at any point in the spectrum of illness. Speculations about how some people infected with HIV or diagnosed with AIDS have died circulate within the gay communities, and psychotherapists at meetings confer anxiously about cases in which they have been confronted with a suicidal patient or lover of someone who is HIV positive.

Because of methodological and other constraints, many questions about HIV-related suicidality have not been adequately answered by research efforts to date. Therapists may be better informed about the risks of suicidality among HIV-positive patients because of available research data and may use these data as justification for making suicidality a normative issue for discussion and exploration. But such research does not help to assess a particular patient's risk for completed suicide. What is gathered from research about gay men in San Francisco (where the risk for suicide may not be increasing, according to one report [Engleman et al. 1988]) may not be accurate for gay men in different economic, geographic, cultural, or ethnic groups.

Other relevant research data come from the studies that look at suicidality in gay and lesbian adolescents. Ramafedi et al. (1991) and others (Kourany 1987; Schneider et al. 1989) have documented that gay or bisexual adolescent boys have three to four times the risk for suicide that their heterosexual peers have. Forstein (1992a) found that, although gay and lesbian teenagers accounted for one-third of all adolescent suicides, the literature on adolescent suicide virtually does not address the issues of sexual orientation and the psychological stressors of being gay or lesbian in a homophobic society. This lack of attention thus reinforces these young individuals' experience of being invisible and unaccepted within society. During adolescence, a gay male may have only begun to develop a gay-affirmative sense of himself and may still be unconsciously conflicted about his sexuality; if during this stage he is also faced with HIV infection—an illness that is inextricably related to his sexuality—he could be at an increased risk for suicidal ideation.

Further, research directly comparing seropositive gay men who are suicidal with nongay patients who have other life-threatening illnesses may be misdirected because the base rate of suicidality in the populations compared may be different. Cabaj (see Chapter 19) further reports on research data that suggest a possibly higher base rate for substance abuse in gay men, another predisposing factor for suicide that might confound any comparison between HIV-infected gay men with other people at risk for HIV infection.

Factors That Increase HIV-Related Suicidality

Although the available research data are epidemiological and do not address psychodynamic or psychosocial factors that increase the risk for HIV-related suicidality, much has been learned from clinical experience at HIV-antibody testing sites, crisis intervention teams, and ongoing psychotherapy with individuals, couples, and groups. The following is culled from the author's own 12 years of experience working with gay men concerned about HIV, as well as from the literature (Forstein 1984; Goldblum and Moulton 1989; Thomason et al. 1988).

Several factors may increase suicidal risk in HIV-infected gay men:

1. A prior history of psychiatric illness—especially depression, panic disorder, psychosis, bipolar disorder, anxiety disorder, or a severe characterological disorder (particularly one of the borderline or narcissistic disorders).
2. Acute crises—particularly when the patient is diagnosed as HIV positive, when laboratory data suggest a decline in immunologic function (e.g., with decreasing CD4 counts), when an acute medical problem arises that requires major interventions such as hos-

pitalization or home or clinic intravenous infusions, or when a major medical problem is diagnosed for which the patient does not believe there is a ready and successful treatment.

3. Central nervous system dysfunction—impulsive, self-destructive behavior can occur when there is disinhibition (e.g., as with infection or neoplasms in the frontal lobe of the brain, delirium caused by change in metabolic function, decreased oxygenation of the brain because of pneumonia, or toxic effects of medications (see also Chapter 6).

4. Acute or chronic disinhibition or increased anxiety secondary to the abuse of chemical substances (see Chapter 19).

5. Sudden loss of job, home, financial status, or invisibility as a gay man within a specific social network. For many gay men, an economic catastrophe is an unexpected outcome of becoming infected, and is experienced as a shameful event and a narcissistic injury. This new crisis also can reactivate early feelings of not being entitled to an equal place in the world.

6. Catastrophic loss of one's social support system (the gay family) or rejection by one's family of origin upon disclosure that the patient is gay or infected with HIV.

7. Exacerbation of physical discomfort or physical pain, with a disbelief or distrust that appropriate treatment will be offered or is even possible.

8. Inadequate psychological resources, particularly in terms of managing increasing anxiety and dependency needs. This inability to cope is exacerbated by the patient's uncertainty about his future health and anxiety about being accepted by the gay male community after being identified as HIV positive.

9. A single loss or repeated losses of friends and lovers to AIDS-related illnesses; the loss of a relationship that signals rejection and engenders a fear that the HIV-positive patient will never find someone to love him again.

10. Unsettled sexual identity, particularly among adolescents, who are unsure about their sexual orientation and associate coming out with dying from AIDS-related illnesses.

11. Real or perceived rejection or withholding by medical providers, who represent the larger societal values that stigmatize gay men;

this furthers exacerbates the internalized homophobic beliefs that may translate into self-destructive impulses.

Clinicians are often confronted with patients for whom one or more of the above issues are important and may become acute along the continuum of HIV-related concerns. This continuum might be conceptualized in four phases, during each of which specific dynamic and behavioral issues can increase suicidality: 1) during the pretest phase, 2) during the HIV-antibody testing process, 3) after determination of HIV-antibody status, 4) during the course of HIV infection and immunologic decline. For example, for the gay man who carries the unconfirmed fear of being HIV positive, clinical evidence has suggested that his anxiety could engender profound psychological consequences and encourage significant risk-taking behavior, suicidal ideation, social withdrawal, sexual dysfunction, and unbearable anxiety. For the gay male who knows he is seropositive, there are always psychological ramifications.

Thus I have reconsidered the notion of there being a truly asymptomatic state. We cannot ignore the psychological impact of HIV on those it affects. It is as though we separate the brain and mind from the rest of the body when we talk about HIV-positive, asymptomatic individuals. I suggest the use of the terms *physically (or somatically)* versus *psychologically* symptomatic. Any psychotherapist working with a patient concerned about HIV infection knows that there is no such thing as a truly asymptomatic patient if his mental state is considered. For example, suicidality in a gay man newly diagnosed as HIV positive may be of such magnitude and seriousness that it appears to be out of proportion to the immediate threat to the self's integrity or the prognosis at that time. One could hardly describe this individual as asymptomatic. Even when an individual finds the strength to grow psychologically from the trauma of finding out about his serological status and manages to successfully integrate that knowledge, there may be symptoms and emotional consequences for him.

Suicidality is also a clinical issue for seronegative gay men who find their serological status psychologically painful and disorganizing (see Chapter 20). The discovery of a seronegative status may have profound psychodynamic meaning for an individual who was better prepared to handle the diagnosis of being infected. Being positive puts to rest the fear of finding out one is positive. Finding out one is negative cannot put to rest the fear that one remains vulnerable to and must continue to be vigilant about the possibility of becoming positive. The psychological resources required to maintain a negative status are enormous and often not well appreciated. This observation is supported by reports (e.g., de Wit et al. 1993) that more than 25% of gay men who are highly motivated to participate in a seroconversion study sometimes engage in high-risk, unprotected anal intercourse.

Sometimes finding out one is seronegative does not make sense to the gay male in whom the outcome was presumed to be otherwise, such as in the following case example:

Case 2

Mr. B, a 24-year-old gay man, had lost four friends and prior lovers to AIDS within a short period of time. The men he had been closest to had all been infected and become sick over the previous 2 years. Mr. B had been vigorous in his efforts to take care of three of his friends, simultaneously putting off his own testing. However, he was convinced that he was positive. Too busy with his friends' care, he was more concerned that sometime in the future, when he got sick, no one would be there for him. After the death of his last friend, Mr. B went to his physician for HIV testing so that he could find out his CD4 count and begin to prepare for his own illness and death. When his test came back negative, he assumed it was wrong and proceeded to be retested several times, always with the same result. Increasingly distraught, Mr. B became convinced that the whole medical system was intent on keeping the truth from him. When he finally allowed for the possibility that he had indeed escaped infection, he became profoundly angry and depressed, as he had had the same risk factors as his dead friends. In the midst of his own grief and despair that he would remain alive, he overdosed on a potentially lethal medication. Waking up in the intensive care unit, he was enraged that he had survived. Following psychiatric hospitalization and psychotherapy, he began the long, painful process of coming to terms with his survival.

Suicide as a Truly Individual Decision: Some Theoretical Concerns

Many existential as well as clinical questions may arise in working with people infected with HIV. How do we evaluate and understand when the patient says, "Enough is enough!"? When there is physical degeneration, loss of bodily function, and even the onset of neuro-cognitive dysfunction, empathic understanding often permits others to support the passive wish, if not the active intent, of the individual to die. Is there a psychological counterpart (not including decreasing brain function) to the physical situation in which those not faced with either the fear or reality of a life-threatening illness imbued with stigma, such as AIDS, would agree that to continue to live seems cruel and pointless, and that to die would maintain some sense of ego integrity? What is the psychological equivalent to being on a respirator from which there is no hope of being weaned? When is an individual acknowledged to have given all he can, and granted the blessing of others to "pull the plug"? When does the clinician step back from the ethical, moral, and legal obligation to restrain the patient from harming himself? What is it about human psychology that allows the mind to decide rationally when the body is ready for death but not the mind?

Buie and Maltsberger (1974) addressed the *narcissistic vulnerability* of the suicidal patient. The contemplation of self-annihilation as preferable to life arises in the individual who is incapable of coping with extreme adversity, is unable to accommodate to a narcissistic injury, and has insufficient internal resources to ward off the terror and anxiety of the unknown, dismal future. Death is seen as preferable to a life viewed by the narcissistically wounded individual as horrifying and shaming. Suicide becomes an individual's permanent solution to a problem that others see as only temporary. Intervention in such circumstances is predicated on the belief that, although the narcissistically wounded patient is incapable of coping at the moment and is bereft of internal defenses, others can lend necessary support and psychic resources long enough for the crisis to pass. This approach assumes that there is both a narcissistic injury and the possibility of healing the wound. In the early phases of diagnosis of HIV, or amidst a sudden crisis, such a hypothesis serves the clinician well, and is reinforced by the evidence that, in most cases, the failure of suicide attempts engenders increased ambivalence about suicide in the one making the attempt.

At what point, however, is it possible to concede that the suicidal ideation is not a result of a potentially manageable narcissistic injury or of a crisis that will pass, but a result of an honest, realistic estimation of damage that has no possibility of being healed? At some point in the illness, either for physical or psychological reasons, one might experience a fatal blow to the integrity of the self, eliciting, perhaps, a positively narcissistic attempt (through suicide) to retain some integrity of the self by deciding when life ceases to be worth living. Because this point will most certainly differ from one human's experience to another, one may not agree with another's decision to end life at a certain point.

Psychotherapists working with HIV-positive gay men are faced with the most basic and primitive issues about human existence. What is usually seen as illness or neurosis is complicated by the substantive difference between the patient's view of the meaning of his life and the meaning ascribed to that life by others. Rank (1945) presented one view of the essential paradox of human existence:

> If man is the more normal, healthy and happy the more he can . . . successfully . . . repress, displace, deny, rationalize, or dramatize himself and deceive others, then it follows that the suffering of the neurotic comes . . . from the painful truth. . . . Spiritually the neurotic has been long since where psychoanalysis wants to bring him without being able to, namely at the point of seeing through the deception of the world of sense, the falsity of reality. He suffers, not from all the pathological mechanisms which are psychically necessary for living and wholesome but in the refusal of these mechanisms which is just what robs him of the illusions important for living. . . . [He] is much nearer to the actual truth psychologically than the others and it is just that from which he suffers. (pp. 251–252)

Who, then, decides what the value of life is to any particular individual who is faced with an unbearable truth? Even in the absence of physical pain or immediate psychological distress, the individual may decide that his remaining life, however long, is without intrinsic value to him. He may perceive suicide as hastening the confrontation with the inevitable in order to prevent what he believes to be a potential dissolution of the self, with the time interval between that moment of decision and the moment of death an unnecessary delay, an embarrassing and unnecessary flailing against finitude.

The countertransferential denial of the possibility that life has ceased to have intrinsic meaning to another individual is probably necessary to sustain the hope and value in living for those who remain alive. Thus there is a chasm, existentially and spiritually, between the individual who wants to die and the individual who wants to live. To sustain the self's integrity right up until the moment of natural death, one must have the capacity to ultimately contain the essential aloneness that is part of the human condition.

Psychotherapists, medical providers, and society itself may cringe when faced with the individual who determines that life has ceased to have value. We interpret the wish to die as a weakness, a failing, a capitulation to the narcissistic injury. Even when there is no hope for recuperation or for a reversal of illness, we search to find meaning in the life that is left to live, no matter how painful it may be. In the absence of any psychological reason for holding on to life at any cost, we look to spiritual reasons to justify the pain of continuing to live. We search aggressively for a way in which to understand that decision to die as an aberration, a momentary loss of reason.

This dilemma is complicated by the experience and research that supports the contention that suicidality is often a transitory state. Suicidality is often reduced when the individual is able to recompensate and become, according to Rank's formulation, less neurotic or less enmeshed in crisis. What happens, though, when the neurotic vision of the essential meaninglessness of a particular individual's life is irrepressible? Becker (1973), a cultural anthropologist, wrote cogently about this:

> We might call this existential paradox the condition of *individuality within finitude*. Man has a symbolic identity that brings him sharply out of nature. He is a symbolic self, a creature with a name, a life

history. He is a creator with a mind that soars out to speculate about atoms and infinity, who can place himself imaginatively at a point in space and contemplate bemusedly his own planet. This immense expansion, this dexterity, this ethereality, this self-consciousness gives to man literally the status of a small god in nature, as the Renaissance thinkers knew.

Yet, at the same time, as the Eastern sages also knew, man is a worm and food for worms. This is the paradox: he is out of nature and hopelessly in it; he is dual, up in the stars and yet housed in a heart-pumping, breath gasping body that once belonged to a fish and still carries the gill-marks to prove it. His body is a material fleshy casing that is alien to him in many ways—the strangest and most repugnant way being that it aches and bleeds and will decay and die. Man is literally split in two: he has an awareness of his own splendid uniqueness in that he sticks out of nature with a towering majesty, and yet he goes back into the ground a few feet in order blindly and dumbly to rot and disappear forever. It is a terrifying dilemma to be in and to have to live with. (p. 26)

The psychotherapist must wrestle along with the patient with the question of not whether, but when and how to face this existential paradox in the context of HIV infection. Shakespeare's Hamlet, experiencing the terror of knowing what has come before and what will continue to poison his life, excludes others from his struggle:

> To be, or not to be: that is the question:
> Whether 'tis nobler in the mind to suffer
> The slings and arrows of outrageous fortune,
> Or to take arms against a sea of troubles,
> And by opposing end them.

(*Hamlet*, act 3, scene 1, lines 56–60)

As with Hamlet, the "cast of thought" may not suffice to make the fear of the "undiscovered country" greater than the fear and anxiety of what any particular gay man feels about the value of his life. In the context of psychotherapy, the decision to maintain the relationship with the therapist must be seen as an important statement about the ambivalence of the individual in deciding to take his life, or as the wish to receive permission to die from the therapist as a transference figure for the parents or deity that gave the patient life. In the absence of this ambivalence or need for permission, the individual who is really at peace with his decision to commit suicide has no need for the continuing therapeutic relationship, as illustrated in Case 3:

Case 3

Mr. C was a 35-year-old professional who had been in a relationship for 10 years until his lover died from an AIDS-related illness. As he himself became sicker with AIDS, Mr. C pursued psychotherapy to mourn and understand what he felt about the rest of his life. He was healthy enough to continue working, but feared losing his job in the near future because of fatigue and the persistent medical problems that occupied the majority of his time.

Mr. C had been alone for 2 years since his lover's death. He had tried to date and get close to another man, believing that, based on their conversations, his lover would have wanted that. In psychotherapy, Mr. C openly discussed his belief that he would join his lover after death, and thus he felt no real urgency to find intimacy with another man. He was grateful for the life he had had, but realistic about his future. Mr. C talked often about the mystery of life and the losses and opportunities he would never have. On balance, even though he had been angry about the abrupt intrusion of AIDS into their lives, Mr. C had come to embrace his fate not happily but as an inevitable part of his life. In therapy he spoke of his great affection for the therapist, acknowledging the help the therapeutic relationship had been during the mourning period for his lover and being especially grateful for the respect that had been granted his relationship with his deceased lover.

Mr. C talked openly about the wish to have his life come to a close before he got to the point his lover had reached—in constant pain and totally dependent on another. He saw death as a new beginning, not as a cowardly way out. He understood that the therapist could not give him permission and might not approve of his decision, if he made it, to end his life. He decided to terminate therapy, making sure that the therapist did not believe that he was experiencing any untreated depression or was not angry at him. He was particularly concerned that the therapist should not feel responsible for anything that might happen to him after terminating therapy and thus left several messages on the answering machine several weeks later that he was doing fine.

After 4 months, Mr. C was found dead in his apartment from a carefully researched cocktail of pain medications, aspirin, and alcohol. The therapist was convinced that he suicided only after making sure that enough time had lapsed to prevent anyone from being legally responsible for his death.

This patient took great care to make his suicide a rational choice, a decision he made alone and within a consistent spiritual framework. He saw the truth of his future as unacceptable, and owned total responsibility for his death, as he had for his life. By comparison, the patient in Case 4 initially wished to use suicide as a vehicle for his rage at being gay, anger at his parents, and disappointment in himself for the way he had lived his life.

Case 4

Mr. D was a 33-year-old graduate student who started psychotherapy prior to finding out he was HIV positive. His initial goals in therapy were to find a way to separate more from his parents and give up his casual sexual experiences for an ongoing relationship with a man with whom he felt safe for the first time in his life. Although he suspected that he had been exposed to HIV, having not engaged in safer sex even after learning about AIDS, Mr. D's diagnosis of being seropositive created a considerable crisis in his life—not in terms of suicide, but in terms of trying to decide if he should continue in graduate school or return home to his parents and simply let them take care of him.

Much of Mr. D's therapy work during the 2 years before his diagnosis had been about his early life. Having had some mild and reparable congenital deformities, he had been quite dependent and enmeshed in his relationship with both his father and mother. His mother, who abused alcohol, had psychologically absented herself from his care except when he required some medical intervention and she could perform concrete functions. Mr. D's work in therapy allowed him to reconnect with his parents as an adult, opening up a discussion about his childhood in a positive and healing way.

When Mr. D was diagnosed as HIV positive, his parents wanted him to return home with them so they could take care of him, but he refused. Mr. D acknowledged that if not for his therapy, he would have given up his education, friends, and hope to find safety in regression with his parents.

Mr. D became quite active in AIDS work, functioning as a spokesperson for AIDS, and became more active in both his medical and psychological treatment. The focus of his therapy changed from the future life he would never have, which he mourned, to his anger and rage at society for not attending to this epidemic. He became more focused on externalized stigma and blame than on his own poor self-image and fear of dying.

Mr. D's illness progressed rather rapidly, making him quite dependent on his therapist and medical providers. He continually asked the therapist to make decisions for him about school, his boyfriend, his parents, and his medical treatment. His worst fears about becoming cognitively impaired began to come true, and he experienced some significant neurological impairment, making him unable to live independently. Again he fought the urge to return to his parents, allowing his friends to help him create a support system that allowed him to live semi-independently in an apartment. His parents, who visited him frequently, were extraordinarily supportive and compassionate, and often met with the therapist with Mr. D's permission.

As he became more bedridden, and therapy had to be moved to his apartment, Mr. D's fear and rage began to reemerge. Nevertheless, the therapeutic relationship allowed for the interpretation of these feelings in both an existential and historical context. For the first time, he talked about wanting to die in order to avoid the embarrassment and shame of regressing once again, as he felt he had done all his life prior to therapy. He began to ask for permission to take his life and in fact tried to stick his fingers in an electric outlet, but was too fatigued to do so. Although he had enough medications at his bedside to kill himself, he demanded in a rage that his father inject him with something lethal.

Through therapy, Mr. D was able to see that his shame at being gay, being sick, and feeling unlovable (that his parents' love for him was out of their own guilt over his early childhood illnesses) made him feel desperate. He could not stand feeling so impaired, knowing that it was probably only a few weeks or months until he would die. He saw wanting to die as courageous, sparing his friends and parents the agony of his dying. The therapist affirmed the wish to die, acknowledging that he and Mr. D's family and friends were ready for his death, but stating that Mr. D could not ask them to take his life; to ask someone else to take the ultimate responsibility for his life, while he was still able to do so, was an essentially hostile demand intended to leave the pain behind in the guilt of someone else who would help him die. Although his parents had brought him into this world, they did not feel it was their place to take him out of it, although they could love him if he chose to end his life. All were in agony about Mr. D's dilemma of wanting to die and yet felt unable to do anything about it, a paradigm for the powerlessness Mr. D had felt most of his life.

The therapist asked Mr. D if he knew what medications he was taking and what they were doing for him. That began a conversation about why he was continuing to take pills to prolong life if he was so sure about wanting to die. Mr. D discontinued all but two medications over the next day, stating that he wanted to see his therapist before discontinuing his methylphenidate (Ritalin) and dexamethasone (Decadron), which were sustaining his cognitive and cardiovascular capacity. In saying good-bye to his therapist, Mr. D was able to own the responsibility for ending his life in a way that he had never owned the responsibility for living his life. He asked forgiveness for torturing his parents and therapist with his requests for help in dying, and thanked the therapist for allowing him to make his final act his own choice. Although he felt at this point he could bear living until he died, he wanted to have one opportunity in his life to make his life his own, and in that decision he found freedom.

Mr. D spent the next day with his family and friends around him, laughing and remembering, and then instructed them all to leave his room, but requested that his parents stay in his apartment. He ordered the nurse to stop giving him the methylphenidate, which allowed him to involute psychologically and cognitively, and left instructions that the dexamethasone should be stopped 24 hours later. Once the steroids were stopped, his adrenal glands could not compensate and he had, as expected, massive cardiovascular collapse.

The intellectual choice Mr. D had made to stop a life-sustaining medication was as active a decision to end his life as if he had jumped off a bridge. In his final act, Mr. D had consolidated much of what he had struggled with in therapy over the previous 4 years.

When suicidality occurs in the patient who is seronegative or physically asymptomatic, it is automatically considered acute and treatable as it is difficult for others to comprehend how someone who is not sick would find death preferable to life. But for some individuals, the degree of fear (more appropriately termed terror), the amount of loss, or the degree of pain they must tolerate without any promise of relief is so great that treatment is not possible or desired by them. Someone in despair must be able to use another's hope to sustain the self when all internal resources have been overwhelmed.

Psychodynamic Meanings of Suicidal Ideation

Suicidal ideation in HIV-positive patients can be conceptualized as having either destructive or constructive value to the patient. From a psychodynamic perspective, suicidal ideation must be viewed as a necessary part of the process of coping with the fear or reality of HIV infection. It may serve constructively to bind the anxiety that rises within the individual who is being forced to integrate significant emotions and cognitions as the self attempts to remain whole. However, when a patient is overwhelmed with depression or despair, suicidality may represent a destructive coping mechanism.

Several dynamic meanings may underlie suicidal ideation:

1. *The fear of pain,* either physical or psychological, which may be accompanied by a distrust or disbelief that medical science is really capable of alleviating either.
2. *The expression of control over one's life,* when external or internal forces engender a real or perceived loss of control because of physical weakness, emotional fatigue, or cognitive impairment. It is the ideation itself, and not the possibility of acting on it, that empowers the self to regain or retain control over its integrity. Early on in HIV infection, the threat of loss of control may be more powerful, whereas near the end of HIV-related illness, the experience of losing control (e.g., over one's bowel movements) might precipitate a sense of unbearable humiliation.

3. *The expression of revenge or retaliation,* that is, as an attempt to get back at the world or specific individuals by obliterating the self, with an unconscious or conscious motive to make those left behind feel guilty.

4. *The acting out of thwarted aggressive strivings,* juxtaposing the strength of the individual against the enormity of the universe in order to protest the unfairness of the illness and the profound loss of basics, such as housing, employment, and economic security that lead the individual to feel incompetent, helpless, and bereft.

5. *A distraction from the developmental work that is beginning in therapy,* often in the context of prior characterological defenses and mechanisms for coping with any assault on the integrity of the self.

6. *An expression of anger* that is experienced as too dangerous to direct anywhere but towards the self. Feelings of rage toward medical providers, the therapist, family, friends, lovers, and so on may feel too embarrassing, inappropriate, or dangerous to express outwardly. Facing mortality often precipitates a resurgence of unresolved spiritual concerns; it is as if the individual is protesting against what is perceived as an uncaring or vengeful deity by exercising the one, final power of the individual to take his own life.

7. *An attempt to manage unbearable and overwhelming grief and loss.* Many gay men have lost what amounts to their entire chosen family to AIDS. Their experience is not unlike that of individuals who were the only ones in their family or neighborhood to survive the Holocaust. They begin to see themselves as the walking dead, condemned to spend the rest of their lives in pain and loneliness, and are unable to make any sense of the meaning of a life in a universe in which such things happen. Their yearning to join the dead, whom they view as being beyond pain and anguish, takes away any belief in the intrinsic value of their particular life. Death comes to symbolize an eternal monument to the dead and dying, and is perhaps even interpreted by the self as a noble stand against the world, which is viewed as actively desiring the annihilation of the group.

8. *An expression of unresolved internalized homophobia.* AIDS is seen as the final proof that no matter how the individual understands

his homosexuality, he experiences it as being deviant, perhaps essentially immoral, and as precluding any pleasure or purpose in life.

9. *An expression of unbearable dependency yearnings or fears,* with the individual unable to imagine that he could tolerate being totally dependent on others for his care, especially if he has historically preferred others to depend on him in order to retain power and control over them.

10. *An expression of a profound narcissistic injury* for which the patient has inadequate or malignant defenses.

Suicidal ideation must be distinguished from taking risks that potentially involve danger to the self. Riding in an airplane involves some statistical and real danger to the self, but would hardly be considered a suicidal gesture, unless the degree of risk was clearly unacceptable for the degree of benefit. It may appear that sexual behaviors that potentially lead to death are purposely (albeit unconsciously) self-destructive. Although for some people this may be true, it is also possible that the psychological mechanism used to deny the potential risk of death from AIDS is similar to the existential defense mechanism that allows any human being to proceed with life in the face of ultimate death. The fact that the latency period from infection to illness may be a decade or more allows for an understandable and perhaps psychologically appropriate form of denial in a gay man who may be unconsciously ambivalent about the value of his life. Were gay men to die within 24 hours of having unprotected sex with someone with HIV infection, it would be more apparent that those who continued to engage in high-risk behavior were truly and consciously self-destructive or in total denial about the fact of death itself.

It might be more useful to conceptualize the risk taking in unprotected sexual intercourse as we do the risk taking from skydiving, smoking, or simply driving one's car, where the real risk to one's existence is considered worth the benefits of the behavior. Even though gay men comprehend the risk involved with unsafe sexual behaviors and the number of gay men who take such a risk is higher than the predicted number of gay men who will commit suicide, one has to assume that either gay men are inherently more suicidal or their risky behavior is a manifestation of some other psychological purpose. Likewise, the use of various substances of abuse in the face of HIV infection might be better understood in some cases as suicidal, some cases as extreme risk-taking behavior, and some cases as an attempt to either avoid intense and unbearable feelings or experience an intensity of feeling that is otherwise not available. One might understand a gay man's risking infection from sharing a needle for the benefit of avoiding or engendering an intense affect. Immediate gratification is more universally characteristic of human beings than the delaying of gratification for benefits either not perceived or believed not to exist.

The meaning and intensity of the suicidal ideation may fluctuate throughout the course of illness. The initial intense suicidal beliefs (e.g., I will take my life when I become incontinent or lose my mind) often are helpful to the patient who needs to imagine such ultimate control in order to contemplate the reality of what might actually happen. In a primitive way, the belief that one can take one's own life, and by so doing "cheat death," may initially be an empowering one. Eventually, the fear of being out of control or of losing one's self may diminish as the patient accommodates to the changes, with relative adjustments from, I'll take my life when I am neurologically impaired, to, I'll take my life when it's more than just this neuropathy. Such bargaining may actually be essential for the individual who cannot imagine death without a horrible process of dying.

One purpose of suicidality, especially if acted upon, may be to avoid living in the fullest sense of the human experience. We are both terrified and fascinated by death and pain, and yet some find it unbearable to live life out to the very end. Out of a desire not to be dependent on others, which is a natural outcome of aging, the gay man may reject any signs that his youthfulness and vigor are on the wane. For the man who defines himself as being valuable only if he is desired by others, any decline of the mind or body is unthinkable. Gay men's lack of trust, supported by reality, that no one will really be there for them in their stage of weakness and dependency, fosters the wish to end life before they are, in fact, dependent. They may choose not to live out life, however it may be, but to determine its end themselves. Becker (1973) wrote about the philosopher Kierkegaard's *knight of faith,* who defines what it means to be a man:

This figure is the man who lives in faith, who has given over the meaning of his life to his Creator, and who lives centered on the energies of his Maker. He accepts whatever happens in this visible dimension without complaint, lives his life as duty, faces his death without a qualm. No pettiness is so petty that it threatens his meanings; no task is too frightening to be beyond his courage. He is fully in the world on its terms and wholly beyond the world in his trust in the invisible dimension. . . . The great strength of such an ideal is that it allows one to be open, generous, courageous, to touch others' lives and enrich them and open them in turn. As the knight of faith has no fear-of-life-and-death trip to lay onto others, he does not cause them to shrink back upon themselves, he does not coerce or manipulate them. The knight of faith, then, represents what we might call an ideal of mental health, the continuing openness of life out of the death throes of dread. (p. 258)

Thus to bear the experience of dying, defined at times by decay and pain, is to believe that life, to be fully lived, requires a courage to see it all as a part of the whole. Isolated from the day-to-day realities of death, decay, illness, famine, and despair, which are the daily chores of life in much of the world, a gay man may be unwilling or unable to partake fully in the last phase of his life—dying. Be that as it may, to philosophize about the knight of faith in the course of therapy with a gay man who is HIV positive, and thereby project onto him the ideal of living life through to its end, might be a manifestation of countertransference, churned up by the therapist's own death anxiety.

Clinical Issues

Assessment of Suicidality

Patients inform psychotherapists about suicidality either directly through verbal acknowledgment or indirectly by describing behaviors that can be identified as self-destructive. In interpreting the ideation or behaviors, it is necessary to distinguish a wish to die from a wish to relieve psychic pain in order to live. So-called self-destructive behaviors, although potentially leading to death, may not be intended either consciously or unconsciously to produce that end. This is particularly true in the complex realm of sexual or substance-abusing behaviors that are potentially dangerous, but motivated by deeply rooted, conflictual needs to connect the self to others and to feel alive amidst the rubble and ruins of one's personal intrapsychic and social landscape.

When a patient tells his therapist about a past ideation, plan, or attempt, the therapist's first task is to ascertain whether he is in immediate danger of ending his life, in which case containment through hospitalization or constant observation by competent others is required. Unless the therapist is satisfied that the patient is safe, it will be impossible to explore in any useful way the meaning of the suicidality or for therapist and patient to feel safe within their relationship. A discussion at the beginning of treatment about the limitations of confidentiality and the ethical responsibilities of the therapist to protect the patient is almost always helpful, and in some states is required by statute or licensing boards' regulations.

The therapist must assess whether an underlying cause exists for the sudden emergence of suicidality. A good working relationship with the primary care provider can often allow the therapist to quickly evaluate whether new information about the patient's health has precipitated the onset of suicidality, or whether an underlying systemic or central nervous system medical condition might be contributing to a change in mental status or coping ability. Asking the patient these questions may not suffice, as he may be denying or minimizing the impact of a medical problem.

Any change in the patient's mental state requires ruling out a treatable cause of the depression or anxiety that often accompanies the abrupt onset of suicidality. For the nonmedical psychotherapist, consultation with a psychiatrist may be helpful in evaluating acute depressive or anxious states, as well as if there is HIV-related encephalopathy that is contributing to the change in mental state or the anxiety about losing cognitive control. Only after the patient has been assessed for any organic or treatable causes of his change in mental state can the therapist focus on the psychodynamic meaning of the suicidality and explore with the patient how to understand its purpose and how to manage it.

Therapists must remember that patients sometime suicide impulsively, before acknowledging the ideation to the therapist. This is most often due to acute intoxication or an organic mental disorder that has had an effect on judgment and self-control. When a patient brings suicidal ideation into the therapy, it means that he has some ambivalence about wanting to die. Thus, although the therapist must take the ideation and any suicide plans seriously, he or she must also understand these within the context of an ongoing therapeutic relationship. However, therapists must not be lulled into thinking that because the patient brings the issue into therapy that he will not act on it. Therefore, both the destructive and constructive aspects of suicidal ideation must be explored.

Patients who are depressed or who have an anxiety or panic disorder have a greater risk for suicide than the general population, and these diagnoses are more prevalent in patients with HIV infection. In addition, there is an enormous fear of losing one's mind because of HIV-related illnesses. Patients deserve an aggressive and complete assessment for a potentially treatable or manageable concern. Therapists, at the same time as being empathic toward patients' fears and anxieties about their disease, have an obligation to help them access the most complete medical and psychiatric assessment possible before acceding to the purported rational nature of the suicide. Even when suicide may appear to be reasonable, the therapist must be alert to his or her projective identification with the patient precluding a thorough dynamic understanding of the meaning of suicidality at that moment in the therapy, as illustrated in Case 5.

Case 5

Mr. E, a 35-year-old gay man with advanced AIDS, had survived several bouts of Pneumocystis and meningitis and had been diagnosed with mild cognitive impairment. He had been actively working in the health care field up until several months before becoming disabled because of the increasing fatigue and neurological pain he was experiencing. His CD4 count dropped significantly, and he became more despairing about his future, although he had never been suicidal.

With a new diagnosis of esophageal candidiasis, Mr. E began to talk with me as his therapist about the option of taking his life before he became more impaired. He was reconciled to the fact he was going to die from an AIDS-related illness and had seen too many people die horribly to want to go through that himself. His mental state convinced me that his situation was not so acute as to render him unable to approach his problem rationally. In an attempt to work with Mr. E to put his plan into effect, I offered to try him on a psychostimulant as treatment for his severe fatigue, not intending for the medication to treat any symptom of depression that he might be experiencing. Within 3 days of being on methylphenidate (Ritalin), Mr. E not only felt more energetic, but lost all suicidality, alerting both him and me to the fact that his suicidal ideation had really not been rational, but a consequence of an underdiagnosed depression. In therapy he continued to talk in an existential manner about how the question of suicide was, for him, really a question about how to make sense out of a life with decreasing options and an increasing awareness of his mortality. Rather than wanting to die by his own hand, he wanted to find a way to make his dying a part of his life's work.

Before the above case, I had treated many people with HIV infection and had been fairly aggressive in offering psychotropic medications to patients throughout the continuum of HIV infection. Because Mr. E did not exhibit clear neurovegetative signs of depression and appeared to be able to contemplate clearly the existential crisis he was facing, I colluded with him in avoiding the possibility that the suicidality was not consistent with his philosophical and psychological nature. My overidentification, partly as a gay health professional, with Mr. E probably contributed to my atypical decision to not intervene aggressively. Subsequent to this experience, I have tried to persuade patients to undergo a trial of antidepressant medication, including the use of psychostimulants, before accepting their so-called rational decision to withhold treatments or hasten death. I remind the patient that the option of suicide will always remain; what harm can come from a few days on a psychostimulant?

Countertransference Issues

In addressing the question of suicide, the therapist and patient confront not only the potential death of the patient but also that of the therapist. In so doing, they relinquish the magical fantasy that the therapist will somehow escape the universality of personal annihilation and expose the myth that one is safe from personal death as long as the parent figure (in the person of the therapist) is alive. Thus suicidality may be as much about the inevitable failures that occur in any human relationship as with any individual's wish for self-destruction. Within the context of a therapeutic relationship, these failures may take on archetypal proportions, having to do with the unconscious perception that the therapist (parent) really wishes the patient (child) dead as a consequence of his having been bad or disappointing because he became infected and sick. In an effort to once again please the therapist (parent), the patient (child) may consider hastening his own death to avoid putting the parent through the horror and grief of his dying. This distorted sort of redemption may elicit complex transferential and countertransferential responses.

Therapists, like patients, experience suicidality with various degrees of apprehension. It is easier to work with a patient who is capable of discussing and working through suicidal ideation without having to act on it, rather than work with a patient whose characterological structure makes the action a continual threat to the therapeutic alliance and work. If a therapist is not clear with the patient about his or her limits of confidentiality, or his or her ethical responsibility to protect the patient from himself if he becomes acutely suicidal, the therapy can become disrupted and derailed. Patients may abruptly end therapy if the therapist does not take the threat of suicide seriously, which has the impact of making the patient feel even more alone and suicidal.

Therapists must also guard against conscious and unconscious wishes that a particular patient might take his life. Such a wish may result from various dynamics: from the overwhelming, malignant nature of the characterological disorder of the patient (with the patient's death as a relief for the therapist), to the therapist's overidentification with a patient whom he or she cannot bear to see experience such pain and anguish, leading to the therapist's wish that the patient have a merciful death. Therapists could potentially resonate with the terrible uncertainty regarding the course of the patient's illness, and collude with the patient's anxiety, thus foregoing a potentially helpful intervention. Therapists who have not had a fair amount of experience dealing with suicidality independent of the issue of HIV infection may either overreact and take unnecessarily restrictive actions (such as hospitalizing patients) or underreact and not protect acutely suicidal patients from themselves.

Several factors may decrease the therapist's own anxiety:

1. Experience with suicidal patients who are not HIV infected
2. Clear guidelines for one's own procedures when a patient is suicidal
3. Supervision with peers or mentors who agree to remain involved throughout the process
4. Clarity about ethical and legal responsibilities
5. A therapeutic alliance in which the role of the therapist in acute circumstances is identified and agreed to by the patient before the crisis occurs
6. A separate, safe place for the therapist who is immersed in working with HIV to deal with the inevitable, overwhelming feelings of loss and grief

Therapists who may have just begun working with patients with HIV concerns will benefit from contact with other therapists engaged in the same work. Motivated by compassion and identification with gay men, therapists may not be as clear about who they can work with and under what circumstances. A thorough evaluation and diagnostic assessment of the patient prior to beginning treatment are essential to discern patients for whom the therapist is not appropriate. More characterologically disturbed patients who are HIV positive can be difficult for even experienced clinicians to work with, and may not be appropriate for younger, less experienced therapists without a great deal of supervision. Nonmedical therapists must inform patients with HIV that there may be a need to involve a psychiatrist or other medical provider in the process from the beginning. Also, patients must understand that consultation may be necessary during the course of treatment, and that the therapist needs clear permission to be able to speak with medical providers and other caregivers about his case during periods of crisis or when help is needed in the course of therapy.

Interventions

Faced with the suicidal patient, the therapist is forced to constantly reevaluate the process of therapy as well as the patient's real situation. A patient presenting initially with suicidal ideation will influence the course of treatment and set in motion a series of expectations, fears, and intrapsychic defenses in both himself and in the therapist. A patient who introduces suicidality into an ongoing treatment situation presents a challenge to the work of that therapy as well as the to treatment relationship between the patient and therapist.

Several strategies may be useful for the therapist in working with HIV-related suicidality:

1. Bring up the issue of suicide early on in therapy, preferably during the evaluation phase of treatment. If therapy was begun following an acute crisis, keep the question alive after the immediate crisis is over, clarifying your role as therapist and the responsibility of the patient in addressing the issue.
2. Identify any ambivalence that the patient may have regarding suicide, using the request for therapy as an example of the ambivalence.
3. Discuss the various fears and anxieties that the patient might experience that he may see as sufficient to induce a wish to end his life. Which of these fears can the patient imagine tolerating and why? What past experiences can be brought to bear on the present?
4. During acute suicidality, whenever ethically and legally possible, and without endangering the life of the patient, ensure that the patient chooses what potential action will be discussed next. This models for the patient the ability to see alternatives to death as a means of maintaining control over his life.
5. Explain to the patient that depression is the absence of hope, and that what one perceives as hopeless may be a consequence of depression, not an inevitable outcome of understanding reality.
6. Draw on all available persons within the patient's emotional network. Give the people whom the patient perceives he is hurting by remaining alive the opportunity to state explicitly whether they

feel burdened by the patient's illness to the point that they want him to die. If they do, help the patient see that their need may not be his own, and they may require therapeutic help to work through their feelings. When it becomes necessary, interpret the unconscious wish of others for the patient to die as their desire to relieve his pain and anguish, or perhaps their own, and emphasize that there are alternatives.

7. Encourage the expression of all feelings, especially sadness, grief, and anger, that are appropriate in contemplating the loss of the self. Overtly affirm your willingness to bear those feelings and validate the patient's losses, whether they be physical changes such as the loss of attractiveness, bodily changes that represent a loss of self-image, or spiritual concerns.

8. Encourage the patient to express how he feels about you as his therapist and how he thinks you feel about him. This will permit exploration of transference issues as well as encourage development of the real therapeutic relationship.

9. Encourage the patient to have contact with a medical provider, consultation for psychopharmacological interventions, and psychotherapy consultation.

10. Act decisively at moments of great danger and ambivalence to demonstrate that you are not ambivalent in a crisis. If you are ambivalent, seek consultation immediately. The patient who has not left therapy or separated from the world enough to act on his wish to die continues to have some fundamental connection to life and needs to be affirmed in that connection. This is particularly true when the patient has a medical or psychiatric illness that is treatable. The patient must be told that suicide always remains an option, but that by allowing you into his life, even with acute suicidal ideation, he gives you permission to help.

11. Acknowledge the patient's wish for you as his therapist to be omnipotent, to be able to clarify beyond doubt the meaning of life for him, and his wish that you give him permission to end his life. Therapists must struggle with their own omnipotent fantasies, and refuse the power to hear confession and forgive beyond what one individual can do for another. Crises of faith must be worked through psychologically as well as spiritually.

Surviving Suicide

For the therapist who continues to work with HIV-infected individuals, suicidal ideation is ever present, and completed suicide an expectable occurrence in the course of one's career. In spite of clear and vigilant therapeutic strategies, competent consultation, and unending self-examination, a patient will sometimes decide to take his life while in therapy or soon after.

Surviving a patient suicide is emotionally exhausting and professionally disturbing for a therapist, even if all that could have been done was done or if the patient really rationally chose to end his life. Therapists are inevitably left with an unconscious sense of incompleteness and doubt about their own participation in the process that led to death. Therapists who are overwhelmed by grief themselves or overburdened by too many patients with HIV concerns may find themselves without the time or support of colleagues to deal with the suicide. It is imperative that the therapist who survives a patient's suicide get consultation and ongoing support for several months after the event.

More worrisome is the therapist who feels that there is no residue from the death of a patient, even if cognitively and emotionally that death seems to make sense. Therapists who become indifferent to suicidal ideation or behavior may themselves have an untreated characterological or affective disorder, or may be emotionally paralyzed with unremitting grief, and thereby may be forsaking their professional responsibility.

Conclusions

Working with the suicidality of gay men with HIV-related concerns challenges even the most experienced therapist. The moral, ethical, legal, and strategic questions, although complex, pale in comparison to the existential and emotional issues that concern the meaning of life itself. Each of us struggles more or less consciously with the purpose of our own life and the place we make for ourselves or believe was made for us. Each gay man struggles to find hope and understanding in a world that denies mortality and existential finitude by remaining indifferent to the pain of people across the globe, within a country, within a family, and ultimately within one's self. In times of unbearable sorrow, loss, indifference, and pain, gay men must find ways to cope with the various assaults, external and internal, on the integrity of the self. The struggle to find the hero within who can bear life as it is may require the contemplation of the annihilation of that very hero, a test of the self to understand its place in the eternal, universality of death.

Ultimately, there is a confusion of psychology and spirituality. As Becker (1973) wrote,

> Psychology was born with the breakdown of shared social heroisms; it can only be gone beyond with the creation of new heroisms that are basically matters of belief and will, dedications to a vision. (p. 284)

The psychotherapeutic challenge for the therapist is to be willing to travel toward that heroic vision that sustains the patient throughout his bout with AIDS until the moment of ultimate separation and death. The fact that death may be contemplated or even brought about by the self unnerves us to our core. How do we understand that moment when death becomes treasured more than life itself? We are always left with doubts as to whether a particular suicide is in fact heroic and life affirming. It is only with humility and an acceptance of the role of the individual within the greater universe that therapists dare to engage in the pursuit of any man's individual and final choice for ending his own life. Again, Becker (1973) eloquently stated our dilemma and our task:

> We can conclude that a project as grand as the scientific-mythical construction of victory over human limitation is not something that can be programmed by science. Even more, it comes from the vital energies of masses of men sweating within the nightmare of creation—and it is not even in man's hands to program. Who knows what form the forward momentum of life will take in the time ahead or what use it will make of our anguished searching. The most that any one of us can seem to do is fashion something—an object or ourselves—and drop it into the confusion, make an offering of it, so to speak, to the life force. (p. 285)

References

Becker E: The Denial of Death. New York, Free Press, 1973

Buie D, Maltsberger J: Countertransference hate in the treatment of suicidal patients. Arch Gen Psychiatry 30:625–632, 1974

de Wit JBF, van den Hoek JAR, Sandfort TGM, et al: Increase in unprotected anogenital intercourse among homosexual men. Am J Public Health 83:1451–1453, 1993

Engleman JE, Hessol NA, Lifson AR, et al: Suicide patterns and AIDS in San Francisco. Paper presented at Fourth International Conference on AIDS, Stockholm, Sweden, July 1988

Forstein M: The psychosocial aspects of acquired immune deficiency syndrome. Semin Oncol 1:77–82, 1984

Forstein M: Sexual orientation and adolescent suicide. Paper presented at The Harvard Medical School Continuing Education Conference on Suicide, Boston, MA, January 1992a

Forstein M: The neuropsychiatric aspects of HIV infection. Primary Care 19:97–117, 1992b

Goldblum PB, Moulton J: HIV disease and suicide, in Face to Face: A Guide to AIDS Counseling. Edited by Dilley JW, Pies C, Helquist M. San Francisco, CA, AIDS Health Project, University of California at San Francisco, 1989, pp 153–164

Holland JC, Tross S: The psychosocial and neuropsychiatric sequelae of acquired immunodeficiency syndrome and related disorders. Ann Intern Med 103:760–764, 1985

Kourany RF: Suicide among homosexual adolescents. J Homosex 13:111–117, 1987

Marzuk PM, Tierney H, Tardiff K, et al: Increased risk of suicide in persons with AIDS. JAMA 259:1333–1337, 1988

McKegney FP, O'Dowd MA: Suicidality* and HIV Status. Am J Psychiatry 149:396–398, 1992

O'Dowd MA, McKegney FP: AIDS patients compared with others seen in psychiatric consultation. Gen Hosp Psychiatry 12:50–55, 1990

O'Dowd MA, McKegney FP, Natali C, et al: A comparison of suicidal behaviors in patients in an AIDS-related psychiatric clinic and in a general psychiatry clinic, in Abstracts of the Fifth International Conference on AIDS. Ottawa, Canada, International Development Research Centre, 1989

O'Dowd MA, Orr D, Natali C, et al: More suicidal ideation in ARC and HIV+ patients than in AIDS patients attending a psychiatry outpatient program, in Proceedings of the 37th Annual Meeting of the Academy of Psychosomatic Medicine. Chicago, IL, Academy of Psychosomatic Medicine, 1990

Ramafedi G, Farrow JA, Deisher RW: Risk factors for attempted suicide in gay and bisexual youth. Pediatrics 6:869–875, 1991

Rank O: Will Therapy and Truth and Reality. New York, Knopf, 1945

Rundell JR, Thomasin JL, Boswell RN: Psychiatric diagnosis and attempted suicide in HIV-infected USAF personnel, in Abstracts of the Fifth International Conference on AIDS. Ottawa, Canada, International Development Research Centre, 1989

Schneider SG, Farberow NL, Kruks G: Suicidal behavior in adolescents and young adult gay men. Suicide Life Threat Behav 19:381–394, 1989

Thomason JL, Rundell JR, Boswell RN: Factors Associated With Suicide Attempts in a Mandatory Human Immunodeficiency Virus Screening Program. Edited by Rundell JR. Lackland AFB, TX, Wilford Hall USAF Medical Center, 1988

Chapter 6

Neuropsychiatric Dysfunction: Impact on Psychotherapy With HIV-Infected Gay Men

Alexandra Beckett, M.D.
Peter Kassel, Psy.D.

Neuropsychiatric Dysfunction in HIV Infection

By 1982, clinicians noticed that a syndrome of depression, apathy, and social withdrawal was often associated with the acquired immunodeficiency syndrome (AIDS). Although first seen as a natural psychological consequence of being diagnosed with AIDS, suspicions arose that this constellation of symptoms, then called *subacute encephalitis* or *AIDS encephalopathy*, had an organic etiology. Soon after its discovery, Levy et al. (1985) hypothesized that the human immunodeficiency virus (HIV) affects the nervous system; eventually evidence accrued that HIV infection in the central nervous system (CNS) led to the development of encephalopathy. In 1987, recognizing the prevalence and severity of HIV-related neurological dysfunction, the Centers for Disease Control added *AIDS dementia complex* to its roster of AIDS-defining disorders (Centers for Disease Control 1987). Since that time, the association of organic mental disorders with HIV infection has become well established.

Because HIV infects the brain—thus affecting mood, cognition, and behavior—a knowledge of these effects is of the utmost relevance in the psychotherapy of those infected with HIV. In this chapter we delineate the neuropsychiatric consequences of HIV infection and discuss their bearing on psychotherapy.

HIV enters the CNS early in the course of infection, though the extent to which there are clinical manifestations at any subsequent time is highly variable. Because HIV infects the brain, seropositive patients are vulnerable to a variety of neuropsychiatric syndromes. The most common of these disorders is *HIV-1 associated dementia complex* (HADC; also known as *AIDS dementia complex* or *HIV encephalopathy*). However, the potential complications from CNS infection can include any of the organic mental disorders identified in DSM-III-R (American Psychiatric Association 1987) such as delirium, organic affective disorder, and organic personality disorder.

HADC is either a heterogeneous group of disorders or a spectrum of a single disorder with cognitive, motor, behavioral, and affective abnormalities. The clinical findings of HADC are often subtle and insidious at onset. Forgetfulness and loss of concentration are the most frequent early symptoms (Navia et al. 1986). Patients may complain of attentional difficulties, memory problems, confusion, or mental slowing. Attentional lapses may be manifested as the inability to read a book, follow a television program, or sustain a conversation. Patients may have trouble dividing their attention when several ideas or tasks are presented concurrently. They may experience problems with actions that were formerly automatic (e.g., using a tool) or complex (e.g., making a meal or packing a suitcase). Deficits in short-term memory may result in difficulty complying with medication regimens, appointments, and so on.

Patients may be depressed and may report neurovegetative signs such as loss of energy and appetite and sleep disturbance. Those familiar with the patient may notice apathy, social withdrawal, or irritability, or may report a "change in personality," characterized by heightened anxiety in response to change and the development of a rigid, inflexible character style (Brew et al. 1988). Agitation and anxiety may be present and can become incapacitating. The subtle cognitive and affective complaints that usually characterize early HADC closely parallel those of major depression, and for this reason the clinician will need to make an important differential diagnosis.

Motor impairments, when present, include weakness, particularly of the lower extremities, and difficulty with fine motor coordination. One may see tremor and physical slowing (Brew et al. 1988). Patients may notice difficulty when walking or climbing stairs, deterioration in handwriting, or a slight slurring of speech. Nearly 50% of patients with HADC complain of motor dysfunction (Gabuzda and Hirsch 1987). These motor deficits may result from concomitant spinal cord disease (e.g., vacuolar myelopathy) and not solely from cerebral involvement. The presence of motor impairments when no other neurological illnesses are indicated is an important sign in the differential diagnosis between clinical psychiatric illness, such as major depression, and HADC, as motor impairments are extremely rare in most psychiatric illnesses (Kassel 1990).

The presentation of HADC is occasionally acute and dramatic, with agitation, hallucinations, paranoid ideation, or frank mania (Beckett et al. 1987). In such cases, one often finds focal neurological deficits or evidence of cognitive deterioration supporting the diagnosis of an organic mental disorder.

The course of HADC is highly variable. There may be little or no progression of deficits, and people who are HIV infected can often develop mechanisms for compensating, such as keeping written records or lists, using a pocket calendar, or making out a daily medication sheet. For others patients, cognitive problems worsen to the point of rendering them dependent on others for help with daily tasks. In rare instances, deterioration is much more rapid, with a catastrophic decline to a state of severe dementia in a matter of weeks.

Studies of neuropsychological performance in HIV-infected individuals have provided strong evidence that impairment occurs in a substantial proportion of HIV-infected patients after the onset of marked immunosuppression, constitutional symptoms, or opportunistic infections and malignancies. However, whether neurocognitive impairments exist in otherwise asymptomatic individuals remains controversial. Whereas some investigators have found impairments in a subset of this asymptomatic group (Grant et al. 1987; Lunn et al. 1991; Navia and Price 1987; Poutiainen et al. 1988), others did not find this group in any way different from seronegative control subjects (Janssen et al. 1989; McArthur et al. 1989). The typical neuropsychological profile includes difficulties in fine and rapid motor control, concentration, problem solving, complex sequencing, and verbal fluency (for a review, see Beckett 1990; Brew et al. 1988). Stern et al. (1991) found subtle neuropsychological changes in some medically asymptomatic HIV-infected individuals, associated with both subjective complaints and with neurological abnormalities that were too mild to affect daily functioning; they suggested that such subclinical abnormalities may portend further intellectual deterioration or disease progression.

Diagnosis and Treatment of HADC

HADC results from the pathological effects of HIV on the nervous system. The precise mechanism for this action has not yet been determined. The diagnosis of HADC depends on a careful evaluation that must include neuropsychological testing, a computed axial tomographic (CT) scan or magnetic resonance imaging (MRI) of the brain, and a lumbar puncture for spinal fluid analysis. This evaluation will identify other potentially treatable causes for the deterioration in mental status.

HIV-infected individuals experience a variety of conditions that adversely affect neurological function, such as anemia, hypoxia, electrolyte imbalance, drug toxicities, and opportunistic infections and malignancies. Because the mental status changes directly caused by HIV infection are usually slow and insidious in onset, a rapid or sudden change in mental state is likely to have a secondary cause. Individuals with even very mild HADC may be particularly vulnerable to the added neurological challenge of a declining hematocrit, impaired oxygenation, or the administration of a drug such as pentamidine.

There is no cure for HADC, but there are therapeutic interventions that may substantially alter the course of the illness or provide significant relief for some of the symptoms. These include initiating treatment with antiretroviral agents such as zidovudine (AZT), or increasing the dosage in patients who are already on such medications; vigorous pharmacological treatment of depression; or the use of psychostimulants such as methylphenidate (Ritalin) or dextroamphetamine (Dexedrine) (Fernandez et al. 1988). Recently, interest has been focused on the use of a calcium channel blocker, nimodipine, which is under investigation for persons with moderately severe HADC (Lipton 1992).

Impact on Psychotherapy

Therapists must be cognizant of the potential for neurocognitive dysfunction among their HIV-infected patients. Concerns about whether a patient is experiencing neurocognitive impairment may be present from the outset or may evolve as the treatment progresses, and may have profound implications for the patient, the therapist, and the course of the treatment. Furthermore, although the question of neurocognitive deterioration is often legitimately raised, one may not always be able to provide satisfactory answers regarding severity or etiology, nor accurately predict the course of the disorder. Case 1 illustrates some of the ways that neurocognitive deterioration may affect psychotherapy with HIV-infected gay men.

Case 1

Mr. A, a 35-year-old gay Latino emergency room nurse, was referred for psychiatric treatment because of his suicidal preoccupation, which had worsened since the onset of HIV-related constitutional symptoms and lymphadenopathy. Mr. A had discovered he was HIV seropositive when his lover of 3 years was diagnosed with AIDS. On medical evaluation, his CD4 count was 54.

Initially, Mr. A was severely depressed. He reported anorexia, insomnia, lethargy, and difficulties with memory and concentration. He contemplated suicide on a daily basis, and, although he did not believe that he would actually follow through, he thought about injecting himself with potassium chloride. Mr. A responded extremely well to psychotherapy and antidepressants within 3 weeks, demonstrating a marked improvement in his mood and the resolution of both his sleep and appetite disturbances. The fatigue persisted, and he continued to notice problems with short-term memory and concentration.

Four months into treatment, Mr. A related two incidents from the preceding week that his psychiatrist found particularly disturbing. The first occurred at home: while making dinner, Mr. A set out the ingredients for a salad and stood before them for several minutes unable to conceive of how to assemble them. The second incident took place in the emergency room, where his duties included venipuncture, insertion of intravenous catheters, and administration of medication. One evening, he administered the wrong dose of morphine to a patient with chest pain, giving 20 mg instead of the 2 mg ordered by the physician. Although the cardiac patient showed no adverse effects, Mr. A was distraught because he failed to discover the error until the inventory at the end of his shift. He then reviewed his charts for the previous days and discovered several entries that he characterized as "incoherent."

Mr. A's demeanor—his tendency to ramble, repeat himself, and lose his train of thought—and the recent incidents he had reported alarmed his psychiatrist. Her suggestion that Mr. A might be experiencing organic difficulties was met with disbelief and fear, and Mr. A refused to undergo neuropsychological evaluation. With a disabled and terminally ill lover and no disability insurance, Mr. A asserted that he could not "afford" to be disabled.

The dilemmas that confronted Mr. A's psychiatrist are typical of those that confront therapists treating HIV-infected patients. How could she help this patient? What were her responsibilities to Mr. A? Did she have a responsibility to Mr. A's employer? Did she have a legal or ethical obligation to protect Mr. A's patients? Should she have insisted on a neuropsychological evaluation? How meaningful would such an evaluation have been? And to what end would the results have been used?

The therapist is compelled to confront these issues despite the patient's wish not to do so. Mr. A's psychiatrist was forced to move from a purely empathic stance into the position of one who is challenged to do something—and in the process risk alienating and possibly losing the patient. On the one hand, our knowledge about subtle cognitive failures in the spectrum of HIV illnesses is limited and subject to controversy. Furthermore, it is recognized that depression and anxiety themselves may give rise to cognitive failures. We may therefore be uncertain as to the appropriate approach to take with such patients. On the other hand, any question of impairment, regardless of the etiology, engenders a second question about competency. The therapist is placed in the unenviable position of empathizing with the patient's wish to deny his own limitations while simultaneously needing to point out to the patient where his own safety or that of others is at risk.

Gostin (1991) argued for the need to carefully monitor HIV-infected professionals, as do both the Association for Practitioners in Infection Control and the Society of Hospital Epidemiologists of America (1990), including vigilance for impairment resulting from fatigue or HIV dementia. At the same time, the American Psychiatric Association (1991) has cautioned that use of neuropsychological testing without observation of performance in occupationally relevant tasks may lead to unwarranted restriction of HIV-infected individuals who are not impaired.

In the context of psychotherapy, the therapist should strive to ally herself or himself with the patient in the pursuit of the patient's best interest. Mr. A's psychiatrist worked with him to negotiate a transfer to a non–patient- care position, evading for the moment the question of whether he should tell his employer about his HIV status and diminishing the urgency for a more thorough neuropsychological assessment. With his psychiatrist, Mr. A grappled with questions of how to cope as he became sicker and whether or not he had developed neurological complications. For both patient and therapist, the emergence of the latter issue changed the nature of the relationship. The patient frequently expressed his concern that his therapist was watching for dementia, fearing that she would report him or otherwise deprive him of his independence. The therapist acknowledged her need to be mindful of Mr. A's cognitive difficulties, framing it in terms of a mutually held desire to anticipate Mr. A's needs and limitations and to plan realistically for the future.

Case 1 illustrates several essential principles that guide our work with HIV-infected patients. First, one must establish a working alliance; there must be a shared sense that the therapist and patient are on the same side. Second, it should be clear that the therapist and patient are working together toward mutually agreed-upon goals. One such objective—to maintain the highest level of functioning and best quality of life possible—can be achieved only with ongoing, realistic appraisal of physical and mental assets and limitations. When limitations become apparent, it is necessary for the therapist and patient to develop together a strategy for dealing with them. Finally, the therapist must be familiar with the mental status failures that may occur in patients with HIV infection, and should request further evaluation when concerns arise. This second case presents the complex problems encountered in treating an individual in whom cognitive dysfunction has begun to develop.

Case 2

Mr. B, a 24-year-old Caucasian gay man, became extremely distraught when he was diagnosed as having Pneumocystis carinii pneumonia (PCP). Mr. B had become sexually active at age 15 but had never come out to his family or friends. Though often terrified by the possibility of AIDS, he did not undergo HIV testing and never discussed his fears. Despite the encouragement of his primary care physician and other health providers, he refused to tell his family or friends about his illness. A psychiatrist saw Mr. B in the hospital and followed him weekly after discharge.

At the time of diagnosis, Mr. B was a third-year law student. He managed to graduate on time, pass the bar exam, and take an entry-level job with a corporate law firm. He initially did well in his job, and, though he came regularly to his therapy appointments, he rarely spoke about his illness or even uttered the word "AIDS." After eight sessions, he told his psychiatrist that he felt fine and that he wanted to take a few months off. Three months later, he was brought by ambulance to the emergency room in a state of confusion.

The psychiatrist was shocked at Mr. B's appearance. He had lost considerable weight and appeared quite disheveled. He had been placed on a medical leave of absence because of his increasingly strange behavior at work. He had been irritable with his colleagues and on several occasions shouted at others during meetings. On his last day of work, he had been seen urinating into a wastebasket. Mr. B spoke very little and seemed to have difficulty finding words. His attention wandered and he appeared to be distracted by internal stimuli, though he denied hallucinations. He insisted that he was fine and refused voluntary hospital admission. After 2 hours, during which Mr. B continued to reject a plan to admit himself voluntarily, the psychiatrist committed him to a locked psychiatric unit. Mr. B was subsequently diagnosed as having progressive multifocal leukoencephalopathy (PML), a relentless neurological illness, and died 3 months later.

This case illustrates one of the most difficult aspects of working with AIDS patients: the duty to intervene when neurocognitive dysfunction leads to impaired judgment. Witnessing a patient deteriorate is quite painful, and having to take action that restricts his freedom may be doubly so. Nonetheless, it is within the scope of our responsibility and expertise to identify neuropsychiatric problems and expedite appropriate evaluation and treatment. One is best suited to exercise this responsibility with good training about HIV-related neuropsychiatric diseases, access to neuropsychological assessment, and an ongoing relationship with an inpatient psychiatric service.

HIV-infected patients are increasingly presenting with organic mental disorders. Any such change in mental status mandates a thorough medical evaluation to rule out secondary causes. The differential diagnosis of a presentation such as Mr. B's is lengthy, with potential etiologies including 1) metabolic imbalances, 2) drug toxicities, 3) hypoxia (inadequate oxygenation), 4) cerebrovascular accident (stroke), 4) seizures, 5) opportunistic malignancy (e.g., lymphoma), and 6) infections (e.g., HIV, toxoplasmosis, and cryptococcus). The evaluation most often will involve a neurodiagnostic examination such as a CT scan or MRI and a lumbar puncture. Though PML is essentially untreatable, many of the disorders listed above respond well to appropriate medical intervention. Case 3 illustrates the complicated relationship between psychodynamic issues and brain dysfunction.

Case 3

Mr. C, a 39-year-old HIV-positive Asian American man, had just marked the ninth year of his sobriety from alcohol when he began treatment with a psychologist. His previous therapist had retired because of HIV-related illness. Like many gay men, Mr. C also had lost several previous lovers to AIDS. Following the death of his last lover, Mr. C moved to a new city and began training to be a physical therapist. He derived immense satisfaction from his new career and his political and educational activities within the gay community.

Mr. C grew up in a tremendously disturbed family where his mother and father drank heavily and avoided discussion of any meaningful emotions. Mr. C's older brother sexually abused him and his two sisters over the course of many years. Like other people who have been sexually abused, Mr. C remembered feeling conflicted about his physical relationship with his brother. On one hand, he was confused and aware of fear and rage toward his brother. On the other hand, the relationship provided much-needed contact and a sense of being valued and "seen," despite the terrible cost it exacted. Among the consequences of a lifetime of sad and lonely feelings was Mr. C's serious alcoholism; his substance use was a factor in the major depressive episode in his mid-20s that led to a suicide attempt and a psychiatric hospitalization.

One of the most enduring and painful outcomes of Mr. C's early experience was his profound anxiety and fury when he was not "seen" or acknowledged in his adult relationships. In situations in which he felt overlooked, Mr. C would become deeply saddened and often enraged. His conscious solution to protect himself from this severe narcissistic injury was to avoid fully engaging with another man. Yet time and again, he would find himself becoming sexually and intimately involved with a man and yearn for more, only to find fault with his partner, distance himself from him, and eventually leave the relationship. In spite of these frustrations, however, his work continued to be a source of great accomplishment and pride.

One year into treatment, Mr. C came to an appointment appearing frightened. While working with a client, he suddenly had become unable to recall who the client was or what he himself was doing there. After a time he had been able to resume his work, but the same thing had occurred during his next appointment. A few days later, he had become suddenly disoriented and confused while grocery shopping: he had known he was in a store, but could not figure out where or why. Coming across some neighbors had enabled him to reestablish his bearings. Mr. C continued to experience feelings of derealization, confusion, and forgetfulness over the ensuing weeks and grew increasingly overwhelmed by the complexity of ordinary life. His psychologist referred him for neuropsychological and psychiatric assessment. The evaluation found no focal neurological disorder, but demonstrated moderate impairments in attention, concentration, sequencing, and initiation. Antidepressants and psychostimulants were initiated, and over time Mr. C's symptoms improved.

During this time, Mr. C's increasing fatigue began to interfere with his ability to get through the day. He lost interest in his speaking engagements and political activities, which had previously been the source of much self-respect and enthusiasm, and he found little pleasure in sex. Most significantly, he was no longer able to sustain his rigorous work schedule.

The psychologist noted the inordinate toll Mr. C's work was having on his patient and gently began to question the wisdom of his working and to discuss the potential of Mr. C's retiring. He was especially mindful of providing Mr. C with alternative possibilities to work such as increasing his speaking and political engagements. Initially extremely reluctant, Mr. C ultimately appreciated the necessity for such a change in his life. With much sadness and supported by his therapist's respect and care, Mr. C decided to retire.

This case highlights several aspects of working with HIV-infected patients who have mild-to-moderate cognitive impairments. Although competence was never a concern, important questions had to be raised regarding Mr. C's quality of life. Was his need to continue working compromising potential alternative sources of satisfaction and a declining store of energy? Might his cognitive difficulties and fatigue eventually affect the quality of his work in the near future? In light of his history, would retirement precipitate another depressive episode?

Mr. C's psychologist weighed the answers to these questions with his peer consultation group, Mr. C's primary care physician, and Mr. C himself. Initially, the therapist was concerned that merely mentioning the possibility of retirement would pose an empathic failure and jeopardize the positive transference; Mr. C might ask, If you really loved me, how could you even *propose* this? The psychologist concluded that giving rise to challenging ideas would not in and of itself disrupt the therapeutic alliance. Ultimately, out of his genuine respect and compassion, he was compelled to address these concerns with Mr. C. The next case example illustrates that cognitive dysfunction may confound the assessment of an individual's competence to make treatment decisions.

Case 4

Mr. D, a 31-year-old Caucasian HIV-positive gay man, sought psychotherapy because of severe anxiety precipitated by the onset of constitutional symptoms. Since testing positive a year earlier, he had substantially changed his life-style, giving up alcohol and tobacco and adopting a macrobiotic diet, in the hope that he would remain healthy. His CD4 count on evaluation was 140.

His older brother had died of AIDS-related lymphoma 3 months before Mr. D underwent HIV testing. In the last year of his life, Mr. D's brother developed dementia; he spent months in bed, emaciated, uncommunicative, and incontinent. Mr. D vowed that were he to develop neurological symptoms, he would choose suicide rather than experience a similar protracted, undignified death.

A year into therapy, Mr. D's constitutional symptoms became sufficiently disabling that he was forced to leave work. He aggressively sought out experimental therapies and became increasingly involved in meditation. He raised the issue of suicide and acquired a lethal dose of secobarbital (Seconal) for use in the event that he found his life unbearable. He often felt despondent but was not clinically depressed. Nevertheless, he agreed to several trials of antidepressants, including nortriptyline, desipramine, and fluoxetine, to which he had no discernible response.

In the second year of treatment, Mr. D was diagnosed as having Kaposi's sarcoma (KS). Within the next 3 months, he had a bout of PCP and was also found to have cytomegalovirus retinitis, necessitating surgical insertion of a Hickman catheter and daily intravenous therapy. His KS advanced fairly rapidly. Soon, despite radiation and chemotherapy, his left leg was extremely swollen and painful. He lost 40 pounds, and, though he tried to eat, he found even the smell of food repugnant. Mr. D also began to notice some difficulties with cognitive functions, especially with respect to attention, concentration, and short-term memory, and he appeared physically and mentally slowed down. There were no focal neurological deficits and he improved somewhat with methylphenidate.

Mr. D decided to discontinue all therapies except for methylphenidate and analgesics. His primary care physician was uncomfortable with Mr. D's decision, but ministered to him according to his wishes. Three months after stopping life-sustaining therapies, Mr. D developed a second bout of PCP. He remained at home as long as he was able, but fevers and shortness of breath brought him to the hospital where he requested comfort measures only. The hospital staff were extremely reluctant to comply with his request for supportive care without curative treatment, with some viewing it as an assisted suicide.

His therapist was called to evaluate. Mr. D again asserted his wish to die in comfort, mentally intact, and with dignity. It was extremely important to him not to spend his last months helpless and dependent. Though worn out, he was not depressed; he was coherent and unwavering in his intention. He told his therapist that he had no ambivalence or regrets, and that nothing, short of being cured of AIDS, would alter his decision. He believed he could not look forward to any significant improvement in his health and wanted to die before further deterioration rendered him unable to take his own life. Despite his neurocognitive difficulties, he remained clear minded with respect to the nature of his illness and his circumstances. Mr. D's therapist supported him in his request for comfort measures only. Mr. D died 2 weeks later.

Should the therapist have tried to persuade Mr. D to accept treatment for PCP? Was his cognitive impairment an indication that Mr. D was not competent to make the decision to forgo therapy? What is the proper stance for health professionals, and mental health providers in particular, when a patient asserts that he no longer wishes to struggle with his illness?

This case illustrates the complex legal and ethical problems that have become a part of everyday mental health practice as a result of the AIDS pandemic. We must grapple with how to respect our patients, how to protect their privacy and vulnerabilities, how to help them share intimacies, how to accurately assess their limitations, and, ultimately, how to support them as they approach their death (Kassel 1990). These challenges are too weighty for clinicians to bear alone, and for this reason work with HIV or AIDS patients calls for consultation with others in the field. With the help of several colleagues, Mr. D's therapist was able to affirm Mr. D's competence to make decisions and his right to refuse treatment.

Even if the treatment is lifesaving (e.g., dialysis, surgery, transfusion), state courts have upheld the right of competent patients to refuse such treatment, whether or not they are terminally ill (Emmanuel 1988). The patient is protected against "unwarranted bodily intrusions" and is guaranteed personal autonomy in making decisions regarding his health and welfare (Bopp 1990). The law affirms the patient as decision maker, provided he has the capacity to reason and make judgments, his decisions are voluntary and uncoerced, and he clearly understands the nature of the disease, its prognosis, and the consequences of his choices (Bopp 1990).

Conclusions

Therapists who work with HIV-infected patients must understand the many signs and symptoms of HIV-related neurocognitive disease. This is especially so in light of the fact that HIV-infected patients have an elevated rate of functional and organic mental disorders. For this reason, a differential diagnosis can be complex and confusing, and referral to appropriate specialists is critical. Therapists must also be knowledgeable about the legal and ethical aspects of the illness as HIV-infected persons and their care providers frequently encounter such dilemmas. Finally, it is essential that therapists be supported in their work by peer consultation as they face some of the difficult and complex issues that arise in treating HIV-infected patients.

References

American Psychiatric Association: Diagnostic and Statistical Manual of Mental Disorders, 3rd Edition, Revised. Washington, DC, American Psychiatric Association, 1987

American Psychiatric Association: Statement on HIV Infection and Impairment of Personal, Social, or Occupational Functioning (Draft). Washington, DC, American Psychiatric Association, April 1991

Association for Practitioners in Infection Control and the Society of Hospital Epidemiologists of America: The HIV-infected healthcare worker. Infect Control Hosp Epidemiol 11:647, 1990

Beckett A: The neurobiology of human immunodeficiency virus infection, in American Psychiatric Press Review of Psychiatry, Vol 9. Edited by Tasman A, Goldfinger SM, Kaufmann C. Washington, DC, American Psychiatric Press, 1990, pp 593–613

Beckett A, Summergrad P, Manschreck T, et al: Symptomatic HIV infection of the CNS in a patient without clinical evidence of immune deficiency. Am J Psychiatry 144:1342–1344, 1987

Bopp J: Choosing death for Nancy Cruzan. Hastings Cent Rep January/February:42–44, 1990

Brew BJ, Sidtis JJ, Rosenblum M, et al: AIDS dementia complex. J R Coll Physicians Lond 3:140–144, 1988

Centers for Disease Control: Revision of the CDC surveillance case definition for acquired immunodeficiency syndrome. MMWR 36 (suppl 1):1S–15S, 1987

Emmanuel EJ: A review of the ethical and legal aspects of terminating medical care. JAMA 84:291–301, 1988

Fernandez F, Adams F, Levy JK, et al: Cognitive impairment due to AIDS-related complex and its response to psychostimulants. Psychosomatics 1:38–46, 1988

Gabuzda DH, Hirsch MS: Neurologic manifestations of infection with human immunodeficiency virus: clinical features and pathogenesis. Ann Intern Med 107:383–391, 1987

Gostin L: The HIV-infected health care professional: public policy, discrimination, and patient safety. Arch Intern Med 151:663–665, 1991

Grant I, Atkinson JH, Hesselink JR, et al: Evidence for early central nervous system involvement in the acquired immunodeficiency syndrome (AIDS) and other human immunodeficiency virus (HIV) infections: studies with neuropsychologic testing and magnetic resonance imaging. Ann Intern Med 107:828–836, 1987

Janssen R, Saykin A, Cannon L, et al: Neurological and neuropsychological manifestations of HIV-1 infection: association with AIDS-related complex but not asymptomatic HIV-1 infection. Ann Neurol 26:592–600, 1989

Kassel PE: Psychological and neuropsychological dimensions of HIV illness, in AIDS and Rehabilitation Medicine. Edited by Mukand JA. New York, McGraw-Hill, 1990

Levy RM, Bredesen DE, Rosenblum ML: Neurological manifestations of the acquired immunodeficiency syndrome (AIDS): experience at UCSF and review of the literature. J Neurosurg 62:475–495, 1985

Lipton SA: Memantine prevents HIV coat protein-induced neuronal injury in vitro. Neurology 42:1403–1405, 1992

Lunn S, Skydsbjerg M, Schulsinger H, et al: A preliminary report on the neuropsychologic sequelae of human immunodeficiency virus. Arch Gen Psychiatry 48:139–142, 1991

McArthur JC, Cohen BA, Selnes OA, et al: Low prevalence neurological and neuropsychological abnormalities in otherwise healthy HIV-1 infected individuals: results from the multicenter AIDS cohort study. Ann Neurol 26:601–611, 1989

Navia BA, Jordan BD, Price RW: The AIDS dementia complex, I: clinical features. Ann Neurol 19:517–524, 1986

Navia BA, Price RW: The acquired immunodeficiency syndrome dementia complex as the presenting or sole manifestation of human immunodeficiency virus infection. Arch Neurol 44:65–69, 1987

Poutiainen E, Iivanainen M, Elovaara I, et al: Cognitive changes as early signs of HIV infection. Acta Neurol Scand 78:49–52, 1988

Stern Y, Marder K, Bell K, et al: Multidisciplinary baseline assessment of homosexual men with and without human immunodeficiency virus infection, III: neurologic and neuropsychologic findings. Arch Gen Psychiatry 48:131–138, 1991

Chapter 7

Taking a Sexual History With Gay Patients in Psychotherapy

Joel C. Frost, Ed.D.

Traditionally, all psychotherapists are trained to take a patient's psychosocial history at the start of psychotherapy. Taking a sexual history is one part of a general history, yet clinicians often report feeling especially uncomfortable with this part because in our culture the open discussion of sexual practices has often been considered a taboo. However, with the outbreak of the acquired immunodeficiency syndrome (AIDS) epidemic, a frank, detailed, and ongoing discussion about sexual practices is critical. The psychotherapist must know everything that might put the gay male patient at risk of exposure to the human immunodeficiency virus (HIV). This can be even more uncomfortable for the therapist if he or she has homophobic prejudices or is not familiar with gay sexual practices (Cain 1991; Fort et al. 1971; Karr 1978; Neisen 1990; St. Lawrence et al. 1991; Troiden 1989).

For many psychotherapists, AIDS has significantly altered the way that they approach psychotherapy in general and the discussion of sexual practices in particular. Psychotherapists have had to alter their assumptions and strategies regarding boundaries, interventions, and notions of therapeutic neutrality. Because of the complex sex lives gay patients lead and the nature of AIDS, psychotherapists have become more deeply involved in the day-to-day fabric of and often feel increasingly responsible for their patients' sexual lives. At the same time, the psychotherapist must respect the boundaries of the gay patient, actively educate him about HIV and AIDS to reduce his risk of exposure, analyze his resistance to change, and protect his confidentiality. Therapists often feel a need to protect others in society from the spread of HIV, as well as respect the laws requiring disclosure of HIV status. The psychotherapist operates within a complex world in which the duty to protect and the principles of confidentiality often dictate conflictual actions. On the one hand, the therapist has the primary obligation to respect the patient's confidentiality in order to enhance and protect the therapeutic relationship. On the other hand, he or she can also feel pressure regarding the duty to protect, a principle that arises from the 1976 California case *Tarasoff v. Regents of the University of California*, in which the court ruled that the duty to warn overruled a therapist's obligation to protect the patient's confidentiality when the therapist had sufficient evidence that the patient intended to do harm to another. Some legal experts take the position that *Tarasoff* does not directly apply to HIV cases, as the majority of HIV-infected gay men have neither homicidal wishes nor a specific individual whom they intended to hurt.

Professional organizations have different recommendations regarding these issues, with some leaving the judgment of what is an appropriate action to the individual therapist. The gay community appears to take the stand that the therapist should adhere to the principle of confidentiality over the duty to protect. Many gay men would sue were a therapist to reveal their HIV status without their consent, even if only to the patient's lover. Because HIV is spread via consensual and intimate acts, many believe that sexual partners must take some responsibility for protecting themselves. (For further review of these issues, see Daniolos 1993; Georgianna and Johnston 1993; Totten et al. 1990.)

These changes in the frame of the psychotherapeutic relationship are meaningful in that they apply not only to gay men but to all sexually active patients in psychotherapy. Thus it is important to begin this section with what has been learned about the meaning of sex for gay men and what psychotherapeutic practices have been changed based upon that knowledge. The information presented in this chapter is based on my experience working with gay men in psychotherapy, supervising the work of others, and presenting workshops and consulting to groups of psychotherapists on taking a sexual history.

The sexual history of a gay man is of central importance because sex is one of the main avenues for exposure to HIV. Sexual behavior has many meanings for gay men, and the meaning of their sex lives deserves close attention. The following material is divided into four main sections: the meaning of sex for gay men, preventive measures in therapeutic interventions, alteration of the psychotherapeutic relationship, and the actual content of a sexual history.

Meaning of Sex for Gay Men

Sexual behavior and sexual expression are fundamental aspects of a gay man's identity. In the early stages when he is just becoming aware of his sexual orientation, a male often realizes he is gay when he acknowledges his sexual attraction to another boy or man. This sexual attraction becomes internalized as a part of the definition of his gayness. Sexual practices are an affirmation and expression of his self-identity.

The therapist must understand the centrality of but also the complexity and dynamics of sexual experience for gay men:

> Our clinical understanding must expand to view the patient who is gay as moving toward the development of a positive gay identity. This development includes integrating his erotic orientation, his affectional orientation, a positive sense of self, and a capacity for a healthy relationship; developmental tasks which are similar for all patients. In addition, the gay patient must also work through internalized homophobia to achieve a full and positive sense of identity free of stigma. With homosexuality as an orientation, and gay as a life-style, the developmental tasks go beyond whom a person has sex with to whom a person loves and who a person is. (Frost 1989)

It is the gay man's ability to experience, integrate, and resolve the meanings and dynamics of gay sexual behavior that enables him to move from sexual exploration to affirmation via sex, then to the development of a positive gay identity, and finally to the position of having the ability to love, be loved, and establish a stable primary relationship. These complex tasks are made more difficult by a generally nonsupportive environment.

Effect of Social Stigma, Continuing Trauma, and Homophobia on Gay Men's Sexual Behavior

Gay men often describe in psychotherapy the cruelty they have experienced as a result of others knowing their sexual orientation. They have often been sexually or physically abused, derided by peers, or rejected by their families. AIDS is also cruel, both in terms of what AIDS does to the infected person and what society does to someone who is known to be infected. This background of cruelty and homophobia and the constant fear of others' adverse judgment and blame is a continual source of trauma for gay men. Often gay men fear they will be further abused, even within the context of psychotherapy.

Because of this trauma, there is often a shroud of secrecy surrounding gay men. They either keep their sexual practices secret or expose the behavior and keep their feelings secret. Having to hide so much of themselves and their behaviors contributes to their shame and guilt. Not being able to control or even wanting to control their sexual behavior can further exacerbate a sense of shame and guilt, which can make open disclosure in psychotherapy difficult. Thus it is important to create a safe environment within the context of the psychotherapy in order to facilitate full disclosure.

Dynamics of Sex in Gay Men's Lives

All people use sex in various ways based on their particular underlying dynamics, but gay men often have a particularly complex set of dynamics based on many internal and external variables. Sexual practices for gay men can have many implications. For many gay men, sexual behavior is a statement of their sense of being gay, an affirmation of their right to be gay, an expression of love, a vehicle through which to achieve intimacy, and a repudiation of the felt prohibition by the greater society. For other gay men, sex is a sport, a means of repairing from narcissistic injury. How gay men feel about their bodies is often affected by whether they played sports growing up or were rejected as being too effeminate, uncoordinated, or not aggressive enough to be included. These early experiences can leave a gay man feeling insecure about his body and his experience of his own masculinity, as illustrated in Case 1.

Case 1

Mr. A, a 32-year-old unemployed man, lived with his 41-year-old lover, who supported him financially. In return, the patient had sex with his lover. Mr. A was angry about this, as it made him feel like a prostitute. He was a skinny and relatively unattractive man who had always felt rejected and picked on because of his body type and because he was gay. The only way that he felt any positive sense of himself was that he thought he was great at sex. His only area of competency was his ability at fellatio and receptive anal intercourse; now that he was HIV positive, these types of sex were a problem. He had no other vehicle to help him build self-esteem as he had never felt competent in any other area.

For some gay men, sex may be the only vehicle for emotional expression, for attaining affection or physical closeness, or for establishing a relationship. Gay men often have had no experience with dating and have only learned to meet other gay men via sex.

Effect of Potential HIV Infection on Gay Men's Sexual Behavior

HIV and AIDS have added further complexity to gay men's sexual and affectional lives. The particular history of AIDS in the United States has meant that AIDS is most associated with gay men (Shilts 1987) and intravenous drug abusers. This stigmatizing association with not only gay men but their sexual practices has resulted in an upsurge in homophobia, both within society, as evidenced in the reported increase in gay bashing, as well as within some gay men themselves who remain conflicted about their gay identity. A gay man's very act of self-expression, which comes out of his core sense of identity and out of a desire to love and be loved, can result in the spread of HIV. Sex and love are interwoven with decline and death into the fabric of gay life. A gay man's struggle with shame, guilt, internalized homophobia, and unresolved grief may be played out through his sexual behavior, as he simultaneously searches for a primary loving relationship. Psychotherapy with a gay man, whether he is sexually active or inactive, must include an open, active, and continual exploration of these themes. At the same time, the therapist must bear the responsibility for ensuring that the exploration of issues such as shame and guilt within therapy does not replicate the humiliation that the gay man experiences in society.

Preventive Measures

Psychoeducation in Psychotherapy

With no cure for AIDS in sight, fostering an understanding and practice of safer sexual practices among gay men remains the single most critical way to protect them from contracting HIV. Thus preventive education within the context of psychotherapy is the responsibility of every psychotherapist working with gay men. Psychoeducation is not new to psychotherapy. It is included in the educative stance of a therapist who looks at a patient's basic knowledge, coping skills, adaptive abilities, underlying dynamics, consequences, and alternative avenues of expression. What is new is the imperative demand for action on the part of the therapist, the pressure to initiate such education, not just respond to requests for information. This approach is similar to the active work required with alcoholic patients or drug users. A therapist's passivity and silence can bring the gay male patient one step closer to HIV infection. In this case, the gay activists' motto "Silence = Death" takes on additional meaning.

Education about safer sexual practices is impossible without specific and detailed information from one's patient about his sexual practices. The main thrust of psychoeducation in psychotherapy has two purposes: 1) to inform the sexually active gay male about HIV, AIDS, and safer sex practices; and 2) to assess the dynamic reasons why a gay male may not be implementing this knowledge or even "hearing" it sufficiently so that his risky sexual practices are changed. Although the role of educator is not customary for therapists, it is a critical one for them as their patients may have no other source of safer sex information.

Not gathering a sexual history may actually put these patients at increased risk by allowing gay men to continue to practice unsafe sex. The therapist's collusion with the patient in denying the risk of HIV infection from certain sexual practices may unconsciously be experienced by the patient, who positively identifies with the therapist, as affirming the unsafe behavior. Therapists cannot assume that gay men are being adequately questioned about their practices elsewhere, even by their physicians. Studies have shown that physicians do not always do an adequate job of taking a sexual history; even less often do they gather sufficient information to establish a patient's sexual orientation (Dardick and Grady 1980; Frost 1989; Kelly et al. 1987a, 1987b; Messing et al. 1984; Owen 1986; Royse and Birge 1987).

Focusing on what a patient does not know can allow the therapist to impart new information. However, a patient's lack of knowledge can also have dynamic aspects, which can be uncovered during an assessment. Sometimes a gay man has reasons not to know about HIV, as illustrated in Case 2.

Case 2

Mr. B, a 26-year-old gay man, initiated individual psychotherapy because he was depressed and was having no luck in establishing a relationship. He had moved to Boston from San Francisco, where he had been the "house boy" to an older gay man. Mr. B was now trying to make his own way in the world. He was attractive and dressed provocatively for the therapy sessions. He used drugs and alcohol extensively and engaged in sex with many new partners.

In taking an initial sexual history, it became clear that Mr. B had somehow avoided learning much about AIDS and safer sex. As we became more frank and detailed in the discussions of his sexual experiences, he began to establish a sexualized transference to me. He thought that I was sexually interested in him. His sexual practices increased in frequency and degree of risk. He then began to talk about having been sexually stimulated by his father, and wondered if he had been sexually abused by him. He recalled how his father would tease the family dog when it was a puppy. The father would excite the puppy, get it frisky and playful, and then continually push it away from him in a harsh manner. Mr. B talked about experiencing me much like his father. As we pursued this material, he became angry and sad, but he appeared more in control of his sexual behavior, which was becoming less frequent and less risky. It seemed that he was able to want greater intimacy outside of therapy as he allowed greater intimacy within our work.

Mr. B's not knowing about AIDS and safer sex practices had a dynamic underpinning. My confronting him with detailed questions about his sexual behavior and my educating him regarding the consequences of his behavior were sufficient in convincing Mr. B to practice safer sex. A greater degree of confrontation is required when the patient knows about safer sex and yet has difficulty consistently behaving safely, as illustrated in the next case example.

Case 3

Mr. C, a 48-year-old gay man, had recently been diagnosed as HIV positive. He appeared quite depressed, with vague references to suicidal thoughts and comments about difficulties with his lover. When asked specifically about his sexual practices, he described being unhappy about recent changes in sexual relations with his partner as a result of his physician's telling him that he had to use a condom. Mr. C and his partner were unable to use a condom consistently, and at first they were not clear about why they should. When I was specific about each stage of putting on and using a condom, Mr. C revealed that he would lose his erection when the condom was in place. He then revealed that he had been impotent ever since he and his partner had tried to change their sexual practices and that their sexual relations were a cornerstone to their relationship and to his self-esteem. His impotence occurred only when he was wearing a condom. We were then able to begin to talk directly about his anger, fear, loss of self-esteem, the dynamic meaning of wearing a condom, and ways to have successful, yet safer sex.

Character pathology can also impair a patient's willingness to change behavior. Case 4 illustrates that confrontation by the therapist is critical, but more difficult, with a patient who presents with this type of pathology.

Case 4

Mr. D, a 32-year-old gay man, began psychotherapy because he was depressed following his breakup with a lover. He was a gay activist and had extensive knowledge about AIDS and already practiced safer sex. When he found out that he was HIV positive he was enraged. The depression regarding the breakup evaporated as he settled into a sullen rage about his previous lover. He decided to not tell him about the HIV test results. He then decided that he might want to have sex with him. Indeed, he decided that he might not tell new sexual partners his status. When confronted that he knew better and that this attitude was evidence of his difficulty in resolving all of the new changes in his life, he laughed. He began to talk about how mean a man his father had been and how he had been abused. Mr. D then broke off treatment.

Effective preventive education and exploration of dynamics underlying noncompliance remain the best protection that we have against the spread of HIV. First, patients need to have a basic knowledge of the risk factors of various sexual practices. Second, patients need to be able to assess how well they really understand the specifics of safer sex and to begin to determine their intent or capacity to actually practice safer sex. Third, in the course of discussing sexual behavior, patients often begin to address possible shameful feelings or past experiences (e.g., a history of sexual abuse or incest; see Chapter 18) or unresolved feelings about being gay that might interfere with compliance. Fourth, patients' responses to the therapist's specific questions about sexual practices will expose their attitudes toward sexual behavior that affect their ability to actually practice safer sex.

Issues That Complicate the Psychotherapeutic Relationship

Timing of Taking a Sexual History

New patients. With new patients, it is relatively easy to take an extensive sexual history. New patients experience a sexual history as just one more aspect of a detailed general history. This history can be completed using a written questionnaire, with follow-up questions being asked verbally. Directly discussing sexual material makes it clear that such issues are an expected part of the therapy, lays the groundwork for how open the therapy discussions will be, and also may illuminate areas of discomfort in the intimacy of the therapy relationship.

Ongoing individual patients.   Taking a sexual history with patients who have been in psychotherapy for some time can raise different issues. The therapist needs to think about why he or she has not been asking about sex, something the patient may wonder about as well. They both need to question whether they are colluding in not looking at sexual material and, if so, why. Therapists can model appropriate behavior for the patient to follow in acknowledging any ambivalent feelings, fears of loss, and anger and grief over having to give up certain sexual practices that were formerly part of affirming gay identity in opposition to society.

Ongoing group patients.   The issue of taking a sexual history with ongoing patients also arises with a therapist's group patients, who are often seen in individual therapy by another therapist. The group therapist must address safer sex issues with the group, as well as how the dynamics of the group may have prevented prior open discussions about sex. The therapist must also decide whether to allow the topic to continued to go unaddressed or actively raise the issue of sex in the group. This may be quite out of character for some therapists, which has further implications. The manner in which this material is experienced and discussed will be different depending on the mix of the group, whether it is all gay male, mixed gay and heterosexual males, or mixed gender.

Couples who are patients.   Taking a sexual history in couple's psychotherapy can be complicated. In a heterosexual marriage, the male might be having extramarital sex with another man. In a purported monogamous gay relationship, one or more of the men may be having sex outside of the relationship. Case 5 illustrates the situation in which one partner in a gay relationship has the permission of the other partner to engage in sex outside of the relationship, but the second partner remains unaware that the first is engaging in unprotected sex outside the relationship.

Case 5

Mr. E, a 39-year-old man, came to couple's therapy with his 25-year-old lover. Mr. E was a newly recovering alcoholic patient and was not interested in sex at all. His lover had been having sex outside of the relationship with Mr. E's consent. The presenting problem was in another area. When asked to be specific about his sexual practices, Mr. E's lover reported that he was having unprotected receptive fellatio, although not to the stage of orgasm. Mr. E had not been aware of the specifics of what sex his lover was having because he had been assured that it was always safe. To Mr. E, his lover's practices no longer seemed safe. Mr. E's concerns led us into a more detailed discussion about sex and the anger these two men felt toward each other and at the therapist. The anger at the therapist began to lead to an underlying wish on both men's part that the therapist would be the active and protective father that neither had had but that both had wanted. Mr. E's lover was referred to individual therapy so that he could begin to look into his yearnings regarding fellatio, his denial of risk, and his difficulty with getting angry directly.

Boundaries and Identification

A continual focus on sex and on death as a real and impending consequence of unsafe practices has a way of breaking down denial, both for the patient and the therapist. The consequences of unsafe sex are staggering. These realities make the therapy an especially poignant relationship. What is safer sex? What is acceptable risk? What stance should the therapist take while the gay male patient decides the answers to these questions? Misjudgments and mistakes have profound and irreversible results. The usual therapeutic objectivity and distance often appear to be clinically inappropriate with gay male patients.

Therapists working with gay men show great care and concern as they work within the day-to-day fabric of their patients' sexual lives.

Therapists not only are concerned about their patients' present and future, but also are sensitive to the deep yearning that many gay men have for a sensitive and caring parental figure in their lives. Within this context, it is often difficult for the therapist, who may hold some of the same yearnings himself or herself, to give up some sense of omnipotent control over the patient's ability to protect himself. Therapists can often feel parentlike, and yet, like parents, they cannot control all of the risks for the one about whom they care. Because AIDS is a fatal disease, the relative risks of working with patients on safer sex issues can create a powerful countertransference for therapists.

There but for the grace of God go I. I'm next. I don't know my own status. I've seen this before, and I'm tired of going to wakes. I know the patient's lover—all of these thoughts may race through a therapist's mind when working with HIV-infected gay men. Therapists who treat gay men often know the tragic consequences of unsafe sexual behavior because many of their patients have been exposed to HIV and died of AIDS-related illnesses. These thoughts can affect how involved the therapist wants to become with new patients. (See Chapter 22 on empathic identification.)

AIDS has affected not only the therapist's customary role of neutrality, but also how the therapist interprets the principle of confidentiality. The duty to warn is a very complicated area of concern, yet it is more clearly spelled out in regards to the responsibility of a physician. In its "AIDS Policy on Confidentiality and Disclosure," the American Psychiatric Association has put forth the opinion that if an HIV-infected patient is unwilling to alter his behavior and will not inform his sexual partner of his HIV status, then it is "ethically permissible" for the physician to notify the sexual partner. Thus, partner notification may be seen as required if an HIV-positive patient is having unprotected sexual relations outside of a relationship. The American Psychological Association and the National Association of Social Workers have taken a somewhat different stand, with neither organization endorsing partner notification. It appears that as one moves from a medical to a psychotherapeutic relationship, professional guidelines show a greater tendency to leave the decision to warn to the practitioner's discretion.

A therapist's *Tarasoff* duty often seems clear when applied to HIV-infected patients. However, with all of the confusion, a therapist's feelings in any of these matters can become difficult to manage. As one female nurse said, "I am not sure that I want to know about his sex life. When one patient told me what he was doing, I wanted to strangle him. I didn't know what to say." It is not always clear what stance to take when one knows about a patient's sexual practices, but once one does know, he or she cannot easily "unknow." The therapist's own defenses may be triggered and, if unexamined, may allow a therapist's countertransference to interfere with the patient's treatment, an example of which follows in Case 6.

Case 6

Ms. F, a young psychotherapist in training, was working with a young gay male prostitute in individual psychotherapy. Her supervisor knew little about homosexuality and nothing about active prostitution. Ms. F found that she was not asking any probing questions when the patient made references to tricks. When he mentioned that he was also HIV positive, she began to experience rage at him, with no way to begin to talk about any of this. Thus she tried to avoid knowing what she knew.

Illegal sexual behavior, prostitution, or sexual involvement with underage children or teenagers are all areas that a therapist may wish to avoid exploring because he or she does not want to know about them. Yet some patients are engaged in all of these activities. For example, a patient who is a hustler (male prostitute) may fear that asking to practice safer sex may cause his clients to go elsewhere. The HIV-positive hustler may have an even greater wish to avoid the entire topic of AIDS, and thus he may make no attempt at establishing safer sex with his clients.

Transference and Countertransference Issues

When a psychotherapist initiates material in therapy, the therapeutic relationship shifts and can affect the patient's transference. Therapists use many different styles to teach material or influence the direction for a patient. The reality of HIV has encouraged many therapists to take a directive and confrontational approach regarding such material as sex and alcohol and drug use. Is this approach an example of over-identification? Does it arise from therapists' not working through their countertransference, just as they might do when they do not respond to suicidal ideation? Do they not want to initiate such an exploration because they do not want to face the possible horrors they might hear about? A therapist's motivations are not always clear, especially when the therapist's supervisor is equally inexperienced or unclear.

When patients become clearly suicidal or homicidal, the therapists are in difficult but chartered territory. They have ethical and legal mandates to act. Therefore, when a patient unknowingly puts himself or someone else in danger because of his unsafe sexual practices, therapists are in an equally difficult position. They cannot forget that most intimate sexual acts are consensual and therefore sexual partners must take some responsibility for their own actions. Therapists often feel that they cannot afford to rest on the cardinal rule of neutrality; the spread of HIV is the spread of a fatal disease. They must take a confrontational role, yet they must also consider the moral, ethical, and legal implications and obligations. In Case 7, the therapist takes a confrontational role with his patient and explores the consequences of doing so.

Case 7

Mr. G, a 28-year-old gay man who had not been tested for HIV, assumed that, given his sexual history, he was HIV positive. His psychotherapist knew that Mr. G was not having safer sex and that he regularly used drugs and alcohol, thus further impairing his judgment. Because Mr. G was not concerned on his own behalf, the psychotherapist broke his neutral stance and brought in an article that rated the safety of various condoms. He initiated a frank discussion with Mr. G about safer sex practices—how to decide about condoms, where to buy them, and how to use them. This also led to discussions about intimacy within the therapy relationship, as Mr. G began to question the increased activity level of the therapist. He wondered openly about the nature of the therapist's interest in him. This led to their being able to talk about how anyone could be in an intimate relationship, whether it be a sexual one outside of therapy or a caring one within therapy, and not care about the other person's welfare and well-being.

Learning about a patient's sexual practices may also uncover his intentions to put himself at risk. His behavior can be a result of his suicidal feelings, his feelings of guilt over the loss of others, his unresolved grief, or his anxiety about exposure and risk. Sometimes putting one's self at risk can be a counterphobic attempt to reduce anxiety. Another difficulty is when a patient puts someone else at risk, as in the case of Mr. G.

Case 7 (continued)

Mr. G had been much better at protecting himself and practicing safer sex. His self-esteem seemed to improve, and the psychotherapist thought that there had been some real growth in terms of Mr. G's ability to take responsibility in his life. Mr. G then traveled to New York City, where he picked up a young man, stayed with him for a few days, and had frequent anal intercourse during which the other man was unprotected. Mr. G knew that he was putting the young man at risk because he assumed that he was HIV positive, although his serostatus had not been confirmed. He justified his actions by saying that any man who lived in New York City and did not protect himself was responsible for his own actions. Based on further discussions with his therapist, the next weekend Mr. G went back to New York City he gave the young man KY Jelly and condoms, and discussed their use with him.

In the above example, the psychotherapist was able to explore the patient's sex life because he was comfortable with the idea that an HIV-positive man can choose to continue to have sexual relations. The psychotherapist wanted to be supportive and open about sexual practices to encourage the patient to disclose his ongoing sexual encounters. There are some therapists who might not be as comfortable with an HIV-positive man continuing to have sex. Therapists are not immune to their own shame regarding interest in sex in general, shame in response to their own intrigue with a gay male's sexual practices, guilt regarding particular sexual practices, or homophobia regarding gay sex in general. These are all the genesis of countertransference, as are possible feelings of anger at a gay patient's willingness to put himself or others at risk of exposure to HIV. It is not unusual for therapists to have countertransferential experiences in response to any patient doing anything that increases his risks in life. That sex is at issue only complicates the matter.

Sexual expression is varied, and the therapist may have a restricted view based on the extent of his or her own sexual experiences. No clear set of sexual behaviors constitute a "normal" gay sex life. What is most important is what the sexual behavior means to a gay man in terms of his gay identity, his safety, and his primary relationship. In taking a sexual history, the therapist must be specific. For example, when the patient has sex, does he put on a condom? When does he put it on? Does he know that certain lubricants such as Vaseline or others that contain petroleum can weaken latex condoms? This may be uncomfortable to talk about for both the patient and the therapist, so the situation is ripe for collusion to avoid specifics. Because the ability to follow through with safer sex is affected by the use of drugs and alcohol. Case 8 illustrates how an assessment of these practices is critical.

Case 8

Mr. H, a 25-year-old gay man, had been talking about his sexual practices in psychotherapy. He had been able to alter some of his risky practices and continued to be sexually active but with safer methods. During a discussion of one particular weekend, the psychotherapist understood Mr. H's reference to "Ecstasy" as being to a drug, not to a sexual experience. In asking more about this drug, the therapist found that Mr. H felt especially wonderful and uninhibited physically and sexually while taking the drug. Indeed, while under the influence of this drug, he was no longer practicing safer sex. Mr. H and his therapist were then able to begin to talk about the consequences of drug use on his safety and the possibility of his "living long enough to finish his psychotherapy."

HIV and the Specifics of Taking a Sexual History of Gay Men

How

I give a written questionnaire to every new patient, including a separate section on sexual history. In that section I ask the following questions:

◆ Please describe your sexual experiences. Do you practice safer sex?
◆ Have you always practiced safer sex? Please describe.
◆ Please give your history of sexual experiences with the same sex. With the opposite sex. With both.
◆ Have you been HIV tested? When? What were the results?

I then use the written material as a stepping-off point for asking more detailed questions, such as the following:

◆ Tell me what you know about how HIV is spread. Do you worry that you might have ever been exposed?
◆ How have your sexual practices changed based on what you know about AIDS?

When

I give out the written questionnaire at the end of the first interview session. I use a questionnaire because I want to include all of the categories that have become meaningful to me through my work as a therapist. There are some issues that do not arise easily in discussions, such as income, ethnic and religious background, class, major life losses, meaningful relationships, and the details of sexual practices. I want to underscore that all of these are "grist for the mill."

I begin going over the answers with the patient in the second session, so that we can discuss the dynamics attached to the material, the answers, and the process of providing the answers. This leads into our discussing sexual practices in the same detailed and dynamic manner.

In following this pattern, I have found that the open and frank discussions about sexual practices become normalized or safer. All patients have some taboos, phobias, anxieties, shame, or guilt about their interest in and practice of sex, some to a greater degree than others. I tell them that it is important that we look at what sex means to them personally.

Why

Safer sex is relative. We know that anal sex without a condom is a high-risk sexual activity. We know that allowing a sexual partner to have an orgasm within any orifice is high-risk behavior. Yet the riskiness of some behaviors is less clear, such as of fellatio not brought to orgasm. The discussion of safer sex with a patient turns to one of discussing relative risks—that is, how far each gay male patient chooses to go and why.

If sex has been the only vehicle for gratifying the many needs of a gay man, and if safer sex means changing his sexual behavior, then the therapist needs to attend to alternative methods for gratifying these same needs. The therapist cannot simply encourage a gay man to stop having sex without understanding the underlying needs being met through sex. Case 9 illustrates the type of patient who needs to develop alternative methods for meeting these underlying needs.

Case 9

Mr. I, a 42-year-old gay man, found that he actually did not like men and that his best friends were all women. The only thing he liked about other gay men was having unprotected sex with them. He was angry that this was the only avenue of a male relationship for him. He was also angry because he felt this avenue was blocked to him because of the risk of HIV infection. "I fought so hard to be free of the repression so that I could be sexually active and affirm my identity as a gay man. It is not fair that I can't have this. I don't like men in any other way."

AIDS has affected gay men's sexual behavior in many ways. Some gay men have stopped having sex altogether. Some stop because of their fear of the risk of contracting HIV. Others stop having sex because of shame caused by their HIV status or their sexual orientation. Gay men with AIDS may stop having sex because they feel dirty or lethal. Others are angry that they cannot practice their usual unsafe sexual behaviors, so they will not have sex at all, as illustrated in the following case example:

Case 10

Mr. J, a 34-year-old man who had been diagnosed as having AIDS 3 years earlier, talked about how upset he was at his lover who wanted to have sex with him. Initially Mr. J told his lover that having sex hurt his body, or that he was tired, or that his lover asked at the wrong times. On further questioning, it became clear that Mr. J was very angry that having AIDS limited his capacity to have unprotected anal sex and that he resented the intrusion of AIDS; avoiding sex was a way to avoid his anger. Underneath this anger and resentment was a wellspring of shame, guilt, and fear. Mr. J was ashamed of his body sexually, not physically; he felt differently about his body when sex was involved. He also felt guilty and afraid of putting his lover even remotely at risk. He talked about feeling spoiled and dangerous. As Mr. J began to acknowledge these fears and recognize his hidden feelings about himself, he begin to grieve the loss of the familiar and unsafe sexual practices that he and his partner had enjoyed for years. They were then in a better position to begin to look for what sexual practices they could enjoy together, leading to Mr. J's having an enjoyable sexual relationship with his lover for the first time in years.

In this case, the therapist encouraged and promoted a patient's active sex life. This would not have been possible without his asking detailed and persistent questions about the patient's sexual behavior and feelings. This also would not have been possible if the therapist had not been clear as to whether he thought that Mr. J should be having sex, that is, if he had not resolved his own countertransference about whether an HIV-positive gay man can have safer sex. Even though Mr. J was blocked from certain sexual activities, he was capable of having a more active and healthy sexual life. Resolving this problem with Mr. J required the therapist to be aware of his own countertransference feelings.

Summary

AIDS has had a profound and deadly impact upon gay men. Sex is a central issue in gay men's lives, but is also the main vehicle for the spread of HIV. All gay men who are sexually active are at risk of exposure to HIV infection. Open, frank, and specific discussion about sex must be a part of therapy with a gay man. The therapist must take an active role in initiating such a discussion early in the work. Exploration, confrontation, and education are the tools for understanding the gay male patient's ability to maintain a safer sex life. Every therapist working with a gay male patient must consider how active a stance he or she will take regarding the exploration of sexual material. Not addressing sexual behavior puts the gay male at risk that he may be exposed to HIV, with disastrous results.

References

Cain R: Stigma management and gay identity development. Soc Work 36:67–73, 1991

Daniolos P: How professional associations view confidentiality. FOCUS: A Guide to AIDS Research and Counseling 8:5–6, 1993

Dardick L, Grady KE: Openness between gay persons and health professionals. Ann Intern Med 93:115–119, 1980

Fort J, Steiner CM, Conrad C: Attitudes of mental health professionals toward homosexuality and its treatment. Psychol Rep 29:347–350, 1971

Frost JC: The sexual history in the context of a medical interview, in AIDS and the Primary Care Providers: A Faculty Development Course for Physicians and Caregivers. Edited by Pisaneschi JJ. Washington, DC, The American Foundation for AIDS Research, 1989

Georgianna C, Johnston MW: Duty to protect: the gay community response. FOCUS: A Guide to AIDS Research and Counseling 8:1–4, 1993

Karr RG: Homosexual labeling and the male role. Journal of Social Issues 34:73–83, 1978

Kelly JA, St. Lawrence JS, Smith S, et al: Medical students' attitudes toward AIDS and homosexual patients. Journal of Medical Education 62:549–556, 1987a

Kelly JA, St. Lawrence JS, Smith S, et al: Stigmatization of AIDS patients by physicians. Am J Public Health 77:789–791, 1987b

Messing AE, Schoenberg R, Stephens RK: Confronting homophobia in health care settings: guidelines for social work practice. Journal of Social Work and Human Sexuality 2:65–74, 1984

Neisen JH: Heterosexism: redefining homophobia for the 1990s. Journal of Gay and Lesbian Psychotherapy 1:21–35, 1990

Owen WF: The clinical approach to the male homosexual patient. Med Clin North Am 70:499–535, 1986

Royse D, Birge B: Homophobia and attitudes towards AIDS patients among medical, nursing, and paramedical students. Psychol Rep 61:867–870, 1987

Shilts R: And the Band Played On. New York, St. Martin's Press, 1987

St. Lawrence JS, Husfeldt BA, Kelly JA, et al: The stigma of AIDS: fear of disease and prejudice toward gay men. J Homosex 19:85–101, 1991

Tarasoff v Regents of the University of California, 118 Cal Rptr 129, 529 P2d 553 (1974)

Totten G, Lamb DH, Reeder GD: *Tarasoff* and confidentiality in AIDS-related psychotherapy. Professional Psychology: Research and Practice 21:155–160, 1990

Troiden RR: The formation of homosexual identities. J Homosex 17:43–73, 1989

Chapter 8

Testing for HIV: Psychological and Psychotherapeutic Considerations

Marshall Forstein, M.D.

The advent in 1985 of laboratory testing to determine human immunodeficiency virus (HIV) serological status precipitated debates about the use of such tests. Public health officials, researchers, political activists, medical providers, and mental health clinicians have put forth positions on testing that are often in conflict. As in the story of the six blind men describing the elephant, the result leaves us wanting a comprehensive view of the issue of HIV testing.

In this chapter, I discuss the clinical issues that confront the psychotherapist treating gay men for whom the question of testing arises. The psychotherapist needs to understand the biological as well as psychosocial data that are relevant to testing in order to formulate a practical, behavioral, and psychodynamic understanding in any particular patient's situation.

Historical Overview

In March 1985, the U.S. Food and Drug Administration licensed the use of the enzyme-linked immunosorbent assay (ELISA) test to screen the nation's blood supply for the presence of HIV antibodies. The public health goal was to protect the blood supply and prevent the further transmission of HIV through blood product transfusion. Concerned that gay men in particular would flood the blood banks to determine

185

their serological status, public health officials and government agencies moved quickly to establish the anonymous Alternative HIV Testing system. This system was preferable to gay men because it would not record the names of those who had been tested, as would the blood bank system (Forstein 1985a).

Although by 1985 the acquired immunodeficiency syndrome (AIDS) had been well described, and increasing numbers of gay men (particularly in urban centers) were becoming sick, palliative treatment was basically the only medical treatment available for HIV-related illnesses. Thus began a complex and confusing debate about HIV testing within the gay community and with public health officials. The latter wanted to test everybody with the notion that this would help define the epidemiological boundaries of the epidemic and reduce transmission of the virus; they also felt that people would behave "correctly" once they knew their negative or positive status. Gay activists and many mental health clinicians initially warned that being tested might involve more complicated issues and that gay men should approach testing with caution. Activists argued both sides of the issue. Some claimed that testing would only help make this more of a "gay disease" and allow the government and society to separate gay men from others in terms of health care and civil rights, thus fostering even greater oppression and stigmatization than was already present. Others claimed that although there was no immediate medical treatment, there were psychological and physical benefits from knowing one's serological status, such as the empowerment of the self in order not to be victimized. Some mental health clinicians were more cautious, concerned with the enormous psychological burden that being tested might bring on top of the emotional pain that was already present in the gay community, embodied in the growing number of gay men who were sick and dying.

The debate centered on two different issues: 1) Was testing as valuable for gay people individually as it was for the public health agenda, or would it simply further stigmatize an already oppressed group? and 2) Would the results of an HIV test help those who were infected live their lives and avoid infecting others, and those who were negative stay negative by changing risky behaviors?

Existing paradigms for other sexually transmitted diseases were not helpful in determining approaches to containing the AIDS epidemic. In the absence of a definitive medical treatment for HIV (such as penicillin for syphilis), all sexually active gay men, regardless of serological status, could prevent transmission only through the universal implementation of safer sex techniques. The gay political community, as well as many gay medical and mental health providers, was reluctant to recommend testing, fearing further stigmatization by others and an exacerbation of internalized homophobic, sex-negative attitudes (i.e., the belief that sex is intrinsically bad) in gay men themselves. The hard-won sexual freedom that had been so much a part of gay male development since Stonewall (see Chapter 2) was now being blamed for the epidemic itself, as evidenced in the initial naming of the epidemic as *gay-related immunodeficiency disease—GRID*. Thus testing was seen as a further way to separate gay males from others and "good gays" from "bad gays." Fundamentalist groups had already called for the quarantining of people with AIDS.

Furthermore, mental health professionals posited that there was not necessarily a positive relationship between knowing one's serological status and changing one's sexual or drug use behavior for the better (Forstein 1985b, 1987). Results from studies investigating such a causal relationship have varied (Centers for Disease Control 1987; Klein et al. 1987; McKusick et al. 1987; Ostrow et al. 1989).

The emphasis on HIV-antibody testing within the gay community evolved from two developments. The first was that, with the advent of antiviral medications such as zidovudine (AZT) and other medications to serve prophylactically against opportunistic infections, early intervention appeared to make for better clinical management. The other was that, as more and more gay men became HIV positive and made their status public, that knowledge became identified with self-empowerment and with the opportunity to take control over one's future by determining what medical and psychological care to pursue.

One persistent danger to the gay community was the emerging fantasy that with the development of some treatments for HIV the universal practice of safer sex techniques was no longer necessary. The wish to see the medical establishment as being able to contain any sexually transmitted disease was confusing to many people unsophisticated about the differences between treatments and cures.

Impact of Medical Interventions

The development of antiviral medications, such as AZT, dideoxyinosine (DDI), dideoxycytosine (DDC), and others still being researched, as well as the use of antimicrobial medications to serve as prophylaxes against opportunistic infections, has had profound effects on the care of HIV-positive patients. The debate continues as to how soon after infection (but while the immune system is still relatively intact) antiviral therapy should be started. As more is learned about viral replication within cells, the standard treatment protocols for HIV infection are bound to be modified. Because there are no clear data to support one strategy over another, there is a range of clinical practices regarding the initiation of antiviral medications in the HIV-positive patient. Current practice suggests that an antiviral medication should be prescribed when the patient's CD4 count is below 500. Newer studies indicate that combination therapies, perhaps with three antiviral medications, may actually make the virus less able to become resistant to treatment. But presently, only when a patient has progressed to a more advanced state of immunodeficiency is there more consensus about the benefits of prophylaxis and treatment for opportunistic infections. No current treatments, however, mitigate against the necessity of all gay men having to continue safer sex in order to prevent infection to themselves or others.

The Decision to Be Tested

Tests for Discerning HIV Status

Several tests are used to determine whether an individual has been exposed to HIV. Most laboratories test for the presence of HIV with a two-stage process: the ELISA, which is a very sensitive test, and an antigen-specific Western Blot test. The ELISA, which is cheaper and simpler, is more than 99% sensitive if antibodies are present. The positive ELISA is about 95% specific for HIV without further testing; but with its 5% false-positive rate, especially when applied into millions of tests, there is a need for the Western Blot, which has to be carefully standardized. The combination of these two tests makes the chance of a false-positive test extraordinarily unlikely, especially if the individual tested has engaged in high-risk behavior (Burke et al. 1988; Centers for Disease Control 1988).

The recent (May 1992) licensing of an HIV-antibody test that can be done within minutes, and which is not followed by a standardized Western Blot test, will have a profound effect on how people are tested. In fact it is possible to do this test without even informing the patient. The test, which can administered using a drop of blood drawn during other blood tests, can be done in a physician's office, a blood bank drawing center, or wherever someone has access to an individual's blood and wishes to know his or her HIV status. (As this test has only just become available, its implications are still unfolding.)

Interpreting the results of the ELISA test, even if confirmed by Western Blot, requires an understanding of the natural history of HIV infection. An individual may take 6–12 weeks or possibly much longer to mount an antibody response after infection with HIV. Although most gay men's systems will manufacture antibodies within 1 year after infection, some studies indicate that occasionally the individual will not mount an antibody response at all, or that it may take more than 1 year in some cases. Thus a negative ELISA cannot be said to be 100% accurate. Living with this small possibility of error requires the individual to make choices about behavior without the certainty the test was expected to bring. Couples who use the antibody test to determine the level of risk in their sexual behavior do so without guarantees of protection. For couples who have not been tested, even those who have had a mutually monogamous relationship for at least 5 years, there may be a false sense of security, given the potentially long latency period between infection and manifestation of the disease, which may be more than a decade. This may lead to unsafe sexual practices.

Testing done within the "window" from infection to antibody response may give a false-negative result, engendering a potentially problematic psychological response in itself. Men who have engaged in potentially risky behaviors within the past year and who are seronegative at the time of testing require repeat testing every few months to confirm seronegativity. A gay man's reliance on a negative test result, especially in the face of high-risk behaviors, to confirm that he is not at risk (the myth of immunity) can adversely affect his capacity to maintain safer sex behavior.

Psychological Issues

The psychological motivations behind any individual's decision to be tested may be complex and may change over the course of time and with the individual's changing self-assessment for risk. A gay man may consider HIV testing for the following reasons:

1. Because he is in the process of making developmental decisions, such as continuing education, changing jobs, or entering into a new relationship.
2. As a consequence of finding out a previous sexual partner has become HIV positive or has developed AIDS.
3. When the anxiety of not knowing his antibody status becomes greater than the anxiety he imagines he will have by finding out he is HIV positive.
4. When he is in the throes of grief and the unconscious wish of finding out he is positive may enable him to identify with the lost objects and feel less alone and bereaved.
5. As a means of monitoring his sexual behavior (e.g., using the test to assess the efficacy of the previous 6 months of safer sex activities).
6. As a means of identifying with either a seropositive or seronegative subgroup in order to establish an emotionally supportive network in which to cope with the threat of illness.
7. As part of the decision to become a biological or adoptive parent.
8. As a security measure before applying for certain types of insurance coverage (many states allow insurance carriers to require a blood test for HIV status); this allows him to be anonymously tested before his test results become part of a national insurance register.
9. As part of a couple's decision to expand sexual activities from what is considered safe to less safe. Couples who have been together a

while and are either mutually monogamous or committed, and who are capable of totally safe sex outside the relationship (such as mutual masturbation) may decide to engage in higher risk behavior with each other based on the 99.5% certainty that they are both seronegative.

The decision to be tested may be either a response to a crisis or a result of much consideration over time, but usually evolves in a way that is consistent with the individual's characterological defenses and coping style.

Reactions to Test Results

Effects on Sexual and Drug-Using Behavior

As the AIDS epidemic has entered its second decade, newer issues have evolved. One is how gay men manage the information about their antibody status, whether it be positive or negative, over the long term as opposed to the short term. What is the lifelong effect of knowing versus not knowing one's antibody status on sexual and drug use behavior? How do gay men make behavioral changes, not for the short term in response to a crisis, but over the course of the rest of their lives as they remain at risk for a lethal disease? (See Chapter 21 on survivor's guilt.) There is clinical evidence that the capacity to prevent exposure to HIV may fluctuate over time and that it is influenced by many factors, including loss, grief, self-esteem, and a fundamental belief that one is entitled to a future.

Another factor is the evidence that knowing one's antibody status alone is not sufficient to engage gay men in medical, psychological, or drug abuse treatment. Even gay men who are immersed in an urban, gay-affirmative culture may be inconsistently or ambivalently engaged in their medical treatment. For gay men within the communities of color, knowledge of antibody status does not necessarily lead to participation in medical or psychosocial support systems, but may in fact reinforce isolation and withdrawal from social contact with gay men.

It was not until the AIDS epidemic was into its second decade, and about 7 years after antibody testing became generally available, that a few studies were conducted that looked into the long-term effect that knowing one's serological status had on one's behavior. Even where gay men have a high level of knowledge about HIV transmission and where there are good psychosocial and medical supports for people who are gay and at risk for HIV, there continues to be a significant proportion of gay men who persist in high-risk sexual behavior. Gay men who came out amidst a climate of ignorance, oppression, and stigma are psychologically more predisposed to continuing their risk to HIV infection.

The research to date suggests that there may be significantly different reactions among individuals who find out their antibody status (Centers for Disease Control 1987; McKusick et al. 1987; Ostrow et al. 1989; Perry et al. 1990a). There are indications that individuals who have perceived themselves as being positive or negative and who have already made behavioral changes prior to finding out their serological status continue for the most part to protect themselves and others. Those who believed they were at risk but made no changes in their sexual behavior prior to antibody testing, and then tested either positive or negative, were no more likely to make changes after being tested.

Several important issues emerge from the literature and clinical experience with gay men. In spite of a high level of knowledge about HIV infection and how to prevent transmission, a significant number of gay men who know their serological status (whether they are positive or negative) continue to place themselves or others at risk by engaging in unprotected anal intercourse with multiple partners. A greater percentage of gay men place themselves or others at risk in unprotected oral sex.

Sexual practices are often influenced by the significant, recreational use of drugs and alcohol, which lower sexual inhibitions and diminish cognitively set boundaries regarding what specific sexual acts an individual decides are prudent to engage in (see Chapter 19). Such disinhibition may allow for the acting out of unconsciously contained conflicts. In other men, serial negative HIV tests reinforce the notion that they are somehow immune to becoming infected in the future, thus enhancing the magical thinking of those who find the ongoing responsibility for their sexual behavior overwhelming.

What appears to be important in contributing to the gay man's capacity to make and maintain appropriate behavioral change can be distilled to a few principles, conceptualized by what is known as the "Health Belief Model":

1. He must perceive that he is at risk or has been at risk for HIV infection. If he assumes he is not at risk, there is no lasting motivation to participate in a societal program to limit sexual freedom or drug use.
2. If he believes that he is positive (whether or not he knows his serological status), he must also have the psychological capacity to care about infecting others or about worsening his own condition by becoming reexposed to HIV or other sexually transmitted diseases.
3. He must believe that his behavior change will have an actual, valued effect—that changing sexual or drug behaviors will affect the outcome of his being HIV positive (e.g., will increase his chances for long-term survival) or will protect him from becoming infected.
4. He must be able to find psychological and social supports within his own community for changing and maintaining the appropriate behaviors. One of the problems with most of the intervention studies is that they are generally based in middle-class, educated, white gay male communities in which peer support for "safer sex behaviors" is growing. To extrapolate this to the gay men of other classes, or to gay men using intravenous drugs, or to gay men of color is presumptuous.

Psychological Effects of Test Results on Different Populations

Seronegative individuals. Individuals who test negative may begin to feel that they are immune to HIV infection, assuming that if they have not yet been infected they must be invulnerable to it. Others develop severe forms of survivor's guilt, not unlike that seen in Holocaust survivors (see Chapter 21). Many of these individuals have lost numerous friends and sexual partners to AIDS and may begin to wonder why they have been spared. For some, there is actually an increase in unsafe practices, almost in defiance of their luck to date and in support of their denial of their own mortality. Some men report that they would prefer the fear and anxiety associated with actually being sick and potentially dying than the constant fear of becoming infected; the former alternative could be less problematic consciously and better defended against.

Seropositive individuals.   Individuals who test positive also present with a myriad of responses upon finding out their antibody status. For some, the fact that they are already infected and the perception that they will die from AIDS-related illnesses engender in them a nihilistic, self-destructive attitude. On rare occasions, the thought of "taking others with me" becomes revenge for the anger and betrayal one may feel for contracting this disease. Although this reaction may appear in the early stages of finding out one is positive, it usually dissipates unless there are characterological traits indicative of a preexisting antisocial personality. The expressed rage directed at others derives partly from the stimulation of self-hate in the infected gay or bisexual man as a result of internalized homophobia. In some gay men, the knowledge that they are infected leads to a difficult set of decisions regarding the continuation of sexual activity, including questions about whether and when to tell prospective sexual partners. The more narcissistically entitled the individual is, the more he may project total responsibility onto the partner, denying his own responsibility or participation in the process. This may be an acting out of intense rage and fear at his own infection, sometimes aimed at a future partner instead of at the partner from whom he believes he might have become infected. In this way the infected individual unconsciously transfers his rage toward himself and the man who he assumes did not care about him onto any sexual partner who comes along.

Intravenous drug users.   For gay intravenous drug users who feel morally corrupt and guilty for their addiction and the pain it wreaks on themselves and others, their self-loathing is intensified on finding out they have been infected with HIV. Their positive serological status may enhance their belief that continued chemical dependence is the only available emotional anesthesia. Antibody testing in the chemically dependent individuals may adversely affect their capacity to maintain or initiate sobriety.

Among gay intravenous drug addicts, the accessibility of treatment programs or methadone maintenance is important in evaluating the benefits or dangers of HIV testing. Addicts without access to treatment are motivated by their addiction, not by an intellectual decision regarding dangerous behaviors based on serological status. Although the gay addict may identify with the gay community, his behaviors are driven more by his addiction than by his social network. Without providing expansive programs to treat the drug-addicted populations, testing in and of itself may in fact encourage further usage, increase high-risk behavior, and keep people away from educational and counseling efforts.

Psychologically vulnerable individuals. Another consideration before advising whether or not an individual should be tested is the long-term effect such information will have on the psychological well-being and functioning of that individual. In a study of gay and bisexual men with HIV infection (Perry et al. 1990a) in which the psychosocial distress and well-being of individuals with AIDS, individuals with AIDS-related complex, and HIV positive but medically asymptomatic individuals were compared, the asymptomatic individuals were significantly more distressed than those with overt illness of varying degrees. In addition, many individuals appear to manage the knowledge of their serological status (either positive or negative) quite well in the period immediately following the receipt of this information. Later, however, many develop anxiety or depressive syndromes triggered by the knowledge that they have this lifelong infection that at any moment might go off like a time bomb.

Clinical experience also suggests an increased risk of completed suicide in asymptomatic individuals and a higher incidence of suicidal ideation, precipitated by the panic of finding out test results (Perry et al. 1990b). Suicidal ideation has been reported in patients who receive both negative and positive test results. In those cases where the negative results of a test were expected to put the patient's fear of infection to rest, the underlying delusional depression was not ameliorated by this information.

Antibody testing, regardless of outcome, can precipitate major depression, panic disorder, generalized anxiety disorders, adjustment disorders with significant morbidity, and frank psychosis with obsessional or delusional characteristics. Clinicians working with gay men to determine if testing is appropriate must remain vigilant to the acute and delayed sequelae of testing. Understanding the particular character structure and coping mechanisms available to one's patient should help the clinician understand whether the patient will be able to manage knowing his HIV status, or whether helping him act as though he were positive or negative (both requiring the same safe-sex behavior) might be more psychologically sustaining in the long term.

Individuals with supportive peer groups.   Different subgroups affected by HIV infection may have significantly different reactions to antibody testing. In the gay communities where there are active, open support networks, usually in urban areas with substantial open gay populations, the peer pressure and support for safer sex continues to be the fundamental influence on behavioral change. Encouraging safe, sexual ways of relating has been a psychologically healthy substitute for fear and anxiety. In less positive environments, however, homosexually active men might continue to turn to unsafe behaviors as an anxiety-reducing activity. Further complicating the capacity to engage in safer sex are the complex psychological meanings of safer sex to a gay man in pursuit of intimacy (see Chapter 20).

Psychotherapeutic Issues

Patients may bring issues about testing into treatment at any point in the course of psychotherapy. A gay man may seek psychotherapy to help make the decision whether or not to be tested. Couples often present either with the request that the therapist help them decide whether to be tested or as a result of being tested and finding out that one or both of them are positive. (The treatment of couples with differing antibody statuses poses special challenges, and is addressed in Chapter 14.)

Individuals or couples may present with the expectation that the therapist will make the decision about whether they should be tested based on the initial evaluation. However the therapist, must clarify that the psychological burden that arises from the decision to test is not his or hers to bear, regardless of the outcome of the test itself. The therapist must distinguish between his or her ethical responsibility to explore in sufficient detail (and with a view to the long term) the advisability of being tested at a particular time versus the patient's or patients' responsibility for actually taking the test. For example, a therapist should point out if a patient is in crisis, in acute bereavement, or newly sober, and note the patient's particular vulnerability to adverse psychological sequelae of testing at that time. However, recommending that the particular moment might not be optimal for finding out the results of a test that has long-term ramifications is not the same as suggesting that the test not be done at all (Marks and Goldblum 1989; Rosser and Ross 1991).

Clinicians should always ask themselves and their patients the following questions:

1. How would either a positive or a negative test affect the way the patient lives his life now? What changes in sexual or drug-using behavior has the patient made prior to finding out his serological status?

2. How well does the patient contain ambiguity? Is it acted out behaviorally or managed in an internal psychological manner?

3. Has there been any prior experience in the patient's life to suggest that knowing his antibody status will contribute to his capacity to change behavior if he has not already done so?

4. How does the patient see the meaning of his life differently when he is asked to explore how either a positive or negative test will affect his view of himself and his hopes for the future?

5. Will the patient be able to psychologically engage in and have the resources for the medical and psychological treatment he will need if he is positive? What are his beliefs and feelings about taking medications?

6. Is there a more than theoretical risk for the patient to become acutely suicidal or immobilized by finding out he is positive?

7. Is there an adequate psychosocial network of people in the gay man's life to sustain him in the short and long term?

Mental health professionals should consider HIV-antibody testing within the context of what is known about the relationship between knowledge and behavior (Martin and Vance 1984). As in the case of smoking, not wearing seat belts, using drugs, or becoming pregnant when it is medically ill advised, knowledge alone about the relationship between the behavior and its potentially lethal consequences has never been shown to significantly affect behavioral change. In fact, to significantly affect the chances for altering the dangerous behavior, repeated exposure to education about the behavior's dangers with sufficient internalized capacity and external support for changing that behavior is required. Even when such behaviors are changed, episodes of the dangerous behavior often appear in the future, as evidenced by the number of people who start smoking again even after long periods of abstinence. Unlike smoking, however, where cessation of the activity often reduces the associated risks, making mistakes in the area of unsafe sexual activity or needle sharing may do irrevocable harm.

An individual who knows that he has been infected may respond very differently from one who simply believes that he has or has not been infected. Believing that one has been exposed may allow for one to assume an altruistic posture as well as a self-protective one, based as much on healthy denial as on accepting the possibility of HIV exposure. Therefore, although one believes that he may have been exposed, a healthy amount of denial allows for the simultaneous belief that one might have, just by chance, escaped exposure (Forstein 1988). This capacity to simultaneously juggle two conflicting and contradictory possibilities allows most people to get on with their lives and maintain a future orientation. In a word, it allows for hope. For people who know that they are HIV positive, the possibility and the hope that they might have escaped exposure are taken away. In the absence of a definitive cure for HIV, as there is for syphilis, clinicians must have a healthy respect for the need to maintain some denial in the service of the individual's need to believe in the future.

Countertransference Issues in Treating Gay Men With HIV Concerns

For Primary Care Physicians

Often patients will present to clinicians in such panicked, anxious, or depressed states about their health status that HIV-antibody testing appears to be a way of decreasing anxiety. Clinicians, facing their own anxiety about treating a disturbed patient who may be infected with HIV, might see the test as providing certainty at a time when everything else feels tenuous to both patient and provider. Physicians, who are trained perhaps more than other health care providers to feel that they have to have the answers (and rely on laboratory evidence to find them), often resort to testing as a way of feeling in control of the uncertain situation. Taking the time to sort out the complex psychological issues surrounding testing instead of resorting to the test as a means of allaying anxiety demands a level of involvement in the psychological lives of people that is expensive (i.e., not reimbursed) and labor intensive, but may be crucial for the patient's well-being. It is unfortunate that physicians often lack the willingness and capacity to meet these demands. The denial of the significant psychological ramifications of testing and the impact of having to provide medical and psychiatric care for those who test positive or are at risk for infection, continue to provoke a simple, reflexive posture advocating testing without consideration for the impact on any single individual within the context of his own community and access to services.

Medical providers who cannot or will not take the time to provide in-depth counseling around the decision to be HIV tested have an ethical obligation to refer the patient to a trained HIV counselor. For people who have complicated medical histories, chemical dependencies, or prior mental health concerns, referral to a mental health clinician is necessary to understand and make explicit the purpose of testing from as many practical, medical, and psychological perspectives as possible.

For Psychotherapists

Therapists working with gay men are vulnerable to their own countertransferential issues, which arise from the wish to protect or save the patient or prevent harm. A therapist's wish to alleviate the patient's enormous anxiety about his uncertain antibody status may unconsciously push the therapist to support a decision to test without first exploring the complex consequences that may arise in the patient's particular situation. Therapists who find the management of a patient's sexual or drug-using behavior anxiety provoking may hope that once the patient knows the results of his serological status, he will diminish or end his risky behavior. More worrisome is the risk that the therapist might recommend testing as an expression of his or her anger at the patient who is not protecting himself or others.

The anxiety involved in listening over a long period of time to a patient anguished by his unsafe behaviors may push the therapist to invest in the test as a means of making the danger overt and precipitating a change that verbal therapy has not been able to engender. For some therapists, especially those who are working with several gay men with HIV concerns, the results of antibody testing would help to sort their patients into two groups: those whom they will work with until they become sick, and those in whom they will invest with a belief in the future. The patient whose antibody status is not certain may trigger more anxiety in the therapist. In fact, even when patients have tested negative, the therapist must be vigilant for signs that their capacity to maintain that negative status is not endangered by their increased psychological stress. These stresses may appear in the form of increasing loss, unremitting grief, assaults on self-esteem (which may occur in the form of overt or covert homophobic trauma), rejection by family or peers, or the emergence or recurrence of psychiatric disorders or addictive behaviors.

Conclusions and Recommendations

The questions around HIV-antibody testing will continue to be complex, especially with the advent of new treatments to forestall immunological consequences of HIV infection. There will be an increasing push to mandate universal testing and contact tracing (public health agencies' contacting of an HIV-positive individual's sexual partners) as improvements in treatments come along. When there is a definitive "cure" for HIV infection (although I believe this is unlikely at this point given the nature of the retrovirus), this disease will be handled by the public health officials in a fashion similar to other sexually transmitted diseases. But until there is a qualitative change in what medicine has to offer people infected with HIV, the issues of prevention must remain paramount, both in terms of the individual at risk and for the public good.

The decision to seek antibody testing must continue to be seen as an important and complex individual process. Long-term ramifications as well as short-term concerns must be taken into account, as the consequences of testing may be significantly constructive or destructive. Gay men must be offered as much insight as possible into the ramifications of testing based on their individual psychological constitution, their ability to manage anxiety and ambiguity, and their capacity to find and maintain resources within their community regardless of the results of the test. Realistic aspects of testing must be distinguished from magical wishes and beliefs. Access to appropriate mental health as well as medical care must be determined prior to testing to avoid setting the gay man up for further disappointment and rejection.

Finally, testing must be seen as a complicated process that does not always lead to behavioral change that makes sense. Although the test may appear to be a simple procedure, the psychological ramifications of testing for any single individual may arise out of significant anxieties and unconscious conflicts that require careful, compassionate, and psychologically intricate consideration.

References

Burke DS, Brindage JF, Refield RR, et al: Measurement of the false positive rate in a screening program for human immunodeficiency virus infection. NEJM 319:961–964, 1988

Centers for Disease Control: Self-reported changes in sexual behaviors among homosexual and bisexual men from the San Francisco City clinic cohort. Morb Mortal Wkly Rep 36:187–189, 1987

Centers for Disease Control: Update: serologic testing for antibody to human immunodeficiency virus. Morb Mortal Wkly Rep 36:833–844, 1988

Forstein M: HTLV-3 antibody testing (letter). NEJM October 31, 1985a, p 1158

Forstein M: HIV Antibody Testing. Paper presented at the National Institute of Allergy and Infectious Diseases Conference on AIDS, Boston, MA, November 1985b

Forstein M: Understanding the psychological impact of AIDS: the other epidemic, in The New England Journal of Public Policy. Edited by O'Malley P. Boston, MA, McCormick Institute, University of Massachusetts, 1988, pp 159–171

Forstein M: HIV antibody testing, in A Psychiatrist's Guide to AIDS and HIV Disease. A report of the American Psychiatric Association AIDS Education Project. Washington, DC, American Psychiatric Association, 1990, pp 77–61

Klein DE, Sullivan G, Wolcott D, et al: Changes in AIDS risk behaviors among homosexual male physicians and university students. Am J Psychiatry 144:742–747, 1987

Marks R, Goldblum PB: The decision to test: A personal choice, in Face to Face: A Guide to AIDS Counseling. Edited by Dilley JW, Pies C, Helquist M. San Francisco, CA, AIDS Health Project, 1989, pp 49–58

Martin SL, Vance CS: Behavioral and psychosocial factors in AIDS: methodological and substantive issues. Am Psychol 39:1303–1308, 1984

McKusick L, Coates T, Horstman W: HTLV-III transmitting behavior and desire for HTLV-III antibody testing in San Francisco men at risk for AIDS 1982–1985. Paper presented at the International Conference on AIDS, Washington, DC, June 1987

Ostrow DG, Joseph J, Kessler R, et al: Disclosure of HIV antibody status: behavioral and mental health correlates. AIDS Educ Prev 1:1–11, 1989

Perry SW, Jacobsberg LB, Fishman B, et al: Psychological responses to serologic testing for HIV. AIDS 4:145–152, 1990a

Perry SW, Jacobsberg LB, Fishman B: Suicidal ideation and HIV testing. JAMA 263:679–682, 1990b

Rosser BR, Ross M: Psychological resistant and HIV counseling. Journal of Gay and Lesbian Psychotherapy 1:93–114, 1991

Section II

Treatment Modalities

Individual Treatment

Group Treatment

Couples and Family Treatment

Individual Treatment

Chapter 9

The Psychodynamics of AIDS: A View From Self Psychology

Sharone Abramowitz, M.D.
Jeffrey Cohen, M.D.

An Introductory Overview

Psychoanalytical self psychology offers a compelling explanatory and therapeutic model for working empathically with the intrapsychic crisis facing *people with acquired immunodeficiency syndrome (AIDS)* (i.e., *PWAs*). It provides a useful psychodynamic bridge between the social consequences and the intrapsychic effects of AIDS. Because gay men with human immunodeficiency virus (HIV)–related illnesses face multiple assaults on their self-esteem from the long-term effects of homophobia, the stigma of AIDS, and a wasting illness that compromises one's self-image, self psychology's focus on the narcissistic dimensions of human experience is especially useful in the psychotherapeutic treatment of these men. As a psychoanalytic theory that has explicitly broken away from classical drive theory, self psychology avoids the homophobic pitfalls of traditional psychoanalysis while retaining a depth psychological transference orientation

As first explicated by Heinz Kohut (1971, 1977, 1984), self psychology bases itself on *selfobject theory*. Selfobject theory defines the *self* as an intrapsychic organization that has "stability over time," and

An earlier version of this chapter appeared as "AIDS Attacks the Self: A Self Psychological Exploration of the Psychodynamic Consequences of AIDS," in *Progress in Self Psychology*. Edited by Goldberg A. Hillsdale, NJ, Analytic Press, 1990, pp 157–172.

that "provid[es] one with a healthy sense of self, self-esteem and well being." The term *cohesive self* describes a state of self that remains steady and dependable, providing one with a sense of stability. When the cohesive self is disrupted by rapid changes and narcissistic threats—a *fragmented self* arises (Wolf 1988). Self psychology's self is not fully autonomous; it thrives in and depends on a matrix of *selfobject functions* (Wolf 1988). A selfobject is not a person; in fact, it is neither a self nor an object, nor is it an interpersonal relationship between the self and others. Rather the term *selfobject* describes the intrapsychic experience of a function performed by a relationship to other people, symbols, or ideas. It describes the subjective relationship to an experience that creates and sustains a sense of selfhood (Wolf 1988).

Empathy sits at the core of self psychology's therapeutic technique. The self psychologist strives to view the intrapsychic world of his patient through the patient's subjectivity. The field of observation is from within, not from without. Because of this empathic vantage point, defense is not seen only as resistance, but as the patient's chronic adaptations for maintaining or restoring self-stability. This empathic perspective leads self psychology to view transference beyond the traditional constructs of repetition and distortion. It includes the creative use of the therapist in a selfobject transference. Several types of selfobject transferences have now been defined, but Kohut (1971) originally described three: the mirroring, the alterego, and the idealizing transferences. *Mirroring* refers to the self's need for affirmation and recognition by others. *Alterego* needs (known also as *twinship needs*) contain the experience of feeling an essential alikeness with others. *Idealizing* describes the experience of the self being soothed, protected, and accepted by an admired and respected person, idea, or symbol (Wolf 1988).

In this chapter we first explore the subjective experience of the gay male PWA, with special emphasis on the multiple ways AIDS precipitates a profound destabilizing crisis for the self. We look at how AIDS threatens self-cohesion through its disruptive destruction of body integrity. Next we focus on how AIDS, as a condition associated with profound social stigma and loss, traumatically disturbs fundamental ties between the self and that which provides stabilizing mirroring, alterego, and idealized selfobject functions. Having detailed ways AIDS destabilizes the self, we then explore approaches to helping PWAs restore self-cohesion. We end with a brief discussion of countertransference issues. The psychotherapeutic challenge is to help the gay man afflicted with HIV illness maximize the cohesiveness, firmness, and vitality of his embattled self.

Disruption of the Body Self

Stern (1985) theorized that the sense of core self is first organized around the experience of the body. Through the body, the first reference point for self-organization, a sense of *self-agency* (i.e., having control over one's own physical activity) and of *self-cohesion* (i.e., the experience of being a nonfragmented, physical whole) develops. Kohut (1971) also viewed the body as an integral aspect of the psychological self. He termed the intrapsychic relationship to the physical body the *body self*. The body self, according to Kohut, is the original vehicle for our exhibitionistic needs. Self-esteem derives in part from the smooth functioning and structural integrity of the body, as well as from perceived physical attractiveness and sexual and athletic prowess. Conversely, a subjective experience of defectiveness through disfigurement or malfunctioning of the body is destabilizing to self-organization.

AIDS-related illnesses, like other physical illnesses, threaten the cohesiveness of the body self. When Kaposi's sarcoma (KS) lesions appear, blood counts decline, or weight is lost, the psychological self can feel damaged, contaminated, or out of control. AIDS especially threatens the body self in three ways:

1. Because AIDS can be such a highly stigmatized illness, visible HIV lesions can cause great shame. For example, KS tumors can become a "mark of Cain," causing the PWA to become isolated from much needed social support.
2. HIV-related illnesses often present with vague and diffuse symptoms. Kohut (1971) noted that viral illnesses that present with nonspecific symptoms leave the self prone to fragmentation. HIV-

related illnesses usually involve a multiplicity of organ systems without a well-defined physical locus around which the PWA can organize his sense of self. This could explain why many patients with AIDS-related complex (and its accompanying vague constitutional symptoms) experience a reduction in massive anxiety once they progress to a definitive AIDS diagnosis.

3. The diverse neuropsychiatric effects of AIDS compromise the brain itself, the smooth functioning of which is so integral to a sense of self-competency. The way that the brain organizes incoming stimuli, even if dysfunctionally, will to a great extent determine the organization of self-experience. The PWA with brain dysfunction often demands that others confirm his cognitively distorted experience. This deterioration of mental capacity also impairs the PWA's ability to cope with the many other losses encountered in the illness.

HIV encephalopathy, which includes AIDS dementia, especially threatens the competency and esteem of the afflicted PWA. Basch (1988), drawing from information processing theory, explained how the brain's task is to establish order among disparate stimuli. When functioning well, this neurophysiological function is subjectively experienced as a sense of order and competency. When HIV-related organic brain states cause memory loss, confusion, and other information-processing dysfunction, the brain cannot easily provide the self with a sense of order. The impaired PWA then feels a compromised sense of efficaciousness. This can cause great anxiety and a state of self-fragmentation with its associated by-products of rage, depression, and confusion. The trouble is that these psychological fragmentation products can be hard to differentiate from the worsening symptoms of HIV-related brain disease.

Disruption of Selfobject Bonds

Loss and Grief

AIDS causes staggering losses. The losses range from the concrete (e.g., loss of job, social role, physical attractiveness) to the abstract (e.g., loss of basic security, self-determination, predictability). The diagnosis of a terminal illness, especially for a young adult, directly threatens normal grandiosity and its common (even if illusory) sense of invulnerability and immortality.

Loss causes grief, and the affective experience of grief brings with it wrenching psychic pain that involves the deepest sadness known to human experience. The death of a loved one who provided vital self-sustaining functions for the bereaved individual can traumatically threaten the mourner's most basic sense of self. A feeling that one is falling apart or is lost and adrift accompanies grief and reflects a profound sense of self-fragmentation. As Bowlby (1980) explained it, the grief process (with its communication of psychic pain through crying or wailing, and its intrusive hallucinations and remembrances of the deceased) may partly function as a way to maintain contact with the lost object and at the same time as an appeal for additional support from the living. As expressed in self psychological terms, the grief process can restore self-cohesion by intrapsychically maintaining the selfobject bond with the deceased and by bolstering and reaffirming selfobject ties with the living.

All catastrophic illnesses cause great loss, but the infectious spread of AIDS leaves vulnerable communities bereft to a massive degree. The very lovers and friends a PWA needs to serve self-restorative functions in response to his grief are often themselves dead or very ill. It is tragic that at a time of heightened selfobject need, the PWA must mourn an ever-shrinking selfobject milieu. The result for these PWAs' selves may be profound destabilization. To cope they may withdraw into depression, disavow the affective experience of the loss, numb themselves with chemicals, stay enraged, or remain more involved with their relationships to the dead than to the living.

The danger of self-fragmentation is especially pronounced for the grieving PWA who is also near death. The dying process is a time of extraordinary vulnerability and increased need. As Kohut faced his own terminal illness, he wrote poignantly of maintaining selfobject ties throughout the dying process:

A human death can and, I will affirm, should be an experience that, however deeply melancholy, is comparable to a fulfilled parting—it should have no significant admixture of disintegration anxiety. It must be stressed, however, that in order to enable the dying person to retain a modicum of the cohesion, firmness, and harmony of the self, his surroundings must not withdraw their selfobject functions at the last moment of his conscious participation in the world. (Kohut 1984, p. 18)

As the following case shows, for many dying PWAs Kohut's conditions cannot be met:

Case 1

Mr. A was a 40-year-old gay man whose lover of several years died from an AIDS-related illness 1 year before Mr. A himself was hospitalized. After establishing a sustaining relationship with his lover, Mr. A, who was a recovering alcoholic patient, was able to give up the drinking that compensated for his earlier unmet selfobject needs. When his lover grew very ill, Mr. A's intensive involvement in his care provided a means for Mr. A to stay bonded with him. In this way Mr. A could stabilize his vulnerable self, which was threatened at the impending loss of his lover.

When his lover actually died, Mr. A traumatically faced the loss of a vital sustaining selfobject tie. His fragile self-organization was dependent on his relationship with his lover to provide him with stability. Without his lover, Mr. A returned to alcohol, the self-soothing chemical he had used prior to meeting his lover. A vicious cycle began: each time Mr. A attempted sobriety, his acute grief would return and an intense anguished sense of self-fragmentation would emerge, again leading him to drink.

When the 1-year anniversary of his lover's death arrived, Mr. A was facing his own worsening health. He became extraordinarily vulnerable, and in a desperate attempt to numb his pain, he drank a toxic volume of alcohol, which caused respiratory failure. Although he survived that episode, he was later found dead for unclear reasons.

Disrupted Mirroring

AIDS profoundly disrupts bonds with whomever or whatever provides mirroring selfobject functions. For example, sexuality provides support and a confirmation of worth. AIDS interrupts this important avenue for mirroring. Many PWAs no longer feel very sexual because of debilitation, fear of infecting others, fear of their own exposure to further infections, or perhaps a disenchantment with sex itself because it can be a route of HIV exposure.

For the gay drug user, the drug often serves mirroring functions. As Kohut (1978) wrote:

> The addict craves the drug because the drug seems capable of curing the central defect in his self. It becomes for him the substitute for a selfobject that failed him. . . . The ingestion of the drug provides him with the self-esteem he does not possess. (p. 846)

The self-soothing functions of drug use can momentarily provide the drug user with the sense of acceptance he so desperately craves. When the drug user is also a PWA, illness or the fear of infecting others can disrupt his drug habits. These interruptions can cause escalating anxiety as an already fragile self tries to soberly face the ongoing fragmentation threats of AIDS.

Rejection, motivated by fear or prejudice, by those who once fulfilled selfobject functions (lovers, family, friends, coworkers) may deprive a PWA of urgently needed mirroring at a time of heightened need. The stigma of AIDS also leads many PWAs to reject needed support. Because the self-cohesion of PWAs is threatened by a stigmatized catastrophic illness, their intensified need for attuned mirroring leaves them very vulnerable to feeling shame. PWAs then especially need reassurance that their loved ones do not view them as disgraceful. It is unfortunate that when PWAs come from families or communities where AIDS and its association to homosexuality and drug use are highly stigmatized, these PWAs understandably expect that their support systems will view them disparagingly. This expectation can cause them to feel deep humiliation about their diagnosis. They will then isolate themselves from potential caregivers, just when they most need reaffirming mirroring. By keeping their diagnosis secret, they can at least maintain the memories or illusions of past intact selfobject ties. Rejection by family and community is unfortunately often a harsh reality; but it is equally unfortunate that many PWAs avoid others who, if given the chance, might be quite supportive. This dynamic is illustrated in Case 2.

Case 2

Mr. B, a 22-year-old non–gay-identified bisexual African American, came into the hospital for a workup of a cough. Although he never used intravenous drugs, he knew a former lover had; nevertheless, he was completely unprepared for the diagnosis of Pneumocystis carinii pneumonia (PCP) that faced him. Although he deeply yearned for the comfort of his family, a deep sense of shame arose within him. He imagined his father walking across a street, and his neighbors pointing and laughing at him, whispering among themselves about how his son had AIDS.

As Mr. B's pneumonia worsened, he grew more despondent. Despite the medical staff's frequent encouragement for him to contact his family, Mr. B continued to refuse. Although he longed for the company of his family, his shame left him feeling that he would rather die alone with his father's pride in him left intact. His self-esteem was dependent on keeping alive this vital selfobject bond.

Eventually, when it became clear that Mr. B would not recover from this first bout of PCP, his physicians contacted his family. Despite their deep shock and grief over his condition, Mr. B's family remained lovingly at his bedside until he died.

Disrupted Alterego Bonds

AIDS can deeply undermine the alterego stabilization some PWAs experience as part of a community of peers. For gay men whose self-esteem has been validated by their "coming out" and openly identifying with the gay community, the traumatic loss of a growing segment of their community can be deeply alienating.

Differences in health status may cause splits in a formerly cohesive community: splits between those who have AIDS or AIDS-related complex, those who are HIV negative or positive, and those who remain untested for HIV infection. Estrangement from the community may even be self-imposed. For example, the diagnosis of AIDS may stir up self-blame, self-hatred, and internalized homophobia in some gay or bisexual men. Whereas previously a community of others with the same sexual orientation was sought, aroused conflicts may lead to emotional distancing.

The AIDS diagnosis may reveal an individual's hidden sexual behaviors or drug use. The result can be ostracism by a formerly supportive community. For example, a non–gay-identified, behaviorally bisexual man, once diagnosed, may find himself rejected by family, church, and subculture.

For gay drug users, alterego selfobject needs are also provided by other drug users. Already shunned by society, if others in the drug-using community also ostracize the PWA, he is left deeply alone. The need for alternative support may motivate some PWAs who use drugs into recovery programs, but for most (despite the public health risk) the greater need to maintain tenuous but psychologically vital alterego selfobject ties motivates them to hide their ill status from their community.

Disrupted Idealized Bonds

The seriously ill individual yearns, like a vulnerable child, for omniscient and omnipotent figures to merge with and be protected by; thus caregivers are sought to fulfill idealized selfobject functions. The PWA hopes that his physician, nurse, or therapist will have all the answers. When confronted with the real limitations of AIDS treatments, caregivers often cannot be the idealized parent figures with whom the sick person can merge and experience safety, calmness, and healing. The resulting disappointment can deeply undermine the PWA's self-cohesiveness.

In an attempt to have this vital psychological need met, some PWAs will keep seeking connections to alternative idealized figures. Although some are ethical and legitimate, others can be exploitative and hurtful. If the underlying desperate need for an idealized healer is not understood, it will be difficult to extricate the patient from the exploited relationship.

Similarly, medications and other treatments may also be yearned for as powerful agents that soothe and cure. The stabilization experienced by ingesting, and thus merging with, these idealized treatments may underlie the power of the "placebo effect." However, here too there is no magical cure, only a plethora of limited treatments that often produce devastating side effects. As medications fail and complications progress, protective selfobject needs are again frustrated.

The Paradox of HIV Transmission

Not only does AIDS threaten physiological life and the psychological self, but it does so paradoxically through mechanisms that normally sustain and protect the body and the self. Just as HIV targets the immune system, thus destroying the body's primary defense, it also compromises sexuality, a vital vehicle for maintaining self-esteem. Just as HIV ruins the blood products on which hemophiliacs depend for their physical survival, it also contaminates the intravenous route on which the drug user depends (even if dysfunctionally) to maintain self-cohesion.

Sexual contact, whether in its more primitive and defensive form or in its mature form, is a fundamental route for fulfilling mirroring, alterego, and idealizing selfobject needs. Because HIV infects the body through sexual routes, the person whose selfobject needs were met through unsafe sex must face the difficult task of changing sexual behavior. If oral sex stabilized the self with soothing and merging, or unprotected anal penetration provided a sense of empowerment, then to the extent that self-stability is threatened by abandonment of these unsafe sex practices, the gay man will resist safer sex alternatives. The specific selfobject needs met by the unsafe practices must first be empathically analyzed before safer sex alternatives can be found that also meet those needs.

For the gay intravenous drug user who harbors deep self-deficits, the drug often serves as a substitute for unmet selfobject needs. An empathic appreciation of the archaic selfobject needs motivating drug use is crucial to working with the addicted patient. For example, drug users may share needles not because of the unavailability of clean needles but as a way of establishing intimacy with another. Having sex "while high" (and taking the extreme risk of participating in unsafe sex) may not be just about irresponsibility; instead, it may be that only in a "high" state can core self needs for sexual contact be met. Most addicted people keep using their drugs to prevent physiological withdrawal anxiety, a cause of terrible psychological fragmentation for these fragile people. Unless the selfobject effects of drug use, needle sharing, and drug withdrawal are taken into account, behavioral change will be doomed to failure.

AIDS Recapitulates Preexisting Self Issues

Gay PWAs represent the full spectrum of psychologies, from those with mature and stable core selves to those with preexisting self-disorders and profound narcissistic vulnerabilities. When AIDS enters someone's life it captures them within their unique developmental level, family history, coping skills, and background of other traumas and losses.

As selfobject ties are disrupted, which in turn destabilizes the self, the PWA may experience his current situation as a recapitulation of an earlier inadequate selfobject milieu. A PWA's current fears and vulnerabilities about AIDS can tell the therapist about his reactions to the deficits and traumas of the early developmental environment. For example, the regressed PWA may once again feel like a frightened needy sick child whose family cannot or will not respond to his needs for affective attunement. Fragmenting feelings of terrifying emptiness, hopelessness, depression, or rage may arise. Dependency brought on by illness may trigger old fears of abandonment or neglect by unavailable caregivers. Fears of abuse or being narcissistically used by caregivers who needed the child to be sick and dependent can emerge.

When the early family failed to adequately mirror the self, the vulnerable self may have rationalized that caregivers "legitimately" failed to affirm him because he was fundamentally "bad." AIDS can then feel like a present-day retribution or confirmation that the self is bad, defective, unworthy, and unlovable. This belief may be the core dynamic of internalized homophobia, in which certain gay men experience AIDS as a punishment for being homosexual.

Restoration of Selfobject Bonds: Crisis as Opportunity

In the context of the devastating disruptions AIDS brings, the relationship to the therapist provides the PWA with fundamental and sustain-

ing selfobject functions. The therapist's mirroring, alterego, and idealizing functions are crucial, as is his or her commitment for a long-term
presence. During the life-threatening illnesses associated with AIDS,
the PWA can easily become childlike and operate at an early level of
selfobject need. The reliable provision of these needs and the security
that one will not be abandoned become critical. Again, to paraphrase
Kohut (1984), until the moment physical death arrives, it is vital to
continually provide selfobject functions to help maintain the dying
person's sense of self.

Working with PWAs requires expanding the frame of the therapy.
The therapist often must work with the patient's support system via
family and couple's work, or conversations with the patient's physician, to enable others involved with the patient to better mirror, accept, protect, and strengthen the PWA's threatened self. The isolation,
alienation, and stigma of AIDS requires that mobilization of interpersonal resources be a part of the therapeutic process.

Meeting Mirroring Needs

At the core level, the therapist needs to empathically explore the PWA's
negative self-images of being bad, defective, or unlovable. Supportive-
ly working through these feelings and actively affirming the self will
help to restore self-esteem as manifested in an increased sense of control, choice, and vitality. Losses and selfobject failures that cause painful affects of suicidal despair, rage, grief, guilt, fear, and injuries to
grandiose invulnerability all require understanding and eventual interpretation as to how they impact the sense of self. The legitimate
mirroring needs provided by unsafe sex and drug behavior require the
therapist's empathy so that safer alternatives that also answer these
selfobject needs can be found.

Some PWAs, by adopting the role of caregiver or teacher, receive
valuable mirroring from their patients or students. The resulting confirmation of worth and improvement in self-esteem strengthens these
PWAs. Through writing, teaching, speaking, and counseling, they can
transform a personal ordeal into something of value for others and for
themselves.

Meeting Alterego Needs

Where possible, the therapist must help the patient to strengthen existing, if shaken, ties to those serving twinship functions. The genetics of poor self-esteem and shame need empathic understanding and explaining, so that the isolated and alienated PWA can reconnect to family and community. The PWA can be directed toward community initiatives that can further stabilize the self through participation in a supportive alterego milieu. AIDS self-help movements, 12-step programs, and counseling groups can all combat the devastating consequences of alienation that AIDS often brings with it.

The AIDS quilt, a living national memorial to those who have died from AIDS-related illnesses, serves an important twinship selfobject function for the growing number of mourning Americans. Its hundreds of connected quilt patches tie each singular death into a larger whole. It reminds the bereaved that they are not alone, but are united in their mourning, and at the same time publicly legitimates their grief. The unity that the quilt conveys as a whole, while celebrating the diversity of its parts, has been one of the best antidotes for the terrible and isolating stigma associated with this disease.

Meeting Idealizing Needs

The therapist must first empathically work with the PWA's understandable disappointment in those who were supposed to supply idealized selfobject needs, including the therapist. By remaining caring and present, the therapist usually can restore stabilizing idealization and heal the breach with herself or himself or with another formerly idealized caregiver, such as the patient's primary care physician. As previously suggested, the curative power of the physician and treatments may partially depend on their ability to be idealized; thus restoration of these selfobject bonds is vital. Alternatively, interpretative work validating the legitimacy of idealization needs may help stabilize PWAs and enable them to separate from disreputable practitioners with whom they have been enacting those needs.

Establishing a new or renewed connection with spirituality may serve a powerfully stabilizing idealized selfobject function for the

PWA. Kohut (1984) wrote that the fear of death is not a fear of physical extinction, "but the ascendancy of a nonhuman environment" bereft of selfobjects (p. 18). If the PWA's spiritual orientation allows him to view the body as a vehicle for a self that lives on in a sustaining selfobject milieu of the afterlife, physical death becomes less threatening. Dying becomes a merger with the eternally sustaining idealized selfobject milieu, one's spiritual power.

Bolstering a sense of living in accordance with one's internalized goals and ideals can stabilize the self, thus increasing self-esteem and cohesion. Volunteer work, generosity, reconciliation, and helpfulness can aid the PWA in finding even greater meaningfulness in his current life than he had before his illness. The crisis of AIDS is also a developmental challenge and an opportunity, as Case 3 profoundly illustrates.

Case 3

Mr. C, a 52-year-old gay Caucasian man, had lost 25% of his body weight because of relentless KS. His body was literally wasting away, causing him profound disintegration anxiety. Too ashamed to go to his usual bars, he soothed himself by drinking alone. His many years of alcoholism had left him quite isolated, and now even his one avenue of social support felt unsafe.

On the third anniversary of his beloved mother's death, Mr. C's extreme alienation further escalated. He could no longer tolerate the intense loneliness and psychic pain; he drank a great quantity of his favorite vodka and swallowed a near lethal amount of antidepressants. He was found comatose by a neighbor and was "saved."

While in a special AIDS psychiatric unit, Mr. C pulled out of his depression and began his alcohol recovery with the help of Alcoholics Anonymous. Despite having to go to an AIDS medical unit for palliation of his now terminal KS, he felt deeply thankful that his suicide attempt had failed. His weeks in the hospital allowed him to reconnect with a recovering alcoholic friend whom he greatly admired. Through this relationship Mr. C found "God's will," and knew he had been spared death at that moment in order to help other alcoholic PWAs go into recovery.

Through his idealized selfobject relationships to his friend and to his God, Mr. C could consolidate his previously beleaguered self around a healthy grandiose belief in his ability to help others. Mr.

C's self could then be revitalized and become more alive at the end of his life than it ever had been prior to his illness.

Countertransference Issues

AIDS not only attacks the PWA's self, it can also attack the self of the therapist working with the PWA. In the intersubjective milieu of the psychotherapy process, the therapist's selfobject needs must also be attended to if she or he expects to help the patient's beleaguered self.

Working with a terminally ill patient confronts the therapist with her or his own mortality and challenges her or his healthy grandiosity. The fears aroused can then impair the therapist's ability to support or allow an idealized transference. As the patient grows more ill, angry, and frustrated, he may want to devalue the therapist. The therapist's own sense of powerlessness might collude with this devaluation, instead of the therapist remaining empathically neutral and interpretive.

A further challenge to the therapist's sense of self-competency is the worry that she or he is always missing something "organic" when faced with the complex neuropsychiatric presentations of many PWAs. The symptoms of HIV encephalopathy (i.e., flat affect, verbal slowness, apathy, and withdrawal) can be mistakenly interpreted as a depressive adjustment reaction. The inattention, irritability, or hypomania of early delirium can be misread as the signs of a self-fragmentation crisis. The deterioration of a patient's mental status can be misattributed to worsening dementia or depression when it may be an early expression of a new systemic infection. The need for frequent contact with the patient's medical doctor or the need to work with psychotropics can add to the overwhelmed therapist's sense of intimidation.

Therapists' selves need to feel mirrored (i.e., affirmed, recognized, and appreciated) by their work. If the therapist needs the patient's improvement to confirm his worth, then when the AIDS patient's health deteriorates the therapist may experience this as a narcissistic injury. For some, the PWA's intense selfobject needs may feel depleting or attacking. If the patient then becomes disappointed and angry at the therapist's failure to meet those needs, the therapist may then find it hard to remain interpretive with the patient. Feeling pressured to provide immediate gratification at those times, the therapist may turn to purely educative or supportive tactics. Alternatively, the therapist may become resentful, withdrawn, or retaliative, and then feel guilty for reacting in these ways. If she or he continues to feel self-depleted or injured, the therapist will experience fragmentation products, including burnout, anger, anxiety, and depression.

Many gay male PWAs seek out others like themselves to be their therapists. Via this twinship connection, the hope is that the alienating experience of having AIDS as a gay man can be understood and normalized. This alterego dynamic works also in the countertransference. The gay male therapist may become anxious and fearful about his own AIDS exposure as he works with a PWA, and then react to the patient with discomfort and withdrawal. If a gay male therapist cannot separate his own grief from the experience of resonating with the patient's feelings, or if he overidentifies with the patient, he will not remain attuned to the patient's unique experiences. At the other extreme, if the therapist represses or disavows his own grief, he will affectively become distanced from his patient—a common consequence for burned-out gay therapists who have large caseloads filled with HIV patients.

From the above, it is clear that therapists working with PWAs must find ways to restore their selves. Although work with these patients can be truly fulfilling and challenging as therapists help them to find self-stability, acceptance, and growth, it can also be very draining. Recognizing one's limitations and seeking consultation and peer support are critical adjuncts to working with this most challenging illness.

Conclusions

We hope to have demonstrated the power of the self psychological perspective, with its emphasis on selfobject disruptions and restorations, both as it elucidates the devastating impact of AIDS on the self and as it suggests psychotherapeutic approaches.

AIDS is a crisis of the self, but it is also a challenge and opportunity for growth and development, for a breakthrough to a state of living more meaningfully and authentically. Many PWAs report that having a life-threatening illness and looking death in the face have led to the experience of feeling more fully alive. Helping the PWA seize this opportunity may be one of the most important functions—and gifts—a therapist can provide.

References

Basch M: Understanding Psychotherapy. New York, Basic Books, 1988

Bowlby J: Loss. New York, Basic Books, 1980

Kohut H: The Analysis of the Self. New York, International Universities Press, 1971

Kohut H: The Restoration of the Self. New York, International Universities Press, 1977

Kohut H: Preface to *Der falsche Wef zum Selbst, Studien zur Drogenkarriere*, in The Search for the Self. Edited by Ornstein P. New York, International Universities Press, 1978, pp 845–850

Kohut H: How Does Analysis Cure? Edited by Goldberg A, Stepansky P. Chicago, IL, University of Chicago Press, 1984

Stern D: The Interpersonal World of the Infant. New York, Basic Books, 1985

Wolf E: Treating the Self. New York, Guilford, 1988

Chapter 10

The HIV-Infected Gay Man: Group Work as a Rite of Passage

Shelley B. Brauer, Ph.D.

Although there has been an increase in the attention given to the devastating acquired immunodeficiency syndrome (AIDS) epidemic in the last few years, much less consideration has been given to those who have tested positive for the human immunodeficiency virus (HIV). At this point in the evolution of our knowledge about the virus, it is clear that individuals infected with it can be asymptomatic for years before they develop AIDS. As a result, there is a tremendous amount of anxiety in finding out that one is HIV positive. Attempting to manage the impact that this new medical status has on one's life can be all-consuming. At once asymptomatic yet HIV antibody positive, healthy yet facing the possibility of becoming seriously ill in the future, the HIV-positive individual lives in a twilight zone, in a liminal space between the world of the ill and the land of the well.

Liminality

Murphy (1987), an anthropologist, explored the intriguing notion of liminality by connecting it to his personal experience with physical disability. He used the concept of liminality, as elaborated by Turner (1967) in his essay "Betwixt and Between: The Liminal Period in Rites de Passage," to describe the type of isolation and marginality with which the disabled individual must contend.

Turner's predecessor van Gennep (1960) originally described three phases inherent in all rites of passage: separation, margin (or *limen*, which means *threshold* in Latin), and aggregation. *Separation* consists of symbolic behavior that serves to isolate the initiate from the social group. During the second phase, the initiate is in an ambiguous, *marginal state* outside of the formal, structured social system. In this liminal period the individual is on the "threshold," a transitional being. With *aggregation*, the initiate is reincorporated into the social system, having earned the rights and obligations inherent in the newly emerged state.

In his later investigations of the rites of passage, Turner focused solely on liminal phase of rituals, as he was interested in the nature of transition in stable societies. The transitional aspect of liminality is particularly pertinent to the experience of those infected with HIV. Asymptomatic seropositive individuals are in limbo; they are in essence neither healthy nor sick, yet they are in the midst of a profound alteration of their lives. It is evident in the expressed concerns of those who are HIV positive that the ambiguity and uncertainty with which they must live is unsettling if not completely terrifying. There is obvious uncertainty about the biomedical implications of their new status: How long will the virus lie dormant before it begins to multiply? Will I become diagnosed with AIDS? When? Will I wake up one day and find myself confused or demented? Should I begin to take medication now even though I have no symptoms? And what treatment, alternative or conventional, do I dare take? Because the medical establishment has been unable to give definitive answers and research reports are often contradictory, an HIV-positive person is forced to come to grips with this new status alone and to deduce a meaning out of it that is completely individualistic.

For the HIV-positive individual, there also exists a degree of uncertainty regarding self-concept, interpersonal relationships, and sexuality. Why did this happen to me? How do I relate to other people now? Will I ever be attractive to others now that I am infected? In this liminal state one's values about life in general are questioned. Despite the fact that this period can be anguishing, it can also be a stimulating time because new ways of seeing the world emerge. The liminal state is, however, a structureless realm, without precedent or rules for behavior. This lack of definition and role is disturbing not only to those who are HIV positive, but also to the people who come in contact with them.

In her book *Purity and Danger,* Douglas (1966) stated that what does not clearly fit into social definitions and categories will be regarded in many cultures as ritually tainted or polluted. Lack of clarity is associated with lack of cleanliness, as in the case of Jewish dietary law, which forbids eating pork because of the pig's inconsistent nature (i.e., it has cloven hoofs but does not chew its cud). Turner uses this notion to argue that, because of the inherent contradiction in liminal people being neither one thing nor another, they are expected to be impure. Douglas's idea of pollution may help to account for the fear in the larger society and for the hysteria with which HIV-infected people are treated by others, in spite of the fact that the virus may only be transmitted in very limited and identified ways. This reaction goes beyond the simple fear of contagion; it resonates with a much deeper fear of difference. That which does not fit into socially defined structures is difficult to comprehend, and what we do not understand is disquieting and subsequently disavowed.

The depth of this fear is illustrated by the experience of family members of people with AIDS. Kelly and Sykes (1989) reported that family members being treated in group therapy are often reluctant to disclose that a relative has AIDS, not only because of the shame associated with some modes of its transmission (i.e., either through sexual behavior or through use of intravenous drugs) but also because of their concern about personal repercussions or the possible loss of jobs. "The greatest fear . . . was that people would not understand and would isolate them" (p. 240). The fear of rejection by others by virtue of a mere association with a person with AIDS or HIV infection speaks to a deep, unconscious fear not just of the disease but, more profoundly, of the liminal situation.

According to Turner (1967), who studied the Ndembu ritual, because neophytes are both structurally "invisible" (neither here nor there) and considered ritually polluting, they are often secluded from the rest of the society; if not actually removed to a "sacred place of concealment," they wear masks or paint their faces to make themselves symbolically separate. Similarly, a collective unconscious process underlies the quarantine of HIV-positive individuals, keeping them separate from the rest of society. There has already been a proposition in a California election calling for mandatory HIV testing, and some politicians have argued in favor of various forms of marking and identifying persons who are HIV positive. In Cuba HIV positive people are segregated from the rest of the population, ostensibly to halt the spread of AIDS. Such "solutions" reflect the meanings given to the liminal state of HIV infection.

Three-Session Psychoeducational Group for HIV-Positive Individuals

In Boston, the practical problem of how to help people deal with a new HIV-positive antibody status was addressed by the AIDS Action Committee, the Department of Public Health, and the Fenway Community Health Center. These organizations jointly designed a three-session psychoeducational group program for people who are HIV positive. These semistructured groups focus on education, resources, and referrals. They also aim to reduce anxiety and isolation and instill a sense of hope in the participants. (M. Gross, S. Brauer, R. Carr, L. Ellenberg, A. Feingold, P. Giulino, unpublished manuscript, April 1989 [published by the AIDS Bureau of the Massachusetts Department of Health] provided a detailed description of the nature of the program.)

From my experience as a group leader, I address in this chapter the impact of HIV infection on the individual, as well as the significance of the HIV group from an anthropological point of view. I probe beyond the educational and supportive goals of the program to examine how these groups function within a form of ritual to initiate members into their new roles. The process of assimilating the new status of being HIV positive is compared with the processes in the typical rite of passage. Finally, I discuss themes that surface as members struggle to incorporate emergent identities into their prior senses of self. Although HIV infection is now making inroads into the larger population, the early patients consisted primarily of gay men, and this study examines their experience.

The three-session model, which was first offered in Boston in February 1988, consists of 2-hour sessions held once a week for 3 weeks. Individuals are asked to participate in all 3 weeks in sequence, as 1) each session builds on the preceding one, and 2) the developing group cohesion facilitates greater support for members. The groups are co-led by a health educator and a mental health clinician. This allows for the integration of factual information and emotional responses to becoming HIV positive.

To maintain confidentiality, groups are not advertised publicly, but health and social service providers (including HIV counselors at alternative test sites and sexually transmitted disease clinics and private medical and mental health providers) are informed of the group and asked to refer appropriate individuals. The qualification for joining the group is that a man be HIV antibody positive. No further screening or preregistration is required.

The curriculum developed for the group sessions essentially has not changed since its inception. Roughly, the first session introduces the members to the medical basics of HIV infection, the second focuses on risk reduction, and the third deals with health maintenance. Each session allows time for discussion of any feelings that arise among members.

The Three Dimensions of Self

Even in the short span of the three-session model, a powerful group dynamic develops. The experience of being among others who share the same HIV antibody status creates a tie that allows members to bond quickly (M. Gross, S. Brauer, R. Carr, L. Ellenberg, A. Feingold, P. Giulino, unpublished manuscript, April 1989 [available from the AIDS Bureau of the Massachusetts Department of Public Health]). Members struggle with common issues related to maintaining a cohesive sense of self in the face of a tremendous amount of psychological and social stress. They eventually address three different but related areas within themselves: the physical, the interpersonal, and the spiritual. I have labeled these areas the *three dimensions of self*. Attention to these dimensions becomes an essential part of the initiation process, as members repeatedly make conscious and unconscious efforts to incorporate their new status of being HIV positive into their existing sense of self.

Physical Dimension of Self

The physical dimension of the self is most immediately addressed by group members because it is felt so intimately. They discuss concerns about stress, symptoms, and the dilemmas of treatment, including when to start treatment and what kind of treatment to try. Members contribute their personal experiences with doctors, traditional treatments, and alternative remedies. The sharing of anecdotes serves both individual and social functions. The camaraderie in this type of sharing is important not only for group cohesiveness but also to bolster each participant's sense of self. The goal is to allow the group members to gain as much information as possible in order to make informed decisions about their physical selves.

Interpersonal Dimension of Self

In the realm of the interpersonal self, group members discuss their relationships with family, partners, friends, and coworkers. They address complex decisions regarding who, how, and when to tell about their positive antibody status. Perhaps the most important question members of the group grapple with is *why* they should tell others. For gay men, the process is similar to coming out. If they are already out to friends and family, it means coming out in a different way, this time with the added fear of confronting renewed homophobia or the newer AIDS phobia. Members share their personal disappointments and successes with all of these dilemmas. The power of the group experience is magnified by the fact that most members have kept the information secret from all but a few. A palpable relief pervades the group as members share their experiences. Individual isolation begins to dissolve. Inasmuch as the interpersonal is in the social realm, it pulls the individual into a broader context. The interpersonal realm serves as a bridge, connecting the individual to the larger community and to larger issues.

HIV infection has a powerful impact on identity. During the period when an individual learns he is HIV positive, he undergoes a special rite of passage. He must assimilate information about seropositivity into his self and become initiated into the role of being HIV positive. The group provides a ritual for this process. The common circumstance of being HIV positive creates a bonding and cohesiveness that enable group meetings to move beyond their educational purpose to function as a supportive experience and, I propose, as a transitional ritual. It is striking to observe that members of these groups, regardless of how diverse they are, find solace in being with others like themselves. The commonality of a positive antibody status transcends all other differences, including race, class, and level of education. Murphy (1987) noted that his shared identity with other disabled individuals had more significance than other social distinctions. And Turner (1967, 1969) described relationships among initiates in the African culture he studied as being completely equal during the liminal period of rituals. Distinctions that exist between members of the society before the initiation rite occurs were abolished.

The gay subculture has an elaborate network of unstated rules of behavior. Importance may be placed on how one looks or what one has to the exclusion of other qualities such as who the person is. In other gay subgroups, there may be an emphasis on how politically involved or politically correct a person is. Typically, members from one subgroup do not socialize with those of another. In the groups with HIV-positive members, however, there is a blurring of these rigid boundaries and superficial distinctions. In my experience, this open-minded spirit was seen in the way group members accepted those who were different from themselves. Members listened with equal receptivity to a Hispanic man who had difficulty speaking English, to an emotionally disabled man who lived in a halfway house and had a speech impediment, and to a middle-class urban white man who ably articulated his feelings.

I do not propose that it is simply the fact of being HIV positive that brings these members together so intensely in a short period of time. Rather, becoming HIV positive separates these men from the society at large and from much of the gay subculture, moving the HIV-positive individual into a liminal space, "betwixt and between." It is the phenomenon of liminality that creates the sense of unity with other initiates and gives these groups their power.

Turner left unanswered the question of why a sense of unity evolves from the liminal experience. I suggest that it develops in response to the fear of the unknown. Being on the cutting edge of something new, such as HIV infection, can be alarming in that one feels disconnected from the rest of humanity. It can, however, be enormously comforting to be surrounded by others who share that same predicament. Kohut (1984) described this phenomenon as the *alter-ego* or *twinship* experience. He hypothesized that individuals have a significant need to experience an "essential alikeness" with others, so as not to feel like alien beings. The simple presence of another individual who is sufficiently like another that he or she can understand that other and be understood by the other is sustaining to one's sense of self (Kohut 1984). Whereas the structureless state of liminality arouses fear and anxiety in members, unity arises naturally out of the relief of connecting with others like one's self.

During periods of liminality in rites of passage, relationships among initiates and elders are not equal. Rather, initiates view the leader as a strong figure who imparts traditional values to the initiate (Turner 1967). During initiation rites the elders have complete authority over the neophytes, a practice that, according to Turner, is based more on tradition than on law. Turner identifies this submission to the authority of tradition as a simple fact, but he does not attempt to answer the question of why such tradition evolves in the first place. What is the significance of turning to a higher authority?

In the three-session HIV groups, members treat the leaders as authorities on the subject of AIDS and all related subjects (e.g., What, if any, medication should I take? Can the virus be passed while handling a tea kettle? How should I disclose information to a potential partner? Should I tell my family?). The more ambiguity that surrounds an issue, the more members look for someone to tell them what to do. To address the question that Turner leaves unanswered, I propose that it is the extreme anxiety of not knowing, of actually being in a liminal state, with its inherent lack of definition and structure, that forces initiates to look outside themselves for guidance.

Traditions develop because they hold meaning for those who participate. I suggest that the submission to the authority of tradition during the liminal period in rites of passage stems from the uneasiness of being in limbo. When one is in unknown territory, the anxiety aroused produces a strong need for something outside of oneself to act as an anchor. In the HIV groups, members turn to the leaders for that grounding. This phenomenon may explain the dissatisfaction of some members of leaderless groups for people who are HIV positive. The important role of a group leader does not appear to be related to the leader's particular qualities. Although leaders vary by sex, sexual orientation, and serological status, in most cases group members are not aware of the leader's personal status. Viewing the leaders as mentors seems important in alleviating the members' anxiety. Regardless of who they are, group leaders are relied on for a sense of security during a turbulent time of transition.

The anxiety associated with the liminal period of being HIV positive is not limited, however, to the initiate. It can also be extremely difficult for the leaders of the groups to cope with the anguish that is aroused. There is a natural impulse to want to mend the hurt, to say or do something to help, rather than simply to bear witness to the pain and emotional distress of the HIV-positive members.

This is where the parallel of HIV infection diverges from other rites of passage. In the case of HIV positivity, there are no "elders" who have already been "initiated" and know what to expect. No authority can predict with certainty what will happen to someone who tests positive for HIV infection. Little exists in the way of tradition to act as an anchor, so members are constantly directed back to themselves for answers.

The psychoeducational groups are based on the presumption that people will need to make their own physical, interpersonal, and spiritual decisions about their lives. The best way to help them consciously do this is to give them as much information as possible, to ask questions that stimulate their thinking, and to provide an environment that allows for emotions to be expressed. In this way, as active facilitators of the group, the leaders can serve as "elders," allaying some of the anxiety of the liminal situation. However, the ultimate choices about how to live outside the group must rest with the individual.

Although I advance the argument that being HIV positive is analogous to being in a liminal state during periods of initiation, it is clear, as Murphy (1987) suggested, that neither the disabled nor the HIV-infected individual ever really returns, as the initiate does, to the original state. Short of new cures or miracles, disabled people remain in the twilight zone of liminality for the rest of their lives. They are always on the margins of society. People who are HIV positive, however, do progress into a new state. It can take many years, but in most cases—and perhaps in all—the HIV-positive individual moves on to develop AIDS. Living with the knowledge that this may occur requires another level of integration, for again the self is transformed.

Spiritual Dimension of Self

Geertz (1966), a cultural anthropologist, pointed out that religion helps explain and give order to that which seems inexplicable (e.g., pain, suffering, death). The human search for meaning is an effort to bear unavoidable suffering. Rituals, according to Geertz, focus "upon the problem of human suffering and attempt to cope with it by placing it in a meaningful context, providing a mode of action through which it can be expressed, being expressed understood, and being understood, endured" (p. 20). It is in this context that the value of groups for HIV-positive individuals can be comprehended. Groups bring people together with common concerns and attempt to facilitate communication among members. As such they are "modes of action" that allow individuals to deal with catastrophe. As a ritual, the group gives its members "a vocabulary . . . to grasp the nature of . . . distress and relate it to the wider world" (Geertz 1966, p. 20). Groups also provide an opportunity for members to share anxiety and pain with those who are struggling with similar life circumstances. Thus they allow them to experience an essential alikeness with others and, in this sharing, to be able to endure unbearable suffering.

Other cultures, particularly non-Western ones, accept death and even provide a ritual for the dying person's anticipation of and preparation for death. At the core of Zen Buddhism is the recognition of life's impermanence and the importance of remembering, rather than denying, that one will die. King (1977) described Suzuki Shosan, a Zen monk whose constant awareness of the imminence of death was referred to as "practicing dying," which he had learned during his days of training as a samurai warrior. This constant awareness of the transience of life forces one not only to face and prepare for death, but also to live constantly in the present.

In Western society, it often takes a confrontation with death to make us appreciate life. This new appreciation appears to be one of the most powerful by-products of the HIV groups. If there can be any meaning gathered from facing a positive HIV status, it is the Zen idea of practicing dying. This heightened awareness manifests itself in assuming a healthy life-style in an effort to delay the spread of the virus. At the deepest level, however, members also try to integrate their new status into their sense of self, and attempt to live deliberate, authentic, and complete lives. This is the spiritual dimension of the self that the groups, as a form of initiation and ritual for the living, help to foster.

As new research and future projections about HIV infection and prognosis become available, it is increasingly difficult to keep hope alive in the groups. Diminishing stress, eating well, and thinking positively were believed to be effective preventive measures against progressing to AIDS. That optimism is fading as more information about the virus emerges. However, group members continue to attempt to reframe the meaning of their lives in terms of a positive antibody status. The confrontation with the increased likelihood of untimely death brings their lives into sharper focus. It pushes them to deal with formerly postponed issues. Members become more connected to their spiritual selves, and "living one day at a time" takes on new, profound meaning for them.

A fundamental paradox exists in the parallel I have drawn between the liminality of an HIV-positive status and the liminal periods in other rites of passage. Initiation is an inauguration. Its root from the Latin *initium* means "beginning." It suggests a starting point, a birth. Ironically, when a gay man is "initiated" into the state of being HIV positive, he is one step away from AIDS, which in many ways signifies the end. Therefore this process of initiation is concerned with ending rather than beginning, with death rather than birth. The added irony is that gay men are often healthy and in the prime of their lives when they are "initiated" into the ranks of the dying. In spite of this contradiction, it is useful to think of the transition from being healthy to being HIV positive to having AIDS as a rite of passage. In our Western culture not only are we uneasy around death, but we are especially uncomfortable anticipating it. Instead, our culture's death rituals concentrate on death "after the fact," providing solace to the survivors. Because of its lengthy liminal period, the AIDS crisis provides a new opportunity to create rites of initiation and meaningful rituals not only for those who will be bereaved, but for those who must do the dying.

Summary

In this paper I have compared the process of integrating one's positive HIV antibody status into one's former sense of self with a rite of passage. Finding out that one is HIV positive is a uniquely painful process that requires its own rituals for healing. The three-session psychoeducational groups, as described, provide this.

Viewing these groups as a form of ritual has the following major implications for how they should be developed and implemented:

1. HIV-positive individuals should be referred at the time they receive their test results to groups that can provide i) the experience of being "initiated" in a ritual, ii) information about HIV infection, and iii) the experience of being with others in similar circumstances.

2. The group leaders should regard the HIV-positive state as a form of liminality in order to be sensitive to the anxiety inherent in the "betwixt and between" experience. They can therefore anticipate members of the group experiencing this state, and by addressing it, normalize it.

3. Leaders should also be aware of the roles they may be thrust into as "elders" of the liminal group. It is important to the success of the group that they accept these projected roles rather than reject them through discomfort with this seemingly misplaced authority or because they feel they cannot provide all the answers the group members expect of them.

4. To help group members assimilate their positive antibody status

into their sense of self, attention should be given to each of the three dimensions of self: physical, interpersonal, and spiritual.

Holding groups for individuals who are HIV positive is an opportunity to assist those who need help in negotiating a very difficult rite of passage. Group leaders who are aware of this can help alleviate the pain of members who are truly novices in the realm of HIV infection.

References

Douglas M: Purity and Danger. London, Routledge & Kegan Paul, 1966

Geertz C: Religion as a cultural system, in Anthropological Approaches to the Study of Religion. Edited by Banton M. Association of Social Anthropologists, Monograph 3. London, Tavistock, 1966

Kelly J, Sykes P: Helping the helpers: a support group for family members of persons with AIDS. Soc Work 34:239–242, 1989

King WL: Practicing dying: The Samurai-Zen death techniques of Suzuki Shosan, in Religious Encounters With Death: Insights From the History and Anthropology of Religions. Edited by Reynolds F, Waugh E. University Park, PA, Pennsylvania State University Press, 1977, pp 143–158

Kohut H: How Does Analysis Cure? Chicago, IL, University of Chicago Press, 1984

Murphy RF: The Body Silent. New York, Henry Holt, 1987

Turner V: The Forest of Symbols: Aspects of Ndembu Ritual. Ithaca, NY, Cornell University Press, 1967

Turner V: The Ritual Process: Structure and Anti-Structure. Ithaca, NY, Cornell University Press, 1969

van Gennep A: The Rites of Passage. London, Routledge & Kegan Paul, 1960

Chapter 11

Special Issues in Group Psychotherapy for Gay Men With AIDS

Gil Tunnell, Ph.D.

For gay men newly diagnosed as having acquired immunodeficiency syndrome (AIDS), issues related to their homosexuality can interfere with their adjustment to living with a serious illness. Group therapy not only can assist group members in working through these issues, and thus facilitate their adjustment, but also has the potential to promote a healing resolution of deeper, conflictual issues members may have about being gay and having AIDS. Realizing this greater potential of group psychotherapy is difficult, however, as these issues appear so emotionally formidable that they are avoided by group members in a variety of ways. Paradoxically, if group members do not grapple with these issues, a serious risk develops that the group will disintegrate as its members become increasingly dissatisfied with the group's inability to confront difficult issues.

I have argued elsewhere (Tunnell 1991) that three particular characteristics make living with AIDS much more difficult than living with other chronic conditions: 1) the extreme stigma associated with AIDS, 2) the threat of an early death, and 3) a very unpredictable course of illness. These characteristics surface immediately in group psycho-

The author thanks Jim Quinn, Gerald Perlman, Jenna Osiason, and Steve Cadwell for their suggestions on earlier drafts.

therapy discussions. I have also described how difficulties around these issues affect early stages of group formation by seriously threatening group cohesion. In this chapter I identify a second set of factors related to male homosexuality that can further inhibit group development: 1) the stigma associated with being homosexual, 2) the particular difficulty some gay men have with intimacy, and 3) a fear of depending on other people, especially other men.

The two sets of factors noted above are linked in several ways. First, in addition to feeling the stigma of having AIDS, which makes people with AIDS (PWAs) in all risk groups feel contaminated (Kelly and St. Lawrence 1988), gay PWAs bear the stigma of being homosexual. How openly and directly gay PWAs have dealt with their homosexuality often predicts how they will deal with AIDS. If they already feel isolated from others, the AIDS diagnosis only compounds their isolation. Second, in acknowledging that an AIDS diagnosis most likely indicates a drastically shortened life expectancy, gay PWAs are thrust into completing the unfinished business of their lives; integrating their homosexuality more completely into their lives is almost always a piece of this business. When AIDS is diagnosed, gay PWAs can be at different stages of coming out—to themselves, to family members, and to significant others (Martin 1991). The gay man who has had special problems adapting to his homosexuality may find himself with few, if any, emotionally intimate relationships. Even if his family and friends have known he is gay, they may know very little else about his life. Beginning with their struggle to keep their homosexuality secret, many gay men learn early in life not to reveal other aspects of their lives. They become masters at "keeping their own counsel" (Carl 1990, p. 32). Although AIDS may trigger a desire to become closer to significant others, some gay PWAs find this task inordinately difficult because they have had so little experience with emotional intimacy. Third, the difficulty many men have with dependency, a trait that has a long-standing and troublesome association with femininity, can impede gay PWAs' ability to cope with an unpredictable course of illness. They may resist the social support that is, in fact, available to them by adopting a position of counterdependence.

Why is social support so crucial? Social support has been described as the "single most effective resource" for PWAs (Coates et al.

1987, p. 21), whether the support is derived from interpersonal relationships, self-help groups, or group psychotherapy. The benefits of organized support groups for individuals diagnosed with cancer and other chronic illnesses have been documented (e.g., Spiegel et al. 1981); however, AIDS is different from these illnesses in the ways previously noted. And although the unique characteristics of AIDS and the special issues related to homosexuality complicate group treatment, group psychotherapy may well be the psychotherapeutic treatment of choice. The difficult issues will inevitably emerge in the group, and the interpersonal experience inherent in group psychotherapy can provide a more effective resolution of those issues. However, to promote a more healing resolution, the group therapist must actively listen for, and engage the members to focus on, these particular issues. (In a support group, compared with a psychotherapy group, these particular issues might be ignored or minimized.)

Coping With AIDS and Homosexuality: Interrelated Issues

Double Stigma: Being Gay and Having AIDS

Gay people, like any other group of individuals unrelentingly ostracized by society, tend to incorporate others' rejection and develop some degree of internalized homophobia. Long before they develop AIDS, gay PWAs typically have realistic concerns about their deviant status in society, a status that produces feelings of unacceptability (Isay 1989). For gay men who have never seriously confronted their homophobia, an AIDS diagnosis unleashes feelings of unacceptability that were often previously repressed. Carl (1990) suggested that "the diagnosis of AIDS confirms to many [gay men] that they have done something wrong" (p. 122). Even for men who had earlier come to terms with their homosexuality and their own internalized homophobia, AIDS can reactivate their feelings of unacceptability, at least temporarily.

Feelings of being found unacceptable by the mainstream culture are not unfounded for gay PWAs. Segments of modern society have strongly expressed their views about banning or segregating gay men in the military, clergy, and other professions, and about keeping HIV-positive individuals away from "innocent" others. Incidents of gay-related violence are rising, presumably because of both AIDS and the increased visibility of homosexual men in society (Herek and Glunt 1988). The manner in which gay PWAs cope with the societal stigma influences their adaptation to illness. If they accept and internalize the stigma, they may feel such extreme shame that they feel they are not entitled to live, in which case they may not comply with or even seek medical or psychological treatment (Backman 1989).

The double stigma of being gay and HIV positive greatly encumbers the gay PWA's relationships with others by undermining efforts to build intimacy and dependency, qualities that ultimately become critical in the long-term management of a very unpredictable condition. At greatest risk for not adapting to living with AIDS are those men who have never come to terms with their homosexuality. Their internalized homophobia has impacted on their socialization such that they have had little experience in supportive, intimate relationships. The same stigma that interferes with gay PWAs' receiving social support outside the group operates in group psychotherapy in particularly insidious ways. If the double stigma of AIDS and homosexuality is not actively confronted in the group, gay PWAs are likely to remain isolated and severely constrained in seeking and accepting social support.

Effect of Stigma and Shame on the Group Process: Projective Identification

In a psychotherapy group, stigma and shame may motivate members to isolate or distance themselves from others. Such behavioral maneuvers can often be observed, for example, when a particular group member is in distress. For the member who has internalized society's hatred as his personal shame, any support he receives from the group will feel alien. Thus he may either reject the support outright when it is offered (e.g., discount another member's attempt to help) or behave in ways to ensure that support is never offered.

The latter alternative involves *projective identification*, whereby a member projects his own self-hatred onto others and induces them through his contempt to behave in an alienating way toward him. The contempt is seen as an "attempt to rid the self of shame" (Morrison 1989, p. 105). The other individual becomes a container for the member's self-hatred, who temporarily is able to disown that aspect of himself. The process is largely unconscious, although both individuals may be aware of contemptuous feelings toward each other.

In sociopsychological terms, projective identification functions in the group as a self-fulfilling prophecy in which one member unwittingly coerces others to validate his own feelings of unworthiness. Projective identification is ubiquitous in AIDS psychotherapy groups as almost all members begin treatment feeling ashamed from bearing the same stigma. Multiple projective identification processes can easily become established as members collude with one another's projections of contempt.

> Other members too willingly accept a member's distancing, contemptuous behaviors as a validation of their own unworthiness. Furthermore, the distancing, unempathic behavior of the subject provides righteous justification for the object not to persist in providing help or support. Hence, stigma operates both to inhibit others from giving support, as well as to prevent the individual from receiving support. (Tunnell 1991, p. 490)

Projective identification is obviously harmful in group psychotherapy because the member's worst fears become validated (i.e., I am not worthy of support), even though the individual has induced this outcome by his own behavior.

Management of Projective Identification

Group therapists have two basic strategies for managing projective identification. Either strategy demands active intervention on the therapist's part. Not responding psychotherapeutically to the distancing maneuvers will eventually cause group cohesion to become so eroded that the group will be in danger of collapse. To intervene, the therapist can either 1) challenge the member who is projecting his contempt by exposing the projection (i.e., make him aware of how he is, at that very moment, bringing about his own isolation and ultimate rejection), or 2) persist in rallying other members to support the individual, thereby interrupting the projective identification. (Examples of how to encourage members to support one another are given in the section of this chapter in which a model for group psychotherapy is discussed.) Fortunately, many psychotherapy groups will include one or two members who have less internalized homophobia and a lesser degree of shame about AIDS. These men may refuse to collude with another member's projection of contempt. Such group interactions provide rich material for the group and therapist to work through. The therapist must continue to actively interpret the group process in ways that are designed to disrupt the projective identification of shame.

Again, the reason the projective identification of shame and self-hatred must be identified, analyzed, and changed is so that group members come to provide acceptance, rather than rejection, of one another. It is not sufficient for only the therapist to provide acceptance, as patients assume acceptance to be part of the therapist's role. A far more healing experience is provided when other group members accept and support each other. The group's acceptance can provide an antidote to both the rejection the members have felt as gay men and the rejection they currently feel as PWAs. A number of gay men have never felt accepted by the gay community, let alone by mainstream, "straight" society. Through others' acceptance, each individual's self-image becomes gradually transformed from one of loathing and contempt to one of respect and dignity. Walker (1991) similarly described this goal of therapy as being "to change the narrative of shame to one of pride" (p. 9). Other people are essential in helping the PWA accomplish this task, and the therapist's role is to enlist the help of those other members.

Threat of Early Death and Fear of Intimacy

Considerable time must elapse in group therapy before members can tolerate any sustained discussion of death. Until sufficient trust and cohesion develop, the group will avoid talking about death and will seem to the therapist to be in denial. If the therapist prematurely forces the issue, the usual consequences are that either the group's resistance becomes further strengthened or the group complies by having an overly intellectualized discussion about death.

Although the therapist must generally respect the group's readiness to discuss death and dying, it is imperative that the issue be addressed once an actual death occurs. Otherwise, group cohesion will be further threatened when members withdraw emotionally following a loss.

> Out of self-protection against future loss, members become unwilling to risk increased vulnerability by becoming closer to people who may not survive them. As one group member said soon after an early death when members were having unusual difficulty talking, "Look, why should I get involved with people here who are only going to leave me?" Although it is not uncommon in uncomplicated bereavement for survivors to disengage temporarily from social interaction (Worden 1982), bereavement in AIDS groups is necessarily complicated by the fact that the survivors share the same diagnosis and prognosis as the deceased. (Tunnell 1991, p. 484)

Mourning the death of a group member is further complicated in a newly formed group because members have not had much of an opportunity to know the deceased. Although the therapist may be tempted to interpret the group's awkwardness following the death as resistance to the work of mourning, a more accurate interpretation may be that the group members are experiencing the peculiar sadness of losing someone whom they did not have an opportunity to know (Tunnell 1991). This interpretation can lead more naturally to a discussion of the members' own fears about dying before others have had a chance to know them.

Such fears occur in ordinary bereavement. Survivors may undertake a review of their own lives, may resolve to work on unfinished business, and may attempt to construct their lives differently. Following a death in a PWA group, a "life review" takes on special urgency because members know they have the same life-threatening condition. Although survivors' unfinished business in ordinary bereavement can be indefinitely postponed, having AIDS can exert pressure on gay PWAs to respond to unfinished business immediately. These unresolved issues frequently involve the lack of intimate, emotional connections with the people these men care about most. The possibility that the closeted gay PWA may die before his family and friends know about his homosexuality creates intense stress, as remedying the situation requires that he now come out, a revelation he has spent years avoiding because of its stigma. Even if the secret of his homosexuality has been shared with significant others, he may have withheld other personal information—feelings, attitudes, and personal values—that has little or nothing to do with sexual orientation.

The experience of sharing intensely personal information is not the only intimacy that many gay men miss out on over the years. In their socialization, they have often been deprived of simple positive interactions in which they could be affirmed for just being themselves. Some gay men experience special problems with intimacy as adults because they have actually experienced situations in which significant others became distanced from them when they were only being themselves. Fathers especially may have reacted with aloofness and distance when they observed their sons behaving in ways viewed as effeminate (Isay 1989). Consequently, these gay men learn it is not safe to be open with others, particularly other men.

On the other hand, the crisis of dying before one's time can provide PWAs with an opportunity to have a different experience, to feel real intimacy as they finally begin to reveal themselves to others. The psychotherapy group can become a safe environment to experiment with nonerotic, male-to-male intimacy, and this experience can transfer to significant others outside the group. It is this type of intense emotional experience that sometimes leads PWAs to experience a "silver lining" amid the extreme distress of AIDS.

Managing an Unpredictable Condition When One Is Afraid to Depend on Others

The medical course of AIDS is highly variable. Some PWAs can become seriously ill rather quickly, whereas others may have long periods of relatively good health. Either way, anxiety becomes the modus operandi for PWAs, and helping them manage their anxiety becomes a major task for most therapists. Witnessing other PWAs' bouts of illness can precipitate "anticipatory grieving" (Rando 1984) in group members (and in the therapist), a process characterized by feelings of ambivalence about whether one should become close to the ill member or keep one's distance.

> When anticipatory grieving occurs in a group, some members will be pursuing further closeness with the ill individual, while others will be taking distance. Thus, the group therapist can observe what is usually regarded as an intrapsychic process getting played out interpersonally. These polarized contradictions in behaviors and feelings may be very frustrating and uncomfortable to group members and further undermine group cohesion. It is usually helpful for the therapist to make an interpretation of the group dynamic in a way that "normalizes," and thus permits the members to express more directly, their ambivalent feelings. (Tunnell 1991, p. 487)

Such distancing in the service of anticipatory grieving might be expected to occur in any psychotherapy group following a member's serious illness. However, in PWA groups distancing is usually more pronounced as members have the same diagnosis as the member who is currently ill. Thus rather than move toward that member with compassion and concern, other members may remain aloof and distant in an effort to avoid experiencing their own vulnerability about becoming sick themselves.

When members do become sick and miss group sessions, the resulting irregular attendance contributes to members' attaching far greater importance to the therapist than is customary (Tunnell 1991). Rather than relying on one another for support, members may rely exclusively on the therapist as though they believe other members cannot be counted on because they are too physically sick or too emotionally vulnerable to help. During group sessions when members seem aloof to one another, it is particularly important that the therapist not resort to doing multiple individual therapies (Tunnell 1991). It is far more useful for the therapist to inquire about why the men seem so adverse to seeking help from one another, both within and outside of the group's regular meetings. (Unlike traditional psycho-therapy groups, relationships among members outside the group are not discouraged, as long as all members are made aware of them. In fact, if some interaction outside the group has not occurred after 3–6 months, it can be useful to inquire why outside relationships are not being developed.) Frequently, the underlying dynamic behind the seemingly aloof behavior is a fear of dependency.

In American society, all men—regardless of sexual orientation—are socialized into being independent. In situations in which they could use help and such assistance is readily available, many men would apparently choose to struggle alone without assistance than ask for it (Tannen 1990). In American society, there seems to be a pro-scription against males appearing to be needy. This proscription leads many men, when under emotional stress, to seek distance from others rather than closeness. In addition, men, more than women, seem to have greater difficulty witnessing other men in a state of need. They may strongly disapprove of a man's exposing his emotional neediness and, in fact, may not respond with empathy or assistance.

Not only are gay men not immune from the gender proscription against males appearing needy, but some gay men may have even greater difficulty with neediness and dependency because of their as-sociation with femininity. Many gay men report humiliating scenes as children in which their peers or family members called them "sissy" (Isay 1989), often during incidents in which they were displaying at-tributes more stereotypically associated with femininity—nurturance, affection, or dependency (Bem 1977). Therefore, to protect them-selves from the social consequences of appearing too feminine, some gay men develop a strong facade of what they believe is independence and become excessively vigilant about neediness. Their facade of in-dependence is not mature autonomy but rather a defensive position of *counterdependence*. If these men had achieved a more mature auton-omy, they would be freer to choose between connection or separate-ness, depending on their needs and the availability of an empathic other. Instead, their habitual position of counterdependence deprives them of an opportunity to experience connecting with others and hav-ing those others soothe them. Based on their previous life experiences, these man seem to expect that any current expression of vulnerability will lead to humiliation rather than soothing.[1]

In sum, a condition as debilitating and unpredictable as AIDS dramatically threatens male patients' views of themselves as autonomous and independent beings. This threat may be even more significant for gay PWAs who have endured difficult childhood experiences related to their being homosexual—social humiliation and isolation, leading to a resolution never again to connect with others. Learning to manage AIDS requires that the PWA rely on other people. The group can become a special place where such reliance begins, but only if other members do not subject the PWA to reprisals when he expresses his needs and feelings.

A Model for Group Psychotherapy With Gay PWAs

Although it would appear that group cohesion is initially facilitated by the fact that gay PWAs face so many similar issues, I propose that the very nature of these issues works against members' giving and receiving support. The double stigma of AIDS and homosexuality can easily function to keep members isolated rather than connected to others; the difficulties in being close may prevent gay PWAs from ever attempting to repair previously unfulfilling relationships with significant others; and the difficulty many gay PWAs have in relying on others keeps them in an estranged position as they attempt to manage a highly unpredictable and uncertain condition alone. Group psychotherapy is well suited for clarifying these issues for gay PWAs and helping them achieve a more adaptive resolution.

Role of Members in Group Psychotherapy

A suggested model for the primary task of the group is that members help and support one another. Reissman (1965) argued that one of the most therapeutic benefits of a psychotherapy support group is that

---

[1] I give special thanks to Dr. Gerry Perlman for these ideas.

members not only experience being accepted and supported by peers, but also can provide acceptance and support themselves. Although specifying that the primary group task is to support one another implies that the group's function is supportive rather than psychotherapeutic, remarkable behavioral and personality changes can occur within a richly supportive environment. Members themselves may be confused by the distinction between a support group and a psychotherapy group. Although the model suggested here emphasizes active support and empathic listening as the major types of clinical intervention, the goal of the group is primarily psychotherapeutic (i.e., to help the individual members understand the ways in which they resist social support, intimacy, and dependency, and then to create in the group a corrective experience in which members feel supported and emotionally close to others).

AIDS, like any other chronic condition, necessitates some degree of change, whether it encompasses relatively minor behavioral accommodations to the demands of the illness or major personality restructuring as individuals evaluate their lives and configure them differently. In other words, after a serious diagnosis, individuals become to some degree *patients*, despite the attempts of many PWAs to resist that term. After receiving an AIDS diagnosis, they cannot remain the same. Group psychotherapy can be instrumental in helping individuals make the necessary adaptations and at the same time take greater control as a way to manage the illness. For group psychotherapy to be effective in this task, members need only to support one another. However, what constitutes support is different from what members initially may think.

Members should be oriented toward their primary task of simply helping and supporting one another during the group meetings. By explicitly establishing this as the group's task early on, the therapist can challenge members when they are not on task. Such an inquiry will frequently elucidate one or more of the psychological conflicts discussed above. When these conflicts or issues are evoked, the most therapeutic response of the group is to provide support through active listening. Through the listening process, the therapist and other group members witness the patient's experience and help him gain genuine acceptance not only of his AIDS diagnosis and what it may mean to him, but also of who he is as a person. Because of the stigma of AIDS, group members may well be the only ones who witness the PWA's emotional journey through the illness. Active listening, however, is not by any means simple or easy. Because the negative affect that is aroused by listening is so powerful for members and the therapist, they may try to avoid or escape from listening in various ways. Yet when listening can occur, an empathic community is created in which the "unbearable is jointly borne" (Beckett and Rutan 1990). This type of experience helps people heal and grow.

Therapist's Role in Group Psychotherapy

Therapists themselves may have difficulty facilitating this empathic community. One difficulty is when the therapist takes on too large a role in supporting individual members. Rather than inquiring as to why members are not helping one another, a therapist may instead offer direct help to the member in distress. Such a reaction by the therapist is usually not a planned, thoughtful intervention; instead, it is triggered by the therapist's own helplessness as elicited by the group, or the therapist's rather grandiose belief that only therapists, not the group, can help members. The dangers in the therapist's continually being the one who helps are threefold: 1) the group will no longer function as a group; 2) other members will acquire a passivity about helping one another, a passivity that feeds their existing feelings of helplessness; and 3) the therapist will rather quickly become overburdened and possibly burned out (Feinblum 1989).

Being overinvolved, however, is only one way therapists experience trouble. Essentially, therapists seem to err in one of two ways in working with PWAs: they remain stuck in a position that is either too close or too distant from the patient's experience. Both empathy and objectivity are necessary in doing any type of clinical work. A primary difficulty in working with PWAs is that the extreme emotionality of the work causes therapists to forget their training (Tunnell 1991). Therapists may fail either by not maintaining sufficient distance from the emotional content or by not making an empathic connection because listening to the patient is too painful for him or her (Muskin 1989). In such emotionally charged situations, it takes an astute clinician to alternate between empathizing with what an individual PWA is saying and maintaining enough distance to analyze the group process. Achieving distance helps the therapist think about clinical process, but the analyzed process is useless if the therapist has not been engaged with the emotional material. On the other hand, remaining with the emotional material is ultimately not useful if the therapist merely absorbs the patients' depression and helplessness and in turn becomes the passive one (Tunnell 1991). Walker (1991) cautioned that family therapists in particular, who are typically far more active in session than group therapists, may have powerful feelings of inadequacy, ineffectiveness, and helplessness when working with PWAs and their families. In group psychotherapy, too, such feelings are easily induced in therapists.

Either tendency—to be too close or too distant—may stem from therapists' overidentification with PWAs. Many therapists who work with gay PWAs are gay themselves or have strong affinities for gay people and have strong countertransferential reactions to the PWAs' experiences. Gay and nongay therapists alike have issues about death and dying that may lead them to behave in ways that are not helpful to PWAs. For example, it is much easier to distract PWAs from their feelings by attempting to solve their problems or by giving advice. It is more helpful, and ultimately more healing given the difficulties many gay PWAs have in feeling accepted, if the therapist and the group members can ask questions to clarify and support the patient's emotional experience.

Application of Erikson's Theory to Therapy With Gay PWAs

I suggested previously (Tunnell 1991) that Erikson's (1963) theory of personality development offers group psychotherapists both a useful theoretical model for understanding the fundamental issues with which PWAs struggle and a practical model for intervention around those issues. Although Erikson's theory is an account of lifelong individual development, his stages remarkably resemble the intense conflictual issues that PWAs face: trust versus mistrust, autonomy versus shame and doubt, initiative versus guilt, industry versus inferiority, identity versus role confusion, intimacy versus isolation, generativity versus stagnation, and ego integrity versus despair (Erikson 1963). Even when in chronological terms a group member is well past a particular stage of development, a serious illness can trigger earlier developmental conflicts, and some reworking of old issues is usually necessary in his adaptation (Backman 1989).

Listening to PWAs through an Eriksonian filter can help therapists sort out the issues. Many Eriksonian-type conflicts arise simultaneously in a gay PWA, an experience that is most unsettling and disorganizing. Moreover, group members may be wrestling with different developmental conflicts within the group, leading to either impatience or a lack of understanding and empathy. These circumstances require active intervention by the therapist. For the therapist to frame each issue explicitly for members normalizes the experience and helps put the issue in perspective. Simply labeling the issue may be useful as a first step to dealing with it. However, labeling the issue is usually insufficient for change to occur. Here Erikson's theory that other people in the individual's environment are essential in helping the individual progress through each stage is helpful.

Erikson's first two stages (trust versus mistrust and autonomy versus shame and doubt) are particularly relevant because they parallel gay PWAs' issues about dependency and their shame about being homosexual and having AIDS, respectively. In the trust-mistrust stage in early development, trust is acquired through interaction with the primary caretaker. As in interpersonal mirroring (Kohut 1971), the caretaker validates the infant's experiences so that the infant comes to trust his or her own self. In other words, Erikson's theory implies that the individual, whether infant or adult, does not initially trust his or her new perceptions and feelings until others have validated them. In group psychotherapy, through sharing personal experiences with other members and experiencing the group as a safe and trusted forum, the individual member comes to accept his own experiences as valid, leading to greater trust of himself. In addition, as group members validate each other's experiences and come to trust not only themselves but one another, they begin to experience a deepening connection and closeness with one another, thus laying the foundation for group intimacy (Yalom 1975).

Similarly, Erikson's writings about autonomy versus shame and doubt are germane to gay men's struggles with the shame related to AIDS and homosexuality. For gay PWAs who had earlier achieved some resolution about their homosexuality, the diagnosis of AIDS can sometimes reignite issues about shame and doubt versus autonomy. But for those gay men who have never confronted their own homophobia, the diagnosis of AIDS throws them into a profound personal crisis, a crisis that is primarily about shame. Group psychotherapy can be an opportunity for the resolution of this personal crisis. Working through shame-related issues must occur in an interpersonal or semi-public context because shame originates in public (Morrison 1989). Indeed, it is difficult to imagine any individual coming to terms with shame on his own. As a gay man discusses his shame in the presence of others, he unburdens himself of terrible feelings he has kept private for a long time. Other members in the gay PWA group have at earlier times felt the same shame and may resist listening to the member's feelings. The therapist must help members bear what the person is saying. In those moments, members need to empathize actively with the individual and validate his experiences of shame. If the group can provide its own unconditional acceptance of the member's experiences and feelings, it can begin to counter the member's internalized rejection and interrupt the process of projective identification. The therapist's role is to keep the group on task (i.e., to listen empathically and offer acceptance).

In successful group psychotherapy, then, members become catalysts for each other as they resolve their developmental conflicts. Therapists must actively evoke, engage, and resolve these conflicts. A successful group experience not only helps the gay PWA trust himself more and thus become more autonomous in the face of AIDS, but it simultaneously deepens his connection to others and therefore helps him fulfill his yearning for greater interpersonal closeness and intimacy.

Erikson's ultimate life stage of ego integrity versus despair is a metaphor for both the entire experience of learning to live with AIDS as well as the more specific phase during which the PWA achieves genuine acceptance of his AIDS diagnosis and the fact that his life is indeed being cut short. Regarding resolving the final developmental conflict, Erikson (1963) wrote that an individual realizes that life makes sense when that individual reaches an "acceptance of one's one and only life cycle as something that had to be and that, by necessity, permitted no substitutions" (p. 268). When a group member begins to use the language of acceptance, others in the group may become uncomfortable because it seems that member is giving in to death (see Tunnell 1991 for a clinical example of this). However, this kind of discussion should not be viewed as giving in, but rather as undertaking a life review in the presence of the group. Instead of rebuking a member who has reached this stage, the therapist and group members should reassure him that his life has made sense and has been worthy and meaningful. Perhaps more importantly, the group can encourage the AIDS patient to live now in ways that contribute to personal integrity.

Summary

Group psychotherapy with gay PWAs is complicated by both the unique characteristics of AIDS (its stigma, the threat of a premature death, and a highly variable course of illness) and by several issues related to the PWAs' homosexuality (the stigma they feel about being gay, the difficulties they may have with intimacy, and their fears of dependency and femininity). If these issues are not managed effectively in the early stages of group formation, the group itself may disintegrate. Because these issues are all interpersonal, group treatment is ideal because it affords an interactive context in which these issues can unfold and be resolved more effectively. A model such as Erikson's, which emphasizes the importance of interpersonal interaction in helping individuals develop, is ideal for understanding and working actively with the issues that arise in group psychotherapy with PWAs.

References

Backman ME: The Psychology of the Physically Ill Patient: A Clinician's Guide. New York, Plenum, 1989

Beckett A, Rutan JS: Treating persons with ARC and AIDS in group psychotherapy. Int J Group Psychother 40:19–29, 1990

Bem SL: The measurement of psychological androgyny. J Consult Clin Psychol 45:196–205, 1977

Carl DC: Counseling Same-Sex Couples. New York, WW Norton, 1990

Coates TJ, Stall R, Mandel JS, et al: AIDS: a psychosocial research agenda. Annals of Behavioral Medicine 9:21–28, 1987

Erikson EH: Childhood and Society. New York, WW Norton, 1963

Feinblum S: Betty Crocker's burnout bakeoff: a workshop on limit setting, in Time Out: A Stress Management Workshop for Professionals Working With AIDS. Edited by Katoff L, McFarlane R, Richardson S. New York, Gay Men's Health Crisis, 1989, pp 22–25

Herek GM, Glunt EK: An epidemic of stigma: public reactions to AIDS. Am Psychol 43:886–891, 1988

Isay R: Being Homosexual: Gay Men and Their Development. New York, Farrar Straus Giroux, 1989

Kelly JA, St. Lawrence JS: The AIDS Health Crisis: Psychological and Social Interventions. New York, Plenum, 1988

Kohut H: The Analysis of the Self. New York, International Universities Press, 1971

Martin HP: The coming-out process for homosexuals. Hosp Community Psychiatry, 42:158–162, 1991

Morrison AP: Shame: The Underside of Narcissism. Hillsdale, NJ, Analytic Press, 1989

Muskin PR: Failure of empathy. Paper presented at the annual meeting of the American Orthopsychiatric Association, New York, March 1989

Rando TA (ed): Grief, Dying and Death: Clinical Interventions for Caregivers. Champaign, IL, Research Press, 1984

Reissman F: The "helper" therapy principle. Soc Work 10:27–32, 1965

Spiegel D, Bloom J, Yalom I: Group support for patients with metastatic cancer. Arch Gen Psychiatry 38:527–533, 1981

Tannen D: You Just Don't Understand: Women and Men in Conversation. New York, Ballantine Books, 1990

Tunnell G: Complications in group psychotherapy with AIDS patients. Int J Group Psychother 41:481–498, 1991

Walker G: In the Midst of Winter: Systemic Therapy With Families, Couples, and Individuals With AIDS Infection. New York, WW Norton, 1991

Worden JW: Grief Counseling and Grief Therapy: A Handbook for the Mental Health Practitioner. New York, Springer, 1982

Yalom ID: The Theory and Practice of Group Psychotherapy. New York, Basic Books, 1975

Chapter 12

AIDS, Sexual Compulsivity, and Gay Men: A Group Treatment Approach

Michael D. Baum, M.A., M.F.C.C.
James M. Fishman, L.I.C.S.W.

The acquired immunodeficiency syndrome (AIDS) looms as an ever-present threat to all gay men, but perhaps the most vulnerable population is those gay men whose sexual behavior is out of control. Sexually compulsive men may have attended the same safer sex workshops or read the same brochures as the gay male population at large; but these standard educational vehicles, which have served to foster change and to protect the health of many gay men, have failed to reach those who are most vulnerable to infection. Even psychotherapy groups set up exclusively for gay patients can spawn a scapegoating phenomenon towards this subgroup, whose members have become, in the light of AIDS, the new pariahs. The burgeoning 12-step program known as Sex and Love Addicts Anonymous (SLAA) may be too loosely structured and lack sufficient boundaries for a population that has eluded so many efforts to bring their sexual behavior under control.

This chapter is based on the experiences we (M. Baum and J. Fishman) had as coleaders of a group for sexually compulsive gay men. The group was formed in an urban mental health and social service agency for gay men and lesbians. Most of the men who approached our clinic for help with their sexual behavior had exhausted the variety of therapeutic and self-help resources that San Francisco had to offer; many felt desperate. Some were overwhelmed and stymied by the sheer numbers of their anonymous sexual encounters; some felt humiliated and at the mercy of uncontrollable impulses to cruise, to make another sexual conquest; others lacked the discipline to use condoms, to stop and think, to negotiate with their partners, or to walk away. For others, sex had become such a time-consuming preoccupation that they lacked the ability to prioritize their activities, even to the extent that leaving the house to do errands presented them with further opportunities to put themselves at risk.

Had these clients presented themselves to a mental health clinic in 1970, undoubtedly they would have been labeled as infantile, fixated, or narcissistic—the usual labels applied to homosexuals seeking psychiatric help at that time. On the other hand, had they appeared at a gay or pro-gay mental health clinic in 1980 at the height of the gay sexual revolution, they may have found their core compulsivity downplayed or overlooked as purely "recreational" sex. In fact, these patients may have presented only with low self-esteem or depression and may not have attributed their distress to their sexual behavior at all. Until the outbreak of AIDS, the multiplicity of needs and functions that sex fulfilled for gay men went unexamined and unquestioned; the sexually compulsive population had been camouflaged by the social and sexual norms that the gay subculture had endorsed.

Before AIDS, in the 1970s, the freedom of sexual expression was a hallmark for gay men. In response to this newly found freedom, the gay male subculture spawned a variety of institutions dedicated to open sexual expression (Fishman 1984). Recreational sex—including anonymous sex, sometimes with multiple partners—was an accepted and, in fact, a celebrated badge of belonging. Sexual prowess and potency became social barometers used by the emerging gay man in his attempt to define his place in the new order. The sexual recreational activity was often split off from emotional needs, dependencies, and demands.

The arrival of AIDS in 1981 marked the death knell for this notion of absolute sexual freedom. After its initial reactions of panic and denial, the gay male community underwent a major transformation in reaction to the ravages of AIDS (Fishman and Linde 1983). The epidemic has been a catalyst for many gay men to do the hard work of confronting psychological blocks to intimate, committed relationships with friends and lovers. Ironically, as gay men's identities are no longer hinged on mere sexual potency, the very heroes of the 1970s gay culture are now, in the light of AIDS, viewed as some of its greatest casualties.

As with any crisis, the epidemic has brought out both the best and the worst in people. On a positive note, the gay community has placed greater emphasis on the search for safer sex, healthier life-styles, increased awareness of substance abuse, and a turn towards spirituality, community, and intimacy. On the other hand, the fear of contagion has at times resulted in scapegoating and splitting within the gay community. Gay men previously seen as healthy and potent are often labeled as high risk, self-destructive, and out of control. A gulf has been created between those who test positive for antibodies to the human immunodeficiency virus (HIV) and those who test negative. And, in its grossest form, this splitting has taken the form of dividing the community into the "good gays" and the "bad gays." The sexually compulsive gay man often carries the unwanted, projected "shadow" issues of the gay male community at large, much as the gay community at times carries the sexual shadow for the heterosexual community. Thus the sexually compulsive gay man of the 1990s faces both internal and external shame and blame.

The group we describe in this chapter is a microcosm of the AIDS-torn gay community of San Francisco. With a 50% infection rate, the incidence of HIV infection is higher in this city than in any other city in the United States. In our eight-member group, three have tested HIV positive, three have tested HIV negative, and two remain untested. Each member entered therapy with multiple losses from AIDS in their most intimate circle—friends, coworkers, sexual partners, roommates, lovers, and former therapists. The strategies group members have used to cope with these losses have ranged from outright denial, on the one hand, to a newfound AIDS activism on the other. In addition, we have seen emotional withdrawal, social isolation, substance abuse, and dangerous sexual acting out.

Unlike those gay men who have effectively adapted to the AIDS era and have been able to grieve the loss of sexual freedom and move on, the men in our group have fallen through the cracks of the AIDS era support network. The pre-AIDS gay bathhouses, for example, may have functioned as a "holding environment"—a perpetually available community to turn to for instant validation when anxiety, loneliness, or stress proved to be too much. The enticement of this form of validation, however, obscured the fundamental differences in coping styles of gay men. For the more adaptive group of men, the threat of AIDS has shifted the focus away from the gratification of sexual needs, per se, and toward an integration of those needs in a relational context. For other gay men, however, the removal of such a soothing and containing self-organizer has produced depression, panic attacks, and even suicidal ideation.

Education alone has provided sexually compulsive gay men with insufficient support for them to implement fundamental changes in their sexual behavior. Advocates of psychoeducation, SLAA, and safer sex workshops have assumed that all individuals have the requisite motivation, psychic energy, and stamina to give up a treasured coping mechanism. They have failed to predict that implementing such a change would threaten the very psychosexual equilibrium of this particular population. For the sexually dependent gay man, sex serves many of the functions that it provides for the population at large: some semblance of validation and self-worth, an outlet for aggression, interpersonal contact, and a defense against depression, boredom, anger, loneliness, anxiety, and loss. Sexual contact can be a vehicle for owning the body and reclaiming one's sexual or physical side when one has been overvalued for other achievements or undervalued physically. The temporary euphoria of sex can serve as self-medication, a reassurance of feeling loved or lovable, and a reassertion of control or power through one's sexual potency and virility (Fishman and Linde 1983).

But for the sexually compulsive population, sex also serves as an organizer of self-needs. The rituals of sexual compulsivity are more soothing and preferable than facing a core psychic void. The removal of this outlet confronts this population with its bedrock deepest pain, confusion, despair, and feelings of worthlessness. Stripped of a critical defense, these men are expected to find a way to endure, move through, integrate, and transcend this pain without having any tools to do so. The rituals this population practices can sometimes represent a recapitulation to a shameful family secret, often sexual in nature (e.g., incest, parental promiscuity, illegitimacy). They serve a function of preserving homeostasis in an extremely fragile self. As a result, even the pejorative labels of *sex addict* and *sexually compulsive* still provide some point of reference in locating one's identity in the world, especially when the alternative is facing a series of terrifying unknowns, including the fear of nonexistence. As one patient put it, "If I weren't a sex pig, then who would I be?" Another patient stated, "At least when I'm in a toilet looking for sex, I know who I am and where I belong." The danger of acquiring AIDS and getting sick in the distant future pales in comparison with the overwhelming and immediate danger of losing one's psychic equilibrium. For some the annihilation of the ego and loss of self pose greater threats than the loss of life itself. For the sexually compulsive man, high-risk sex feels less cataclysmic than living a life without sex at all.

Even though we have observed a correlation between an early sexual secret and later sexual compulsivity, we have worked with many patients whose early sexual abuse does not manifest in this way. Survivors of sexual abuse display a whole range of symptoms—depression, eating disorders, sexual dysfunction, and substance abuse.

In embarking on this group, the leaders hoped that in-depth, long-term treatment could provide this population with the excavating tools necessary to uncover the wounds, move through the anxiety and pain, and replace a potentially lethal coping mechanism with an opportunity to heal and change.

Contract, Frame, and Structure

Although we perceived the group as a long-term commitment, the structure we chose grew out of an assumption that this population—unfamiliar and fearful of in-depth commitments—would be able to commit to a therapeutic group only in small increments, such as with a renewable, 12-week contract. Their past experiences with loss of boundaries and personal disempowerment led us to conclude that to ensure a sense of safety there had to be the option to stay or to leave;

this option served as a symbol that interpersonal boundaries were chosen rather than imposed. The leaders periodically reminded group members of where they were in the chronological cycle; the renegotiation periods in weeks 10–12 provided rich opportunities for the group members to reflect, assess, and choose whether or not to recommit.

Membership was limited to a maximum of eight individuals, and the group as of this writing has had a stable membership for the past 3 years. The group meets weekly for 90 minutes, and the only procedural structure within this period is a 15-minute "checkout" time at the end of the group when members express how the evening's session has left them feeling.

The group, now in its seventh year, has maintained a multileveled approach to the treatment of sexual compulsivity. Sexual abstinence is not a requirement, and the leadership places relatively low priority on quick solutions to problems or oversimplified answers to complex phenomena. Rather, we state our goals as being the following:

1. To understand the whys of sexual acting out—why and when it happens and what emotions or catalytic events precede it
2. To look at the psychological underpinnings of sexual addiction from a psychodynamic level, especially where sex has become a reenactment of early object relations or is an attempt to counteract those dynamics
3. To use the group as a laboratory for members to talk about their inner state rather than acting out

It is our stated belief that the longevity and stability of the group inherently acts as a holding environment for members.

We neither encourage nor forbid members from exchanging telephone numbers or engaging in extragroup contact. We do make explicit our expectation that any outside contact (whether it positively or negatively affects the group's dynamics) be brought back to the group so that no secrets build up that could undermine group cohesion. Although there is no explicit clause prohibiting sex between members—anticipating that such a clause would result in rebellion or acting out—we have explained the countertherapeutic effects that such behavior would engender. We also have explained that, by abstaining from sexual contact with other members, the group is securing its ability to deal openly and honestly with sexual feelings, rather than feeling compelled to act on those feelings.

Theoretical Approach

The leaders' theoretical perspective integrates Yalom's (1975) interpersonal learning with Beck's (1981) work on leadership roles in groups and the stages of group development; with these interpersonal and group-as-a-whole perspectives we incorporate a psychodynamic frame that is grounded in Kohutian self psychology (Kohut 1971) as well as object relations theory (Mitchell 1988). The group contract gives considerable priority to the use of here-and-now feelings. Members are encouraged to view the group as a microcosm and laboratory for learning about their current interactive patterns and discovering new, more effective ways of relating (Yalom 1975). Beck's research on how certain individuals carry certain issues for the whole group and the need for other group members to "take back" their projections is particularly well suited to a population that has been scapegoated by society at large, by the gay subculture, and by families of origin (Beck 1981; Dugo and Beck 1984). Beck's outline on how to help a group negotiate conflict, power struggles, and differences has been useful, as we have witnessed a heavy reliance on splitting, with the concomitant urge to oust nonconformist or aggressive members. Lastly, we are particularly influenced by the work of Mitchell (1988), who stated the following:

> The centrality of sexual experience for most people . . . and its key role in psychopathology derive not from its inherent properties, but from its interactive, relational meanings. . . . The passion comes not from a build-up of sexual needs per se, but from a kind of suffocation anxiety. In the primary surrender to the object, there is a sense of giving away too much, of one's distinct selfhood being smothered; the counterobject defiance, whether in fantasy, masturbation, or secret liaisons, becomes desperately sought. Often what is experi-

enced as great sexual need reflects a mounting anxiety concerning
a loss of self, and a need for the escape and defiance which the sexuality can provide. (pp. 115, 118)

Thus the leaders' interventions in group interweave the intrapsychic, the interpersonal, and the group as a whole.

Clinical Profile of Group Members

The clinical picture of those accepted into the group emerges as a
remarkably consistent one. Initially, each member displayed characterological impairment ranging from borderline and narcissistic to
avoidant and passive-aggressive. What links members is a pervasive
impulse control disorder, which may also include the misuse of food,
money, and substances. One major defense employed by all members
is massive splitting: splitting between sex and intimacy, aggression
and victimization, and an idealized parent who must remain "good"
and a self-image as the child who must hold all the "bad" for the family
system, thus triggering a lifetime of shame. As a result of extensive
pregroup interviews, the leaders were able to glean in virtually all
members an overpowering sexual secret, although on several occasions the secrets did not emerge until well into the group.

In taking a psychosocial history, we found, in addition to the sexual secrets, pervasive boundary trespassing, inappropriate distance or
closeness, and an early loss or abandonment of a parent or parental
figure. The abandonment may have occurred within the context of
family sexual abuse, when a trusted family member or guardian
betrayed the patient through subtle or gross attempts to make the
child meet the adult's sexual or emotional needs. The patient initially
might not have viewed this sexual contact as unpleasant or abusive.
For example, one member who had been in the group for 3 months
complained that he dreaded going home to his grandmother's house
over Thanksgiving because he would have to share a bed with her.
This patient was 35 years old at the time and did not label such behavior as abusive; rather, he held the belief that something must be wrong
with him for allowing family visits to stir up such feelings of power-

lessness. Another member's scenario went like this: the mother has a boyfriend and her son sleeps in his own room; the mother loses her boyfriend and moves her son into her bed; the mother gets a new boyfriend and her son is ejected and sent back to his own room, feeling rejected and confused. In the case of another member, his parents entrusted him to the care of a female baby-sitter who molested him. When he sought solace and protection from his parents, they denied the incident, rejecting their son and humiliating him in the process. Thus in any pregroup intake we feel it is crucial to take a detailed sexual history, to ask about any unwanted touching, how sex was handled in the family, and to thoroughly explore boundary issues.

Likewise, it is important to ask whether or not patients have engaged in unsafe sexual practices and whether or not they have been tested for the HIV antibody. Although a patient may not report suicidal or homicidal intent, the intake interview can uncover passive suicidal or homicidal ideation. It is especially important to note whether or not the patient is the one who is exposed or is the exposer. The patient who presents as HIV negative but puts himself at risk usually displays passive despair, whereas someone who is HIV positive and knowingly puts others at risk may be cloaking his rage in quasi-political or moral rationalizations (e.g., It takes two to have unsafe sex, or, If it wasn't me, he'd be doing it with someone else). These are sometimes gray areas, and clinicians may vary in their own assessments of what is safe, what is reckless, and what is reprehensible. A delicate balance must be maintained in providing a nonjudgmental, caring interview while also letting the patient know that his behavior could have very powerful meanings and that he may be putting himself or others at risk.

This paradox—providing the safe container while also not flinching from necessary confrontation—arises frequently with this population, whose members also seem to test boundaries and limits with leaders in subtle or sometimes provocative ways. The leaders must have a place to take their own concerns and countertransference reactions, which at times are quite powerful, varying from rage and anxiety to depletion. Group consultation as well as regular meetings between coleaders have proven to be invaluable tools for both tracking group process and for managing the potent countertransference issues that the group provokes.

Transference and Developmental Stages of the Group

The stages of development for this group can be charted transferentially. The earliest stage of the group was marked by ambivalence around dependency and the suppression of aggressive feelings at any cost. On the one hand, what emerged was an overly polite group; on the other hand, feelings about payment, leaders' involvement and limits, or vacations were funneled into reaction formation (e.g., "I don't want to kill you!"), humor (e.g., "Off with your head!"), or acting out via lateness, missed sessions, or seductive or provocative attire and behavior. The massive dependency needs were just beneath the surface but could not be tolerated or openly expressed. Members did not feel it was safe to acknowledge aggressive feelings. The ambivalence that characterized the early phase of the group was illustrated in one member's stalling on whether or not to recontract while at the same time suggesting that perhaps the group could meet for 2 hours instead of 90 minutes. One newly joined group member came 45 minutes late to his first session because he met someone on the way to group and went off to an X-rated bookstore to have sex. He displayed his presenting problem via trying to get the leader to see him as "bad," by inviting punishment and seeking forgiveness; only then could he truly see himself as a full-fledged member of the group.

Once the ground rules were established and norms developed, the next distinct group phase was marked by an atmosphere of extreme competition. Members could not get enough from the leaders: "We're all piglets, and you're the tit," was how one member put it. Our countertransference in this phase was one of extreme depletion, despair, and emptiness. Competition revolved primarily around the question, Who is the most damaged? Sibling rivalry issues were rampant and became crystallized when the leaders announced that three new members would be added at the beginning of the next 12-week contract, thus expanding the group from five to eight members. Although a high degree of sexual tension existed in the group during this stage and members occasionally dressed provocatively, up until this juncture no attempts at intragroup sexual contact had been reported. However, the one time in 6 years sex between members occurred was the night before adding these three members. When the family jumped from five to eight, two of the original members disclosed in the newly expanded group that the previous evening they had embraced each other "like an octopus" and that this had led to sex. The leaders had to contain the overstimulating feelings that emerged and hold in check the wish to respond punitively. The interpretation that these two members may have been expressing anger and despair at possible abandonment with the addition of "triplets" to the family provided the group with insight into the threat that adding new members presented.

Frequently during this phase the members expressed the wish to flee from the group, doubting the efficacy of feeling and expressing their pain. The despair underlying this wish to flee was rising to the surface and was terrifying for them. The leaders were required to actively assure the group members that this excavation was indeed the work that needed to be done and not a sign of fragmentation. The notion of life without the identity of a sex addict was frightening and overwhelming to contemplate. "What if I became master of my own ship?" one member asked during this phase. Sometimes it was safer to regress into old behaviors rather than face the void of a series of unknowns.

Simultaneously, the group began to own and express its aggression. Because so many members experienced severe violations or the misuse of aggressive feelings in the home, extreme anxiety was felt whenever anger surfaced directly. The sexualization of aggression gradually receded as members began to trace the sources of their sexual acting out (after a group session, for example, or right before or after a leader's vacation) and to understand the connections between sexual dominance and the hidden wish to assert control in the group, in a relationship, or with a family member.

Permanent Coleadership

The introduction of a permanent coleader, coinciding with the addition of a new eighth member, has stabilized the group in many ways and deepened a sense of cohesion and trust. This is best exemplified by the group's use of transference and object splitting. By bridging this split, both transferentially and intrapsychically, members have made a profound shift in object relatedness, resulting in a transition from a lower to a more higher level of functioning. It is also worth noting that the group could only seriously grapple with the threats and challenges of AIDS, incest, and sexual abuse when it felt secure enough and trusting enough of its container. The container's safety was exemplified by a stable group membership and by trusted, tested leaders. Furthermore, the leaders, in order to pass these tests, had to be willing to confront each other openly with their own parallel process regarding the uses of power, safety, rivalry, and trust in their own relationship.

The Aggressor and the Victim

We have seen two clinical profiles emerge in the group that represent common coping styles in relation to themes of aggression and victimization. The aggressor, emerging from a family background and childhood of repeated violations and made to carry the "bad" for the family, internalizes the aggression and crystallizes the dynamics via increasingly dangerous acts to himself or others. The victim likewise has endured early abuse, but responds to familial pressure to carry the "bad" by identifying as helpless and powerless, thus splitting off his own rage and aggression.

Although aggression is manifested in both typologies, there is a striking difference between the overt use of power by the aggressor versus the covert maneuvers of the victim. The aggressor often presents as engaging in relationships; his power advantage is casually minimized and, when challenged, defended. These relationships may range from the sexual to the professional, from the social to the political. For the sexually compulsive aggressor, the behavior may be unsafe sex, sex with a minor, or sex in which he potentially infects another. An exploration of the aggressor's power and position reveals he is unconsciously reenacting the original abuse he experienced from the perspective of the abuser. In the dynamics of the split, the aggressor cannot see how he exploits the less powerful because he has not been able to own or integrate his past position of victimization.

In contrast, the victim may initially present as the "healthiest" member of the group. He frequently is nurturing of others in the group and in his life, and may coast along in this role for months or even years. The outer picture may be one of financial success, an abundance of social and relational opportunities, and few apparent needs from the group. However, his nurturing persona functions as a defense against his overwhelming self-needs, deprivation, and invisibility. His resentment at the profound neglect, exploitation, and abandonment experienced in his childhood is sublimated and he becomes that which is expected of him—the model boyfriend, the model employee, the model group member. This is a reenactment in vivo of his family role. His skill at nurturing others and in presenting a need-free state masks a profound inner sense of victimization. Beneath his massive attempts at helping others lies the cry, But what about me? This cry, with its underlying despair and rage, is split off into unconscious sexual exploits where he demands, withholds, or controls sex in a shamelessly aggressive manner. In his sexual relationships, he is at last in control and on top, and at times exhibits sadistic overtones. For him, aggression is only available during sex.

Whether it is disowning one's aggression or victimization, the therapeutic work ultimately must include the reintegration of this split. As a way to illustrate these two typologies, we present the following case examples. Case 1 illustrates the aggressor role.

Case 1

Mr. A, a successful professional, presented with the problem of frequent unsafe sexual practices dangerous to himself and others. He reported many humiliating childhood events in which he was ridiculed for being unathletic, uncoordinated, and "freakish." However, he recalled a pivotal first sexual experience at age 6 when his female neighbor had him stimulate her genitals and breasts. This sexual exploitation continued for 1 year. For several years into the group, he reported this as a positive experience that had been sexually exciting—a way to "own the body" and find the one way it could work. When leaders questioned or explored the potential for abuse inherent in this act, Mr. A repeatedly denied there was any trauma or exploitation involved.

In group, issues of power and abuse surfaced for Mr. A explosively. Although he had not been tested for HIV, he was at high risk for being positive because of his sexual history. He could not admit that his having unsafe sex and putting others at risk was in any way abusive. "It takes two to have unsafe sex," he would respond. When challenged by group members, he continually defended his actions, accusing the group of imposing unfair moral judgments on him and stating that he felt victimized by this. In a dramatic effort to reach Mr. A, the group leaders uncharacteristically began a session by expressing deep concern about Mr. A's continuing unsafe sexual practices, addressing both the health risks these behaviors posed for himself and partners, as well as the inherent underlying aggression in such acts and attitudes. Mr. A vehemently defended his actions, but the group and the leaders did not back down from the confrontation. Eventually, Mr. A's combativeness ebbed and he became more reflective. At this point, another group member came to his defense and disclosed his own unsafe sexual practices. In a moment of insight, and only by observing the denial of another, Mr. A was able to break through his own denial. This session marked a turning point for Mr. A on many levels.

Because the leaders' intervention was well timed and occurred at a stage of deepening trust in this group, Mr. A managed to eventually experience the interaction as caring, containing, and illuminating. A connection was made between his confusion in putting the responsibility elsewhere in his current sex life, and his adopting the blame and shame experienced when he himself had been abused sexually as a child. During this same session, Mr. A was able to recount the pain and abandonment he felt as a 6-year old when he had attempted to tell his parents about the abuse. Expecting parental protection and intervention, he met with derision, rejection, and blaming.

Mr. A's inner confusion between abuse and victimization seemed to be a product of his inability to own his former victimization, his need to idealize his parents at any cost, and his employing the defense of identification with the aggressor. As an adult, by inverting the victim's role into the aggressor's role (i.e., by turning passive into active) he adopted a pattern of irresponsible sexual behavior while claiming, "It's not my fault." This adamant denial represented his attempt to redress a traumatic childhood grievance—that of childhood sexual innocence and lack of culpability. Thus another split—that of Mr. A's having to contain all the "bad" for his family whereas his parents remained all "good" and even saintly—began to give way to a greater tolerance for ambivalence towards his parents and to a more forgiving attitude toward himself. Learning that he did not need to be "all bad" helped him accept responsibility for specific behaviors in his current life that were abusive toward himself and others. The anger and its attendant guilt, previously unexpressed toward his parents for their neglect and scapegoating, had been rerouted into this sexual arena—hence, the sexualization of aggression. This aggression was directed toward both the other and the self. Once he could work through this anger and reintegrate it, Mr. A no longer needed to use sex as a weapon.

Mr. A was finally able to link his rejection with his acting out, his aggression with victimization, and his fear of intimacy with sexual compulsivity. Later on in the group when he had to face a major health crisis, Mr. A was able to use the group by exposing his deeper vulnerability and his need for others rather than resorting to the dangerous behaviors he had once used as a defense. He could expose this vulnerability both because of the safety of the container and because he no longer was carrying the baggage of being "all bad" and deserving of punishment and neglect.

If Mr. A represents the "bad" boy in the group, Mr. B embodies the exact opposite—the "good" boy who is caught between protecting a powerful family secret, at the expense of his own needs, and exposing those needs and jeopardizing the family's equilibrium.

Case 2

Mr. B was the younger child of two in a family in which both parents competed with the other for the affections and attention of the children. Initially in the group Mr. B could only idealize his mother and remembered being her confidant and best friend. Meanwhile, his older brother was the identified "problem child" in the family who received all the parental concern and focus. Although Mr. B received strokes in his family for maintaining a facade of having no needs and for being in control, his older brother was his nemesis who merely had to "cry wolf" for his parents to come to his aid.

In his romantic life, Mr. B played the nurturing provider who inevitably found himself angry or disappointed when his own needs went unnoticed. Typically, he then acted out sexually, withdrew, or found a new boyfriend. In group, Mr. B reenacted his family dynamic by outwardly deferring to "problem members" with more blatantly dangerous behaviors, while at the same time inwardly accumulating frustration and resentment. In turn, other members participated in keeping him in the good-boy role, pointing to his relatively higher professional status and his current relationship as proof of his relative health.

As Mr. B began to identify his group role and express his insistence that he needed to be heard, the leaders validated his perceptions that his group position mirrored his family position and that, in the therapeutic family, he needed to be able to shed that role and find more direct ways to deal with his neglect, anger, and disappointment. By knowing he was being held safely by the "good" leader, whom he said resembled his father, he could confront the "bad" leader whom he feared as he had once feared his manipulative and intrusive mother. Unlike his parents, who had vied for his affections, the leaders encouraged the working through of the transferences. By experiencing a family in which, for the first time, he was permitted to express his woundedness, Mr. B began to uncover a traumatic series of incestuous encounters with both parents that had occurred during his adolescence. In so doing, Mr. B was able to reintegrate his repressed feelings of rage and sadness, which he had sublimated into his good boy persona while directing all unacceptable aggressive impulses into acting out sexual behavior. One concrete by-product of owning the split-off feelings of need and anger was that Mr. B was then able to maintain an intimate relationship with another man and to transfer his newly acquired communication skills into this relationship, rather than leaving the relationship or acting out sexually. Although he occasionally relapsed into his old style of burying his resentments and adopting a false self, Mr. B was able to recognize these patterns and resume authentic communications.

Value of Group
Treatment and Coleadership

The sense of the group as a new family is palpable in that for all eight members the group is the first sustained commitment they have had, in spite of major disappointments, injuries, and de-idealizations. Each member has his own version of splitting and uses transference to members and coleaders as a way to heal these fractures. By tolerating emptiness and hopelessness in the move toward deeper intimacy, members have been able to transfer this newfound capacity for relatedness to their outside jobs and relationships. Another by-product of this shift has been a significant decrease, and in some cases complete abstinence, of sexual acting out, including unsafe sex. As sex in public bathrooms, dangerous or anonymous encounters, and risky or self-destructive and impulsive behaviors have gradually receded, many "firsts" have occurred: dating, developing new friendships, actualizing a talent, achieving financial stability, and drawing appropriate boundaries with family members. We feel the success of the group lies in our ability to broaden the problem from a mere monitoring of sexual activity to encompassing the broader issues of commitment, expression of needs, and self-esteem.

In order to contain all the emotional currents and countertransferences, the coleaders participate in a weekly consultation group, which has helped immeasurably. We have had the opportunity to explore content and process group themes; we have also found an all-important vehicle to build coleadership alliance. A crucial part of our work has been confronting parallel process issues, such as competition, sibling rivalry, and periodic splitting into the aggressor and victim roles. In being able to identify power issues between leaders and to work through our feelings about these roles, we have become more effective in empowering the group members to do the same.

AIDS in the Group

We had expected that, given the high incidence of AIDS in San Francisco and given that this was a group of gay men whose sexual behaviors were self-defined as out of control, AIDS-related issues would be frequently explored. Although unsafe sex and periodic losses were tangentially addressed in the first few years of the group, AIDS did not surface as an in-depth topic until several years into the group. For AIDS to be explored in the group, members were required to face some of their most primitive fears of abandonment, annihilation, and frag-mentation—all the ingredients that make intimacy and commitment so frightening, particularly for these men. Furthermore, for one who holds as his anthem, My body never worked for anything except sex; finally I found something I'm good at, to now confront the potential threat of physical deterioration and the loss of sexual potency risks profound anxiety and decompensation.

By facing AIDS directly, opportunities have been created for the group to work together amid an overwhelming threat; to separate out loss from abandonment and pain from annihilation; and, ultimately, to survive and grow closer within these losses. It has truly been an accomplishment for members of the group-as-a-family to decide for themselves what appropriate boundaries they need while simulta-neously maintaining intimacy and vulnerability. These issues have been tested through several members' declining health, hospitaliza-tions, unexpected health-related absences, and noticeable physical de-cline, and through the confrontation of issues related to death.

The multiple losses from AIDS-related illnesses have created a narcissistic blow to group cohesion. During the height of accumulated group loss, the group regressed to a much earlier stage of develop-ment. Several members reported marked increases in sexual acting out, both as a form of self-medication in the face of impending loss as well as a means of sending the leaders the message, I still have my needs, too. Others insisted that AIDS only impacts the individual who has the disease rather than the whole group: It's not my issue. When can we deal with me? This insistence is a form of denial and a defense against loss. The leaders have had to make a concerted effort to con-nect AIDS and loss with sexual compulsivity. The inability to face anger, sadness, dread, or intimacy in the face of such loss is a prime example of how members turn to sex as a defense and as an escape.

As leaders, we too have had weeks when we dreaded going to group because we felt overwhelmed, guilt-ridden about not doing enough, or fearful that our "family" was falling apart. Outside consultation has proven critical in our reestablishing a sense of direction, steadfastness, and self-forgiveness. We have had to struggle with how to maintain the therapeutic frame yet adapt it to the realities of the illness. For example, the leaders kept the group informed about the impending death and subsequent memorial service for one group member. Although this was a bonding experience for the group, another member who was becoming sicker himself from an AIDS-related illness, accused the leaders of "dropping the ball" and of not doing enough for the first member. In short, he perceived that we could not protect either of them from their eventual death.

For the self-effacing member who downplays the legitimacy of his own needs, AIDS offers an opportunity to evade or confront his deepest issues—loss, abandonment, and lack of control. Earlier on in the group, we observed that one "codependent" member acquiesced to another member who had AIDS: My issues pale compared to yours; you go first. In this instance he was replicating his family dynamics whereby he deferred to the needs of the identified patient but inwardly felt neglected. In contrast, when the group had advanced to a deeper level of intimacy and that same member had time to assert and explore his own issues, his deference to the person with AIDS no longer needed to be viewed as a form of avoidance; in fact, he was replacing a dysfunctional family dynamic with a new ability to interact, grieve, and be part of a meaningful group process.

The exploration of the impact of AIDS on the group has provided an opportunity to deal with grief in a multitude of ways. The unexpected and unpredictable intrusions of AIDS have triggered intense conflicts and acting out as well as provided the group with its most profound moments of tenderness and caring.

Conclusions

Compulsive sex is a complex and multidetermined phenomenon that overlaps with the functions of sex for the population at large. As one by-product of the tragedy of AIDS, a population has emerged that can be characterized by its excessive dependence on sex in an attempt to maintain self-cohesion. This population reports the experience of being "held captive" by its sexual dynamics. By exploring the various meanings that sexuality serves, therapists can assist these patients in gaining an understanding of their dynamics and, ideally, achieving greater control and responsibility in sexual, interpersonal, and intrapsychic realms. We have found that a renewable, 12-week contract provided the safe container in which to do this work. We believe that in-depth group psychotherapy can lead to fundamental psychic change and integration.

References

Beck AP: Developmental characteristics of the system-forming process, in Living Groups: Group Psychotherapy and General Systems Theory. Edited by Dirkin JE. New York, Brunner/Mazel, 1981, pp 316–332

Dugo JM, Beck AP: A therapist's guide to issues of intimacy and hostility viewed as group level phenomena. Int J Group Psychother 34:22–45, 1984

Fishman JM: Responding to crisis: the changing nature of gay male sexuality. Bay Windows (published by Alyson Publications, Boston, MA) 2(16), 1984, pp 10–12

Fishman JM, Linde RJ: Informed consent: making appropriate choices about AIDS from an informed perspective. Gay Community News 10:8–9, 1983

Kohut H: The Restoration of the Self. New York, International Universities Press, 1971

Mitchell SA: Relational Concepts in Psychoanalysis. Cambridge, MA, Harvard University Press, 1988

Yalom ID: The Theory and Practice of Group Psychotherapy, 2nd Edition. New York, Basic Books, 1975

Couples and Family Treatment

Chapter 13

Home to Die:
Therapy With HIV-Infected Gay Men in Smaller Urban Areas

Bruce J. Thompson, M.S.W., Ph.D.

A s the acquired immunodeficiency syndrome (AIDS) epi-
demic continues into the 1990s, it has been predicted that an
increasing percentage of the human immunodeficiency virus (HIV)–
infected population in the United States will be not from the major
urban epicenters with which AIDS was associated during the 1980s,
but from smaller urban areas. For example, the Institute of Medicine
and National Academy of Sciences (1988) predicted that up until
1991 New York and San Francisco would account for 40% of all AIDS
cases, and that after 1991 these two cities would account for only 20%
of the cases. The National Commission on AIDS (1991) indicated that
the cumulative number of deaths in the United States from the first
decade of the epidemic (1981–1991) will more than double in the first
2 years of the second decade; researchers also emphasize that gay men
will remain dominant in the statistics, at least in the short term (Dilley
et al. 1991).

One result of this epidemiological profile is that, as the 1990s proceed, the smaller urban areas, which have not developed the AIDS
service networks of the larger urban centers, will be faced with increasing demands for services. Many of those people with AIDS
(PWAs) who will appear in these new caseloads will be gay men who,

275

for a variety of reasons, have returned to their family of origin's home as a result of infection or illness.

In this chapter I examine the phenomenon of gay men with HIV-related illnesses returning home to their families of origin, with a particular emphasis on the issues that might predictably emerge in the psychotherapeutic treatment of these men. Although there are potentially a wide range of precipitants to the decision to return home, they usually include a combination of practical, reality-based concerns and intrapsychic-interpersonal psychological concerns. Gay men will negotiate the tasks involved in returning home and adjusting to the changes that this creates for them and their families in a variety of ways, depending on the psychological intactness and adaptability of the individual and the family. Using three case examples, I explore specific situations and clinical responses.

HIV and the Family

The stressful impact of HIV disease on the family has been well documented (Cates et al. 1990; Frierson et al. 1987; Kelley and Sykes 1989; Moynihan et al. 1988; Pearlin et al. 1989; Stulberg and Buckingham 1988; Trice 1988). Most of the literature to date has emphasized the parallel process in the experience of the PWA and his caregivers, particularly with both working through the forceful affective concomitants of serodiagnosis, illness, and approaching death. This literature has built on studies of other chronic and life-threatening illnesses, suggesting that there may be some universal themes for families dealing with young adult members who are physically traumatized or who may be approaching death (Mallick 1979; Moynihan et al. 1988; Steinglass et al. 1982).

However, it has also been pointed out in the literature that the social stigma and blame surrounding HIV infection and social hysteria about contagion may contribute unique dynamics to the interaction between many PWAs and their families. These external sources of distress can very easily exacerbate the anxiety, feelings of helplessness and hopelessness, terror, and isolation that frequently accompany the course of HIV-related illnesses. In one small sample study, Trice

(1988) found that 84% of mothers who devoted full-time care for substantial periods to their sons with HIV-related illnesses showed a cluster of symptoms normally associated with posttraumatic stress disorder. In addition, when a PWA returns home, he is very likely reentering a family system that is "out of sync" with his own process in confronting the reality of HIV. Although this discrepancy has been alluded to in the literature on HIV in rural communities (Rounds 1988a, 1988b), it may also typify smaller urban areas that have not been greatly affected by the epidemic to date. As compared with families from the larger urban epicenters of HIV infection, families in smaller urban areas may have less formalized and institutionalized resources to rely on as well as fewer visible role models for caring for a loved one with an HIV-related illness. They may also have experienced less consciousness raising about HIV in general. Most families are likely to react to the returning member in a manner that will most effectively maintain the equilibrium of the family system. As Herz (1980) noted, "Since anticipated or actual death disrupts the family equilibrium, family members react automatically in a fashion that will be least disruptive and upsetting to themselves and to each other" (pp. 223–224).

Normative Developmental Events for the Family and the PWA

The literature has also emphasized the ways in which HIV infection has accelerated adult developmental tasks for those who are confronted with the possibility of a shortened life expectancy. This literature has frequently focused on themes addressed by Erikson (1982)—themes of intimacy, generativity, and integrity, and their opposites (i.e., isolation, stagnation, and despair). For those gay men who are returning home, at whatever point along the HIV-related illness continuum, their normative adult developmental issues frequently collide with the regression and narcissistic vulnerability that is expected in dealing with terminal illness. At times the regressive aspects of the personality may overshadow gains that have been made through consolidated adult differentiation from the family. The degree of oscillation between regression and consolidation will likely reflect both the patient's lifelong developmental achievements and his pre-morbid functioning in general.

In addition, the gay man who is ill with an HIV-related illness will usually be returning to a family system at an advanced point in its own developmental life cycle (Herz 1980; Rhodes 1977), and his family may already exhibit some of the "attendant strains" (Pearlin et al. 1989) that will predictably compete with his own wishes and needs. For example, in some families parents may be in the process of rees-tablishing their intimacy with one another after all of the children have left home; in others, the parents' focus may have shifted to the returning member's siblings who are raising families of their own. It is not unusual for the HIV-infected individual in his 30s or 40s to be returning to aging parents with their own physical limitations and their own anxieties about illness and death.

Furthermore, in addition to attending to its own developmental tasks, each family will exhibit its own characteristic dimensions of enmeshment and disengagement (Hoffman 1981) and its own cul-tural style. Some families might engulf their "son in need" with an overdetermined devotion that is lacking in boundaries; others might be cold and distanced, unable to cross the boundaries in any way that will permit compassion and warmth. The returning family member, particularly the individual who has been away for many years, may have suppressed some of these family characteristics in his wish for the idealized family of his childhood to care for him and to bear some of the burden of his diagnosis and physical and emotional distress. Whereas under usual conditions reencounters between adult children and their families of origin might hold the promise of further consol-idation and individuation (Oldham 1989), they are a challenge to the returning family member who is infected with HIV, particularly if he has idealized expectations either that "nothing has changed back home" or that "things back home must have gotten better by now." Reunions are even more complicated when there has been an avoid-ance or distancing between the individual and his family because of issues surrounding the son's gay life-style. An extreme, though not uncommon, example of this might be the gay man who returns to his family to reveal both his sexual orientation and his health status simultaneously. The extent to which he has been seen either as an extension of his parents' hopes and dreams in life or as a repository of their shame and guilt also provides further potential complications to the process of returning home.

Consolidation and Loss: Unfinished Business

The following case example illustrates the difficult challenge of maintaining a consolidated sense of self in the face of the losses AIDS delivers:

Case 1

Mr. A, a 40-year-old Portuguese immigrant who had come to the United States at age 10, had attained a high level of professional accomplishment as a secondary school teacher (*senor d'etud*), a position that carried considerable prestige within his family and community of origin. He was seen as being a teacher who was particularly helpful to newly arriving immigrants' children.

In early 1986, Mr. A began to feel sick, presenting with a recurrent bouts of constitutional symptoms of HIV-related illnesses, but without opportunistic infections indicative of AIDS. By the beginning of the school year, his increasing debilitation made it impossible for him to work and resulted in increasing depression. He experienced recurrent and painful candidiasis and shingles during 1986. In 1987 he developed persistent anemia secondary to antiretroviral therapy; he received bimonthly transfusions for the anemia, and he was also maintained on a psychotropic regimen of lorazepam (Ativan), triazolam (Halcion), and amitriptyline (Elavil). From 1986 until his death in 1991, he continued to slowly decline but had long plateaus of relatively comfortable functioning.

Mr. A was referred for psychotherapy by his primary care physician in 1987 for help with acute depression and anxiety and for ongoing support. I saw him once a week for therapy. In 1989 he participated in a support group for 10 months with other gay men dealing with HIV-related illnesses. After he was hospitalized for Pneumocystis carinii pneumonia (PCP) in June 1991, I continued seeing him once a week at his home.

Before becoming ill, Mr. A taught and lived about an hour's distance from his family in a city where he had bought a house and had a social network of gay friends. He usually visited his family once a week. As the most educated and successful member of his immigrant family, Mr. A was emotionally very important as the object of both his family's pride and envy. His illness initially resulted in severe disequilibrium for the family system. When it became clear to him in 1987 that he was not going to be able to continue teaching because of increasing fatigue and the need for regular transfusions, he stopped working, sold his house, and moved into a unit in the tenement that his parents owned and in which they lived in a small, working-class New England city. His unit was across the hall from his parents' unit. His two sisters lived in neighboring towns and were in and out of the parents' home regularly with their children. Mr. A had a brother who had been severely disabled from alcoholism for all of his adult life and who lived in the cellar of the tenement. The family was moderately enmeshed, a style that may have served them well as they made their way in a new country. Mr. A's family had discovered his gay sexual orientation many years before his illness, but never discussed it; Mr. A did not attempt to integrate his gay self-identification with his role in the family. His parents spoke only Portuguese.

At the beginning of our work together, Mr. A was extremely angry, depressed, and distrustful. However, as an alliance developed over the first year of therapy, his anxiety decreased (except when he experienced acute medical episodes), and his trust of me and his other care providers increased. His depression, which had both reactive and endogenous components, continued with more severity during setbacks in his health. From the beginning he was clearly struggling with multiple losses (i.e., health and stamina, career, home, and standing in the community), his self-esteem was very fragile, and he experienced his disease with a mixture of shame and a long-standing sense of defeat about life.

During his 4 years of therapy, Mr. A worked consistently on these issues. One major focus of his work was the gradual confrontation and working through of issues related to his family of origin. In addition, he concentrated on adapting to his multiple losses and negotiating immediate crises, particularly those related to disease progression and practical issues of insurance, eventual applications for Medicaid, supplemental security income, and so on.

The work related to his family centered on his unresolved feelings of anger and shame about his mother's alcoholism and psychiatric hospitalization at the time of their immigration 30 years ago and about his father's periodic violence within the family over the years. It also centered on his feelings that both parents had always been ashamed of him for his sensitivity. He was able to identify some connection between what he viewed as his parents' disgust about his homosexuality and his own inability to integrate his sexual orientation with other aspects of his life. The work also focused on the rage and shame he felt toward his alcoholic brother and on his alternating anger and admiration of his two sisters.

After moving back home, Mr. A gradually renegotiated a more comfortable relationship with his parents, who were then in their 70s and beset by their own failing health and worries about death. He was able to confront his terror that they would die before him and leave him alone. He was able to distance himself emotionally from his brother and to be more sad than enraged about him. He continued to split his sisters, experiencing one as the idealized caretaker of him and his parents and the other as selfish and uncaring. He had a warm relationship with his six nieces and nephews, ranging in age from 2 to 17, who were more affectionate toward and important to him following his move home. He did not have many friends who visited him. This was related partly to his not being honest with his family over the years about being gay and partly to his not telling most of his friends about his diagnosis and his gradual distancing of himself from them at the beginning of his illness.

The clinical work with Mr. A involved 1) helping him mourn his multiple current losses, particularly his professional activities and his own home; 2) helping him work through issues related to earlier developmental experiences and renegotiate his relationships in his family; 3) increasing his tolerance for the hopelessness, helplessness, and uncertainty that accompanied his progressive physical decline, particularly assisting him with both the containment and expression of affect about this; and 4) helping him maintain his self-esteem by encouraging him to continue pursuits that gave him pleasure, including writing and traveling (when possible), and focusing on his adaptability and accomplishments. These treatment goals incorporated aspects of *life review therapy* (Borden 1989) and, as such, were aimed at increasing his integrity and consolidation. Working through his predominantly masochistic reaction to his illness ("I deserve to have HIV") and his shame about his homosexuality ("I guess I can now be gay in my family as I'm going to die anyway") was an important part of the work from the beginning. During the last 6 months of his life the locus of the work shifted to the hospital and home, and its focus shifted to the more immediate issues related to death. It included more focus on spiritual issues and preparing to die, such as questions of self-termination and how he wanted to say good-bye to his family and to his health care providers. Even though he was receiving palliative medications, repetitive reassurance that he would not experience physical pain was an important part of the work.

My initial coordination (case management) of home care between Mr. A's primary care physician, family, and community agencies also became part of the work at this time. Regularly scheduled home visits provided more opportunity for contact with family members. A hospice agency in his home city was able to provide him with routine home nursing care and his parents with counselors fluent in Portuguese.

Mr. A's experiences clearly illustrate the struggle to hold on to adult consolidation and autonomy in the face of the regressive pulls resulting from debilitation and being forced by circumstances to go home. Having succeeded in differentiating himself from his moderately enmeshed family, the necessity to move back in with them was a powerful stimulus for opening old wounds and, ultimately, for working through as many of his long-standing psychodynamic issues as possible. Because we were able to establish a stable treatment alliance and because Mr. A had a highly developed intellectualized style, which served his psychological adaptation and survival extremely well, he was able to respond positively to a cognitive treatment approach. Mr. A was able to accomplish some of the normative developmental tasks of mid-life, even with the reversal of roles with his parents and even in the face of all of the losses he experienced as a result of his HIV-related illnesses. He was able to put his own "stamp of approval" on his accomplishments, particularly his ability to meet the extreme challenges that were presented to him by life in general and by living with HIV-related illness in particular. He made significant gains in working through his shame, anger, and self-hatred. He stated that he was at peace with himself and his family just before his death, which took place at home with most of his family present.

Returning Home to Dying Parents

In the following case example, the patient's experience with returning home illustrates some of the same inherent issues as found in Mr. A's case. However, the physical and psychological vulnerability of both the patient and his family in the next example resulted in a very different outcome.

Case 2

Mr. B, a 40-year-old man who was the middle child of three siblings and his parents' only son, returned to his parents' home in a small New England town after living in a large West Coast city for 12 years. While trying to break into the world of professional acting, Mr. B had supported himself in a series of positions as a waiter, much to the chagrin of his self-made, emotionally distant, wealthy father. His parents, both in their early 70s, lived in the house where Mr. B had grown up. His younger sister, who was very involved with the parents, lived nearby with her husband in the same community. The other sister, who was emotionally more distant, lived in Florida where she was raising her own family.

While in California in 1987, Mr. B was diagnosed as being HIV positive. In 1989 he decided to move home to live in an apartment over the garage of his parents' home. At this time Mr. B had multiple infections, including toxoplasmosis, cytomegalovirus, thrush, and shingles. He drove across the country alone, although he was very sick, planning to let his family know about his diagnosis when he arrived home. He was sure that he would get better medical treatment at home than on the West Coast.

On examination by physicians in Boston, the diagnoses of his multiple infections were confirmed. In addition, he was diagnosed as having probable HIV-related encephalopathy and depression. It was also discovered that he had a low tolerance for zidovudine (AZT). Multiple medications were prescribed for his opportunistic infections, and desipramine (Norpramin) was prescribed for his depression. His medical expenses were paid by private health insurance, which had been maintained for him over the years by his parents.

Mr. B was referred to me by his primary care physician and

began seeing me for psychotherapy once a week in November 1989, shortly after he returned home. Through sporadic contact with his family before his return, he knew that his father had been having some neurological problems. When he arrived home he discovered that his father was scheduled for an operation for a brain tumor resulting from metastatic prostate cancer. Consequently, at the beginning of our work together, Mr. B was very anxious about his own condition, about his father's poor prognosis, and about the strain that both of them were putting on his mother, whom he idealized for her ability to persevere through so many crises

During the winter and spring of 1990, Mr. B's condition stabilized and he was able to purchase a car (with financial help from his mother), work part time in a retail position, and reconnect with some friends and relatives. During this time his father was recuperating from his surgery and gradually regaining some functioning, but still had a guarded prognosis. Mr. B's work in therapy focused primarily on his stormy history with his father and his feelings of intense regret for "never making more of life." He devoted himself to gardening and pruning the family property during this period; he would then become enraged at his father for not noticing the work he had done. This became a useful metaphor in therapy for Mr. B's feelings that his abilities were always devalued and underappreciated in the family, particularly by his father. Confronting these feelings allowed Mr. B to address more directly his longing that he could have had a better relationship with his father when he was a boy and to begin to grieve for what had not occurred between them. He felt that there was nothing he could ever do to please his father, whom he experienced during his childhood as either absent or ridiculing. His work on these issues enabled him to begin to forgive his father and to make tentative moves closer to him in the role of caretaker, fixing him meals or feeding him. Even with these progressive steps, resistance predominated in the treatment, the alliance was weak, and there was a narcissistic and repetitive quality to the sessions. Some of this may have been attributable to Mr. B's increasing neurological impairment.

During the fall of 1990, both Mr. B and his father began to deteriorate rapidly, with his father requiring a second operation and Mr. B being admitted episodically to the hospital for infections, high fevers, a collapsed lung, and severe diarrhea. During this period, Mr. B's symptoms related to encephalopathy also seemed to increase, although his depression seemed to wane. He was no longer able to work, had an automobile accident and eventually was not able to drive, and experienced increasing fatigue between hospitalizations. Also during this period his mother was admitted to the hospital several times for cardiac symptoms.

In December 1990, his mother died of a heart attack. Mr. B, who was in the hospital with beginning symptoms of mycobacterium avium complex, was given a day pass to attend her funeral. He was alternately in the hospital or at home with hospice care during the several months following his mother's death, which left him very depressed. His father was also at home with hospice care during this period and his younger sister was providing overnight coverage for both of them. As time went on, his sister appeared increasingly depleted by the rapid deterioration of her family, the loss of her mother, and the ongoing demands of her father and brother. Mr. B's father died on Mr. B's birthday, 4 months after the mother's death. Mr. B was again given a pass from the hospital to attend his father's funeral. Following this, Mr. B's condition steadily declined. His dementia caused him to become very forgetful and threatened his safety to the extent that his sister did not want to continue to care for him at home, even with hospice support. There was some question of placing him in a residential facility for homeless people with HIV disease in a nearby city, but Mr. B refused to be admitted.

During this critical period, there was a change in Mr. B's ability to continue his work with me. Although he expressed a desire for me to follow him when he was in the hospital, he would usually be too tired or too depressed to talk. Furthermore, he made it clear that he did not want to see me at home. I let him know verbally and in writing that I was available if he wanted to see me. I also made it known to his medical treatment team that I was available if he wished to see me. He did not respond, and there was no formal termination to our work together. Mr. B died in the acute setting 4 months after his father's death.

Mr. B's first year of therapy had focused on helping him 1) mourn the changes in his physical functioning, including sexual functioning, changes in appearance, and the loss of his dreams of success as an actor; 2) identify his feelings about his father's rejection of him, particularly in the context of his father's approaching death; and 3) identify and manage the stress that he was under, particularly as it was compounded by the extreme disappointments and further losses that faced him after his return home. Mr. B was able to approach these tasks intellectually and defensively only. His choice to not continue our work might be seen as adaptive, particularly in the context of his self-sufficient style. However, it might have been too threatening to be dependent on anyone at a time when his parents, whom he had returned home to depend on, were dying and he was moving closer to his own death. His narcissistic defenses against affect may also have resulted in his avoidance of an alliance and of the longings that are part of the therapy relationship. Increasing neurological dysfunction also may have attenuated his ability to use psychotherapy at the end stages of his life.

Old Conflicts Revisited

This next case illustrates what happens when early developmental events that were never completely resolved reemerge in the context of a new crisis.

Case 3

Mr. C, a 24-year-old bartender, moved home to a small New England town from a nearby city in August 1987, 5 months after he was diagnosed as having Kaposi's sarcoma (KS). He was referred to me for psychotherapy by his primary care physician for help in obtaining compliance with his medical treatment plans and to decrease his acting out. At the time of his diagnosis, Mr. C was started on experimental treatments for his KS, but he removed himself from these protocols after several weeks. His medical condition was becoming more complicated and, at the time of his return home, he was diagnosed as having toxoplasmosis and was scheduled for a bronchoscopy because of the possibility of PCP.

Mr. C presented as a crisis-ridden young man much in need of supportive treatment. He was very receptive to twice-a-week work for the first few months. He then tapered to once-a-week therapy until his death in December 1988.

Mr. C's medical condition gradually worsened during the last year of his life to the point at which his body was covered with lesions and his breathing was so labored that he carried a small oxygen tank wherever he went. Even so, he was in denial about the seriousness of his illness and would consistently overextend his activities, particularly in the gay community and especially in the bar where he had formerly worked.

Mr. C's family at home consisted of his father, stepmother, and a half sister, age 15. His biological mother lived in the city with his stepfather and another half sister, age 17. He had two full brothers and a sister who were all older and living on their own. His return home, progressive neurological symptomatology, and crisis-ridden and demanding behavior placed immense emotional strain on his family. For example, Mr. C caused two car accidents within 1 month at the end of 1988 after using cocaine. Although his stepmother was able to set limits on Mr. C's behavior, her strengths were challenged by the reinvolvement of the biological mother, who waged a continual contest to win the affection and custody of her "baby" before he died. Long-standing marital and family conflicts, some having begun 20 years ago, reemerged as Mr. C's illness progressed and as he assumed the responsibility for "bringing the family together before it was too late."

Just before his final admission to the hospital where he died, Mr. C was alternating his living arrangements between the homes of his biological parents. It was necessary to work with Mr. C in a variety of settings, including my office, the two parental homes, and the hospital. It was also helpful to see his biological mother, his father, and stepmother separately. In the beginning the work with the parents included a constant focus on education about HIV, including discussion of their immediate concerns about being infected and their need to know Mr. C's prognosis. As time went on, the work revolved around both Mr. C's and his parents' containment and toleration of affect. His father was only slightly able to put his feelings into words without prolonged periods of crying, and his biological mother was only slightly able to examine some of her guilt and shame related to her son's homosexuality and his infection with HIV. Mr. C was only slightly able to decrease his acting out, which was based on his terror at being so sick, and to talk about his feelings of abandonment stemming from his parents' divorce.

Because there were always medical and practical crises to be dealt with, some of this work was assisted by task management. For example, as Mr. C's neurological functioning decreased and he became more regressed, dividing tasks between the two biological parents (such as getting him to his various appointments) seemed to be useful in helping them work through some of their strong feelings. Because they refused to be in the same room together, even Mr. C's hospital room, this approach had its complications. However, it did become clear as time went on that Mr. C was still torn over his parents' divorce and that the early trauma of this event had been revived for him. His unresolved longing to have his parents reunited (and to feel cared about by both of them) and his orchestration of the family's acting out of his wishes and fears may have given Mr. C some sense of mastery at the end of his life. He died relatively at peace at the hospital, stating that he felt like he had "given it his best shot." His parents were finally able to attend his very elaborate funeral together.

Summary

In this chapter I have illustrated some of the expectable psychotherapy issues that arise in working with gay men with HIV-related illnesses who have returned to their family of origin's home. I have suggested that therapists outside of the large urban epicenters of HIV infection may begin to see more gay men who are moving home and their family members as time goes on. The use of developmental theoretical frameworks in approaching practice with these men and their families may help therapists appreciate the ways in which normative, expectable developmental tasks for the individual and the family can be radically complicated by the diagnosis of an HIV-related illness.

As the above case examples have suggested, the best predictors of adjustment to the complications presented by HIV may be the relative psychological health and adaptability of the individual and the family before the diagnosis. Certainly when there is significant unresolved shame about homosexuality, when other family members (particularly parents) are sick or dying, or when old family conflicts are revived following the return home, the adjustment related to the return home is more complex, as is the psychotherapeutic work. A dual focus of attention within the treatment to long-standing and immediate psychological issues and to practical concerns is essential to the work. This dual focus may require therapists to reformulate their practice to include more family involvement, to make more home and hospital visits, and to provide case management functions as needed. As might be expected, these changes in the parameters of practice require being familiar with the medical course of HIV infection and HIV-related illnesses, being willing to work in an interdisciplinary way with the medical team in following the patient as the disease progresses, and staying familiar with community resources. Because of the increase in time and energy that this work requires, it may be necessary to be realistic about the number of HIV-infected patients one can work with at any one time. The intensely emotional nature of working with men who are going home to die presents the therapist with fundamental psychological concerns.

Fueled by the urgency and uncertainty inherent in HIV infection, patients seeking help in dealing with the internal and interpersonal concomitants of returning home can evoke very powerful transference and countertransference issues in the treatment relationship. For example, when the return home results from a failure of the patient's support system or primary relationship, issues of dependency and abandonment typically characterize the treatment relationship. When the family is unable to accommodate the patient's return home or when a delicately balanced arrangement between the patient and family fails after the return home, anger and disappointment usually characterize the treatment relationship. When there has been a history of disappointment in the relationship between the patient and his family, the treatment alliance may be fragile, and mistrust and splitting may characterize the relationship. I have found that the countertransference is predictably more complicated under the following three circumstances: 1) when patients or family members are more like me and members of my family, 2) when illness or death within my own friendship or family systems are competing for my emotional energy or attention, and 3) when the patient or family members have reacted masochistically to HIV infection, believing that they deserve in some way to be infected.

Although countertransference issues are predictably intense for all therapists engaged in this work, my experience suggests that gay therapists doing this work may be presented with particular challenges. The consolidation of gay adult identity usually entails cultivating one's own home in the world—a home that is frequently tied to hard-won differentiation from one's family of origin and the establishment of one's family of choice. Ongoing empathic attunement within this work requires the therapist to be able to tolerate the range of emotions that surrounds the regressive pulls to his or her own family of origin. In addition, this work obviously and powerfully confronts us with continual intimations of our own mortality. Although supervision and support systems can be useful in managing these feelings, it may be the joining in the emotional and existential journey of these patients that gives this work its particular challenges and rewards.

References

Borden W: Life review as a therapeutic frame in the treatment of young adults with AIDS. Hlth Soc Work 14:253–260, 1989

Cates JA, Graham LL, Boeglin D, et al: The effects of AIDS on the family system. Families in Society 71:195–201, 1990

Dilley J, Helquist M, Marks R: Report from the international conference: hope and apprehension. Focus: A Guide to AIDS Research and Counseling 6:1–8, 1991

Erikson E: The Life Cycle Completed. New York, WW Norton, 1982

Frierson RL, Lippman SB, Johnson J: AIDS: psychological stresses on families. Psychosomatics 28:65–68, 1987

Herz F: The impact of death and serious illness on the family life cycle, in The Family Life Cycle: A Framework for Family Therapy. Edited by Carter EA, McGoldrick M. New York, Gardner Press, 1980, pp 223–240

Hoffman L: A family model, in Foundations of Family Therapy. Edited by Hoffman L. New York, Basic Books, 1981, pp 284–304

Institute of Medicine and National Academy of Sciences: Confronting AIDS: Update 1988. Washington, DC, National Academy Press, 1988

Kelley J, Sykes P: Helping the helpers: a support group for family members of persons with AIDS. Soc Work 34:239–242, 1989

Mallick M: The impact of severe illness on the individual and the family. Social Work in Health Care 5:117–128, 1979

Moynihan R, Christ C, Silver LG: AIDS and terminal illness. Social Casework 69:380–387, 1988

National Commission on AIDS: America Living With AIDS. Washington, DC, U.S. Government Printing Office, 1991

Oldham JM: The third individuation: the middle aged child and his or her parents, in The Middle Years: New Psychoanalytic Perspectives. Edited by Oldham JM, Liebert RS. New Haven, CT, Yale University Press, 1989, pp 89–104

Pearlin LI, Semple SJ, Turner H: The stress of AIDS are giving: a preliminary overview of the issues, in AIDS: Principles, Practices and Politics. Edited by Corless IB, Pittman-Lindeman M. New York, Hemisphere, 1989, pp 279–289

Rhodes S: A developmental approach to the life cycle of the family. Social Casework 58:301–311, 1977

Rounds KA: AIDS in rural areas: challenges to providing care. Soc Work 33:257–261, 1988a

Rounds KA: Responding to AIDS: rural community strategies. Social Casework 69:360–364, 1988b

Steinglass P, Temple S, Lisman SA, et al: Coping with spinal cord injury: the family perspective. Gen Hosp Psychiatry 4:259–264, 1982

Stulberg I, Buckingham S: Parallel issues for AIDS patients, families and others. Social Casework 69:355–359, 1988

Trice AD: Posttraumatic stress syndrome-like symptoms among AIDS caregivers. Psychol Rep 63:656–658, 1988

Chapter 14

Psychotherapy With Gay Male Couples: Loving in the Time of AIDS

Marshall Forstein, M.D.

The acquired immunodeficiency syndrome (AIDS) epidemic has had an irrevocable impact on all gay male relationships. In this chapter I focus specifically on treatment issues for gay male couples in the age of AIDS. Although there is some discussion in the literature about how male couples function (Blumstein and Schwartz 1983; Carl 1990; Forstein 1986; McWhirter and Mattison 1984; Mendola 1980; Silverstein 1981), little attention has been given to how gay men enter into and maintain relationships or how they cope with the threat or impact of human immunodeficiency virus (HIV) infection within their relationships and in the context of their social network.

Although men have been having sex and living in loving relationships with other men throughout history, it is a relatively new phenomenon for male couples to work toward equal acceptance and legal status in society as overt couples. Even within the gay male community there has been great ambivalence and a wide range of thinking about how gay couples should define and constitute themselves and how closely they should mimic their heterosexual counterparts. As part of the development of a paradigm of the gay male identity in the United States, there has been a tension between gay men who want to be thought of as no different from their heterosexual counterparts (except for their choice of sexual and affectional partners) and those who believe that there is something inherently distinct manifested in sex-

293

ual ideology concerning issues of fidelity and monogamy, and in the psychological and emotional realm concerning issues of autonomy, connectedness, and commitment. This tension is evident in the debate about whether gay men should be allowed to couple with legal as well as religious sanctions, or to have and raise children.

As the AIDS epidemic exploded, homosexual men were in the process of trying to define gay male identity in terms of sexuality and relationships. During the 1960s and 1970s, this included for many experimentation with multiple sexual partners and anonymous sexual encounters that celebrated the newly asserted right to publicly display gay male sexuality (see Chapters 2 and 20). Outlawed by society and denied access to socially and legally affirmed relationships, gay men found ways to separate themselves from their heterosexual peers, who were themselves moving further toward nontraditional living arrangements and relationships.

In addition to the effects of growing up with an emerging homosexual orientation, all gay men are affected by the male socialization process that occurs from infancy. Growing up male in American society often facilitates the dissociation of behavior from affect, the suppression of feelings of dependency and need, and the affirmation of feelings of independence and autonomy. Gay men also face the task of integrating into their relationships their initial socialization as if they were heterosexual males, and then reinterpreting this in the context of their emerging same-sex orientation (Carl 1990; Forstein 1986).

The feminist movement has had a profound impact on both male and female gender roles. As women struggle to determine what it means to be in a relationship, manage careers, raise children, and celebrate their sexuality with new affirmation of their gender, heterosexual men have had to reconsider what it means to be male. These gender role changes have had an affect on the power dynamics within relationships, regardless of whether the relationship is between individuals of the same or opposite gender. Apart from the greater tendency for gay male couples to be overtly, perhaps even deliberately nonmonogamous, nonmarried heterosexual couples and gay male couples of the 1980s and 1990s may be more like each other than not.

The AIDS epidemic has further changed how gay men feel and think about relationships. They are challenged to initiate and foster relationships within the era of gay rights on one hand and amid the catastrophic, epidemic destruction of gay male life on the other. Each new generation of young gay men faces real threats to life in the forms of AIDS, hate crimes and other violence, and the internalized threat to self-affirmation and loving others resulting from societal antihomosexual bias and rampant homophobia. Many same-sex–oriented men continue to split off sexual drive and behavior from emotional and affectional yearnings and avoid relationships with men openly identified as gay. They may engage in furtive or one-time sexual contacts to reduce the sexual tension that makes them anxious about their sexual longings, and then retreat back into invisibility within the larger heterosexual society. Often these men do not believe that a relationship with another man is possible, or at best see it as only fleeting and impermanent.

That more and more gay men continue to struggle and forge relationships in the face of these hardships is a testimony to the intrinsic and powerful drive not just to be sexual, but to relate, connect, commit, and love someone of the same sex. Often gay male relationships are thought of as being motivated by only sexual desire. Instead, the extraordinary desire to love, to share a dream of a future, to build a family of friends and sometimes children, even in the time of AIDS, speaks to the fundamental affectional needs and yearnings of gay men.

How Gay Men Define Their Relationships

Gay male couples define themselves as being coupled in several ways (Forstein 1986):

1. Two men living together and committed to a long-lasting relationship most like a heterosexual marriage
2. Two men living apart in the same geographical area but considering themselves mutually committed to a long-lasting and emotionally bonded relationship
3. Two men living geographically apart but considering each other the primary person to whom each is responsible and emotionally committed

4. Two men, one or both of whom may be heterosexually married, whose lives are emotionally committed to each other but who outwardly, for a number of reasons, must maintain the facade of a heterosexual marriage

For therapists who are not familiar with the variety of ways in which gay men construct their relationships, any appearance of their relationship being different from the heterosexual marriage model might create discomfort. Assumptions by therapists as to the degree of commitment, love, and stability of a male couple based on the way the couple defines itself, establishes a home, or deals with sex or money can undermine an objective view of the relationship and collude with society's antihomosexual bias.

Clinical Issues

Gay male couples seek psychotherapy for several reasons, many of which are similar to those of heterosexual couples: sexual problems, crises, family of origin issues, financial and power dynamics, and attempts to further the degree of intimacy within the relationship and yet maintain the autonomy of the individuals. In addition, gay male couples sometimes seek help to work through the internalized residue of homophobia or the differences in how public or "out" each member of the couple is. They may seek overt affirmation for a relationship for which there may not be other supports. For some gay couples, they may have no experience of other male couples with which to compare their relationship, and thus use the heterosexual models from their own families of origin as the basis of understanding for themselves.

McWhirter and Mattison (1984) described *stage discrepancy*, which is the conflict that arises when two men in a relationship are developing with different expectations and needs at a particular point in the life of the couple. These authors noted six developmental stages, each with particular characteristics:

◆   Stage one—blending (year 1)
◆   Stage two—nesting (years 2 and 3)

◆ Stage three—maintaining (years 4 and 5)
◆ Stage four—building (years 6 through 10)
◆ Stage five—releasing (years 11 through 20)
◆ Stage six—renewing (beyond 20 years)

The extraordinary stress of living within the HIV epidemic often creates a major shift in how these developmental stages evolve for and are resolved by any particular couple. The unrelenting threat of potential infection in each sexual act with a seronegative partner, the unremitting grief of continual loss of loved ones, and the apparent disinterest by the federal government to take significant action against this ravaging epidemic profoundly affect gay men throughout the daily fabric of their lives. As Stein (1988) wrote,

> Whether issues related to physical illness, death, or grieving are present for a particular couple, all gay men have been influenced by the specter of this dreaded disease, and male couples can, therefore, be expected to present routinely with concerns related to fears of disease, to altered patterns of sexual behavior, and to changing needs and expectations in relationships. (p. 18)

Gay men present with a broad range of concerns relationships that have been affected by HIV. Essentially, these concerns break down into couples who are dealing with similar HIV status (negative or positive) or dissimilar HIV status (one negative, one positive) as they consider becoming involved in a relationship, dealing with the developmental stages of defining themselves as a couple, or moving through the inevitable growth and life-stage changes that may be significantly influenced by the AIDS epidemic. In presenting for therapy, these may manifest overtly or covertly in

1. Men who have been in a long-term relationship who suddenly face the diagnosis of one or both of the individuals as being HIV positive or becoming sick
2. Men who have been in an ongoing relationship and are trying to decide about whether to be HIV tested in order to negotiate safer sexual behavior

3. Men who have been recently coupled and find out about one member's HIV positive status, which threatens the stability of the relationship
4. Men who have recently met and know that their HIV serological statuses are different
5. Couples in which both members are HIV negative, and their support group is being devastated around them, raising issues for them as survivors

Although there are many issues that might be explored, in this chapter I specifically focus on those that are related to HIV. These concerns must always be viewed in the light of all other concerns facing the couple, such as the possibility that each couple member has been split off from his family of origin, initially because of his unacceptability to his family as a gay person and second because of the added stigma of his being HIV positive.

There are several overarching issues that HIV infection may crystallize within a couple's relationship. Regardless of their serological status, gay men often experience changes in their awareness of time and of the future and in their fundamental beliefs about the nature of life itself. Spiritual concerns, which may have been forsaken because of the enormous conflict surrounding homosexuality within most religions, may be reawakened with some urgency in an attempt to understand the inordinate loss and anger that HIV infection and homophobia create. The need to confront the end of their lives at a time when they should be planning for a future together can precipitate significant crises within couples, can result in members of a couple coping with the existential and spiritual issues in different ways. Sexual vigor within a relationship may be affected by the unconscious intrusion of the association between sex and death, experienced as a constant reminder of the potential for losing the loved object. Young people who fall in love usually have many years to integrate the reality of "till death do us part." Every orgasm, fraught with increasing vulnerability within an ongoing relationship, becomes truly symbolic at some primitive level of what the French have called *la petite morte*. To fully abandon one's self to one's sexual desire and open one's self up to a lover (in the midst of this epidemic) may engender inhibitory defenses of significant magnitude.

All of this must be viewed within the context of trying to live an affirming, gay-identified life within a homophobic society. During a gay man's growth and development, society initially traumatizes him as deviant, unacceptable, and repulsive. Later, his love for men is rejected and devalued at every turn. Some gay men see a gay relationship as their only safe haven, and may put unreasonable expectations on their partners. These may include a self-enforced isolation. As Carl (1990) pointed out, some gay men have been so successful as a traditional male that they find it hard to let others help them. Such men may also be less able to nurture another with the same degree of giving that women have demonstrated in caring for others.

The threat of being infected or infecting others with HIV; the realities of living with a chronic, usually debilitating and fatal illness; and the emotional impact of living under siege present enormous challenges for any gay male relationship. HIV has changed the normal course of life events. Some must now work hard to affirm their right to remain seronegative in the face of an infected partner, while at the same time remain intimate and emotionally connected. Others must negotiate life with a new set of parameters: a potentially shortened life span, the presence of illness at a time of life that would be typically free of illness, and a heightened awareness of mortality that affects all aspects of individual psychological function. Normal psychological defenses, appropriate for a certain stage of life, may become impossible or dysfunctional in the context of developmental concerns that are out of phase with the crisis engendered by HIV.

Many gay men, afraid of exposing themselves to HIV and feeling unable to negotiate the normal tasks of becoming intimate with another person, use the epidemic to avoid establishing intimate relationships. Others, denying the reality of AIDS, immerse themselves in sexually intense relationships without ever addressing the possibility of health risks with a partner by either assuming that the partner is negative or taking a nihilistic stance as a manifestation of internalized homophobia or unresolved feelings of grief and loss. Although the following case example presents the issues from therapy with an individual, it raises a number of typical concerns with which couples present:

Case 1

Mr. A, a 25-year-old gay-identified man who was in the process of coming out, came to psychotherapy to work on issues about his sexual identity and issues concerning his family that arose out of a difficult parental relationship. Having had only one same-sex experience in his teens, he was overwhelmed with how easily available sex with other men was for him now. He was working in a less-than-satisfying job, well below his aptitude, and living with his mother who had relied on him as the man of the house since his father's death 5 years earlier. Mr. A had tried to talk to his mother about his homosexuality, but had been rebuffed, with her telling him that he should see a priest and get over it. Through a personal advertisement, Mr. A met a 28-year-old man with whom he developed an intense infatuation. This man represented all of the physical and personal characteristics Mr. A believed he lacked.

During the initial session, Mr. A spoke about his difficult childhood and his feelings of being homosexual within the context of his family and church. He painted a landscape of superficial happiness with emotional deprivation stemming from the narcissism of his parents and their inability to empathically support his unique strengths and talents, which lay not in the areas of athletics and business like his older brothers' did, but in the fine arts.

As part of the evaluation, the relationship with the new lover was explored to assess Mr. A's character strengths and weaknesses and his psychological capacity to handle coming out in the age of AIDS. What Mr. A acknowledged somewhat offhandedly was that his lover was athletic, masculine, and self-confident, and had been HIV positive for 3 years. The lover had been direct about his seropositivity from their very first meeting, during which they had engaged in sex using condoms and avoided the exchange of semen.

Mr. A then disclosed that several weeks into the relationship his lover began to complain about using condoms, stating that as the penetrator, he had less sensation than he would like. After promising Mr. A that he would withdraw before ejaculating, they then proceeded to have unprotected anal sex, with Mr. A accepting this out of a wish to please his partner and avoid what he would perceive as inevitable rejection if he didn't comply. He shared with his therapist that the lover had told him in a passionate moment that he really loved him and that he would never let him become infected.

Trying to contain his feelings about what the patient was participating in, the therapist explored the patient's baseline knowledge and information about HIV, which turned out to be quite good and accurate, but which had not been effectively integrated into the patient's capacity to modify risk behavior. The therapist suggested that long-term psychodynamic therapy might not be possible if the patient was consciously unconcerned about preserving his life. In the process of exploring how Mr. A understood the behavior of his partner to be an act of love, Mr. A's underlying confusion about sorting out his complex feelings of anger, aggression, and sadness he had faced in the relationship with his father was revealed. Over the next few sessions, hostility in the name of love was identified as a repetitive theme in his relationships with many male figures in his life. This precipitated an acute state of anxiety and fear that he might actually have been infected, which stressed Mr. A's relationship with his lover and ultimately fractured it.

Although this case illustrates many issues that arise in individual therapy with gay men, it points out the problems in sorting out what it means for different people to define themselves as part of a relationship prematurely and without a clear understanding of the relational dynamics. The extraordinary need for gay men to be accepted by other gay men may often facilitate a dissociation of knowledge and behavior in the area of sexual activity. The therapist's questioning of Mr. A about what being loved and being in a relationship meant to him, questions originally asked in the context of assessing the lack of an empathic, loving connection in Mr. A's relationship with his lover, allowed Mr. A's denial, which was fueling destructive behavior to be broken down. Furthermore, for gay men who had been traumatized in early childhood (see Chapter 18), there may be complex meanings behind the unsafe behavior that emerges only within the context of a relationship in which emotional attachment develops.

For those who manage to cope with their fears and anxieties about becoming close to someone and then finding out they might be HIV infected, there may be a tendency to start or stay in relationships that are not appropriate, gratifying, or psychologically healthy for them. Relationships that have been ongoing but that are destructive may be maintained out of fear of having to become sexual and intimate with new partners whose HIV status may not be known.

An awareness, however, that the potential threat of HIV that exists in the world outside the relationship may have the effect of encouraging some couples to seek therapy to work through problems that previously might have led to a precipitous breakup. In the past, with an easy availability of sexual partners, gay men may have been more likely to seek new partners instead of understanding and adapting to normal changes in sexual behavior within an ongoing relationship. Unaccustomed to feeling vulnerable and intimate, gay men may fail to understand that familiarity and emotional vulnerability may engender defenses that may be manifested as sexual inhibition and withdrawal. Often even fairly new relationships have been forced to cope with enormous burdens of loss through death of friends in the immediate social network that has served as a surrogate, "chosen" family. In addition, the fears and anxieties of HIV that intrude directly into the relationship may trigger defenses against potential loss, which may lead to a premature sense of emotional intimacy.

Through their roles as caretakers and primary providers of emotional sustenance throughout the course of their friends' illnesses, gay men have matured and developed enormous capacities to tolerate anxiety and ambivalence. They have translated their experiences into skills that allow them to acknowledge conflict within a relationship, value the fundamental structures that have kept them together, and seek help to resolve their problems rather than separate from each other.

HIV-Negative Couples

Couples in which both members are HIV negative may seek therapy to deal with the impact the AIDS epidemic has on them as individuals and as a couple. The continual loss of friends to AIDS-related illnesses may precipitate an ongoing, sometimes unacknowledged, grief reaction that erodes the sense of healthy entitlement for one or both members of the couple to enjoy life and look forward to the future. One effect of so much bereavement is the social isolation the couple is forced into because the couple has literally lost an entire network of friends. This enormous loss may force reconsideration of previously held values, in both the physical and spiritual realms, throwing the couple into an existential crisis. This may manifest itself as a sense of growing apart if the partners are not able to share and help each other grieve.

Another common issue is a loss of sexual desire by one or both members of a couple as an unconscious attempt either to join with those ravaged by the epidemic or to avoid feeling guilty about being seronegative after having engaged in much of the same risk-taking activities as those who are ill and dying. The therapist can help the partners examine their relationship within the context of the loss of life and the sense of doom within the gay community. The therapist might reframe the perceived distance in their relationship not as pathological but as an attempt to ward off magical fears that if they enjoy their life together too much they will be punished at some point. Alternatively, the therapist could frame the distance as an attempt to modulate what might be perceived at an unconscious level as too much intimacy and pleasure at a time when others are fighting for life itself.

Sometimes the discovery of seronegativity in both partners may revitalize the sexual relationship with a renewal of commitment to remain mutually monogamous. For couples who have not been monogamous, the negative HIV status may confirm that whatever sexual behavior is happening outside the relationship appears to be safe. Therapists, however, must not automatically assume that a seronegative test result proves the safeness of one or both partners' sexual activity. The seronegative couple continues to have the burden of remaining uninfected amidst the epidemic. They may be envied for the sexual freedom others assume they experience together as a consequence of their negative status. Furthermore, when they turn to peers for support during times of stress, their difficulties may overtly or covertly be deemed unimportant in the context of the epidemic.

HIV-Positive Couples

Couples may be forced to deal with HIV as one of the initial barriers to forming a relationship. A couple in which both members are HIV infected may feel a pressure to grow and develop at a pace out of phase with a normal perception of time because they believe that their lives will be shortened. This may occur unconsciously or consciously and may be experienced by each member of the couple in different ways, depending on the individuals' capacity to tolerate the perception of mortality at a time of life in which the denial of death would be more age appropriate. At the beginning of a relationship, HIV-positive men may believe they are so fortunate to find another person to love that they avoid dealing with conflicts or basic incompatibilities out of fear of jeopardizing what they believe is their last chance for romance.

Other couples may find out that both are positive after beginning the relationship. The longer the couple has been together before this information becomes apparent, the more opportunities they may have had to work through other significant issues together, such as loss of a job, death of a family member, or some other life event that stressed their relationships and tested their commitment, love, and ability to support each other. Facing major assaults on the integrity of one or both members of the couple may prepare them for the extraordinary pain and difficulty HIV may engender. For couples who have been together a significant time, there may be unspoken questions about who might have infected whom. In the face of feeling overwhelmed and victimized by HIV, the couple may be at risk for perpetrating emotional or even physical abuse on each other (see Chapter 18) or for acting out sexually outside the relationship in an unsafe or self-destructive way.

At various times, one member of the couple may seek more intimacy or distance than is tolerable to the other in an effort to cope with increasing dependency needs or the loss of self-esteem and autonomy secondary to the physical changes brought about by his worsening medical condition. When both members are HIV positive, there are lurking questions, sometimes not overtly addressed, about who will become sick first, who will survive longer, and who will be there to take care of the one remaining. The illness in one or both partners can destabilize existing power, control, financial, and emotional dynamics within the relationship. Some gay men fear the incredible responsibility they feel towards their partner, voicing doubts as to whether they are strong enough emotionally to really help the other. Their self-doubt is exacerbated by internalized homophobia. In some cases where couples came together before the AIDS epidemic, there may be tremendous shame and guilt about not having maintained a monogamous relationship. This self-punitiveness may derive from confusion about their motivation for having taken risks while in a relationship when they had full knowledge about HIV transmission. Case 2 illustrates some of the complex and often unconscious forces that contribute to a man's taking risks in the face of knowledge about HIV.

Case 2

Mr. B, a 29-year-old gay man, and Mr. C, a 34-year-old gay man, had been in a relationship for 6 years. Just prior to their fifth anniversary, Mr. C became acutely ill and was hospitalized with meningitis. Both men became concerned that this was a manifestation of HIV infection, having both felt they had been at risk because of their sexual behavior before meeting and during a difficult period in the third year of their relationship when they had been apart for about 5 months.

When the diagnosis confirmed their fear, a cascade of events followed, with Mr. C undergoing an exhausting battery of medical tests in order to determine the stage of his HIV illness and protect him from opportunistic infections. By the time Mr. C was diagnosed as having AIDS, he had a significantly impaired immune system, leading doctors to inform Mr. B that his partner was at imminent risk for another major illness or neoplasm. Totally caught up in Mr. C's illness, the couple paid little attention to the possibility that Mr. B was also infected. Mr. B himself entered an initial state of denial about this possibility in order to attend to Mr. C's needs.

Once his condition was stabilized, Mr. C himself opened the subject of Mr. B's risk for HIV. Although they had practiced almost exclusively safer sex during their relationship, there had been rare instances in which each of them had been relatively unsafe when they had been apart. It was at this point that the couple entered therapy to address the precipitous changes in their lives, which included loss of one of their incomes, a fear of being rejected by peers and families, and the emerging anger that was making it difficult for them to communicate.

What was immediately clear was Mr. C's doubt that Mr. B would want to stay with him and be burdened by his illness. Exploring that led to Mr. C's fear that if Mr. B turned out to be infected also, that he would blame Mr. C. Therapy helped to put all the issues out on the table and offered an opportunity to explore what was known medically about AIDS, including the issue that just because one's immune system was more impaired than the other's, it was still uncertain who had infected whom. Once the therapist framed their questions in terms of whether they helped or damaged the couple's expressed desire to work through these difficulties, Mr. B and Mr. C could move from issues of blame and self-destructive behavior to those of intimacy, commitment, and safety. Even the issue of how they defined their relationship emerged when the therapist reframed the question of commitment and doubt in terms of whether it might be different if they had been heterosexual and one of them had become potentially terminally ill.

Before Mr. C's illness, both men had avoided acknowledging their lifelong commitment. By finally owning their commitment to each other, they were able to look at the potential impact on their relationship that Mr. B's being tested or Mr. C's family wanting Mr. C to return home to them for his care would have.

Eventually Mr. B tested positive, although his immune system was significantly more intact than Mr. C's. Once again Mr. C offered him a way out of the relationship, saying that his family wanted him to come to their home to die. Mr. B was outraged that Mr. C would even think that he could abandon him, and made it clear that he would be the one to care for Mr. C. The therapist injected the reality of legal and health care proxy issues and actively encouraged them to seek legal counsel in order to put in place many of the protections that heterosexually married couples take for granted. The therapist became not only a transference figure for each of the men, replacing the parents who had been unable to affirm and honor their relationship at all, but a real person to them as well, giving practical advice and often sharing his experience about how other couples were handling some of these issues. When Mr. C took another turn for the worse, Mr. B called the therapist and asked him to meet him at the hospital. When they met, Mr. C was able to verbalize his hope that after he died Mr. B could continue in therapy, and that the therapist would make sure that Mr. B would have someone to take care of him.

Therapists working with a couple in which both members are HIV positive may find themselves becoming a permanent part of the dynamic between the two men. Especially where the families of origin may have been unable or unwilling to offer the type of support during the illness that might have been offered had the couple been heterosexual, the therapist is often drawn into the relationship in a way that requires a reframing of the therapeutic relationship and careful management of the inevitable changes in the boundaries to include pragmatic help with medical and psychosocial problems. An extraordinary intimacy often develops as one or both of the partners become more ill, requiring the therapist to visit them at the home or in the hospital, sometimes seeing patients more dependent, vulnerable, and physically exposed (because of hospital dress) than in the office. Engaging the couple in a dialogue about expectations of the therapist before either member becomes sick will prepare both the therapist and couple for these changes in the therapeutic frame.

The healthier member of the couple will sometimes experience a sense of urgency to live his life more fully, becoming ambivalent or even angry at his partner for becoming sicker. The therapist must understand that one partner is seeing his own future mirrored in the slow demise of the man he loves, exacerbating what is an existential gap between the two men as the very substance of what made them define themselves as a couple becomes challenged.

One or both members of the couple may begin a process of anticipatory grieving, and the therapist might have to give voice to the anguish of imagining the future loss of self and the other. Upon the death of one member of the couple, the nature of the therapist's continuing relationship with the survivor will become a concern and must be renegotiated. One issue that may arise for the therapist is whether to attend the funeral or memorial service of the deceased member. This might be raised in the context of the therapy when the couple discusses and plans the way in which the death of either one of them is to be handled, and what role the therapist might be expected to play.

When both members of the couple are HIV positive, they may have difficulty breaking up if their relationship is emotionally unhealthy. The emotional burden of dealing with HIV infection and the extraordinary narcissistic injury incurred may make an unhappy couple stay together in spite of any destructive dynamics that might be present. Fears of being alone or of never being loved again and feelings of contamination are sometimes lurking just beneath the surface, and are expressed as a sense of being trapped or feeling hopeless about whatever life might still be ahead. Financial problems, which are most often inevitable during the course of illness, may prevent the couple from considering separation.

Couples With Dissimilar HIV Status

As HIV serological testing became available, couples were faced with the wrenching possibility that the test might yield a different result for each member of the couple. At a time when few effective treatments were available to forestall the onset of disease or boost the immune system, couples often deliberately put off testing in order not to know if they might differ in their HIV status. Knowing their serological status would open up many issues with which they might have been unwilling or unable to deal. Some couples preferred to assume they were both HIV infected in order to avoid introducing into the relationship a potentially destructive piece of information. Assuming little could be done to treat the illness, they chose to act as if they were either both infected or both not infected.

The implications of these couples' dilemma were significant; medical and mental health care providers used the term *discordant couple* to describe a couple with dissimilar HIV status. Although *discordant* has a ring of scientific authority to it, it clearly was not neutral in its suggestion that men of dissimilar status would necessarily have trouble (i.e., discord). The term played into the insidious homophobia internalized by gay men, who were blamed for having contracted HIV infection, as compared with those who were noted by the popular media to be "innocently" infected (e.g., those who became HIV infected through blood transfusions). The term suggested that a dissimilar serological status would inevitably tear apart a relationship.

In fact, there are many clinical implications for a gay male couple with dissimilar HIV status. Depending on when in the course of the relationship it is discovered, and the character of the men and their coping style, the impact of dissimilar status on the stability of the couple can vary tremendously. Couples who had been looking for a way out of the relationship might use this information as the reason to separate, citing fears of infection and limitations on the ability to care for the one who is infected. Other couples use this event in their lives as a way of consolidating the relationship and moving to a higher degree of commitment and connectedness. Helping couples describe and understand the nature of their relationship before and after HIV infection can help differentiate problems associated with the illness from preexisting problems. Fed perhaps by his sense of shame and guilt, the seropositive man may unconsciously find ways to distance himself from his partner, often by withdrawing sexually and emotionally in order to prevent transmission of the virus. On the other hand, the seronegative partner, having contemplated leaving his partner for any number of reasons, may find it impossible to consider leaving the partner who is newly diagnosed with HIV. Afraid of being called cowardly or feeling guilty, the seronegative partner may feel trapped.

Therapists can facilitate the elaboration of all of the couple's fears and anxieties upon finding out one member is HIV positive and one is HIV negative. Some couples describe a sense of having to work everything out more quickly as a result of the distortion of time that the diagnosis of HIV seropositivity often brings. Couples often express a sense that they live in two separate worlds: one for the living and one for those preparing to die.

Both the seropositive and seronegative members of the couple face particular challenges to the existing dynamics of the relationship. The one who is positive may develop rageful envy of his partner, which must be suppressed in order to maintain the relationship. He may develop feelings of envy and of not really being understood. His feelings of increased shame and of being contaminated may manifest themselves in many ways, and the therapist must be on the lookout for these inevitable human responses to a sexually transmitted disease. The one who is seronegative may find himself angry at his partner for becoming infected, sometimes reflecting an unspoken dynamic in terms of their sexual lives. Feelings of being unable to stand the potential loss and of being incompetent to handle the burden of someone sick, and a wish to run away before becoming infected himself, may drive one member from the relationship, as illustrated in Case 3.

Case 3

Mr. D, age 29, and Mr. E, age 31, had been lovers for 5 years when they found out that Mr. E was HIV positive. Mr. D tested HIV negative at the same time. They presented for couples therapy with the request that they work on dealing with the stress and difficulty that had developed in the relationship over the past 2 years, starting the year before they even knew their serological statuses.

Mr. D, whose parents were divorced and whose father was alcoholic and emotionally abusive toward him, was questioning whether they should stay together. Eventually he was able to verbalize that he felt incapable of committing himself to the relationship in the way that Mr. E expected. This included sexual fidelity and a commitment to seeing Mr. E's illness through to the end. Mr. D felt cheated out of the lifelong relationship he had always wanted but feared. He believed AIDS was a cruel irony in the development of their loving relationship, imposing itself on their lives just as they were settling into the long-term nature of the relationship. Mr. D expressed many concerns about how he didn't think he could handle Mr. E's illness and wanted to be able to escape before Mr. E became sick. The couple had become estranged sexually, and Mr. D had begun to explore isolated episodes of sex with other men, leading Mr. E to feel contaminated, repulsive, and unwanted.

In therapy, both members of the couple came to understand that Mr. D feared not contagion but losing Mr. E, and that he was attempting to distance himself before he had to face the potential loss of his lover. As they approached the decision to separate, Mr. E was hospitalized with meningitis, becoming acutely ill and close to death. Contrary to Mr. E's dreaded expectations, Mr. D stepped in and exercised his rightful power of attorney, orchestrating the hospital stay and managing the essentials of dealing with family, friends, and doctors. He was very much in command of the situation. Without having time to ruminate about the possibility of failure, Mr. D had overcome his worst fear: that he would run away at the time Mr. E needed him most. At that time Mr. D even thought how much easier it would be if he were HIV positive, which scared him. Likewise, Mr. E began to get in touch with feelings of anger and jealousy that Mr. D was not infected, and his guilt over thinking how much easier it would be if they both were sick.

During this period, Mr. D found himself taking more risks sexually than he had ever allowed. Although the therapist felt Mr. D had been minimally risky (i.e., had not exchanged fluids), his behavior was interpreted as standing for the ambivalent and complex feelings of wanting to join his partner in illness so he would not be left and for the sense of helplessness he was experiencing in the relationship out of fear and anxiety.

The next year was quite turbulent, with the therapy focusing on how the two men conceptualized their relationship, comparing it with the models they had experienced growing up. Mr. E's parents were still married and felt close after more than 40 years, whereas Mr. D's family had broken apart because of his father's alcoholism while Mr. D was still in high school. The therapist asked them to consider how they thought about their relationship. Were they married? What did that mean? Would Mr. D feel differently if he were married to a woman who was diagnosed with terminal cancer? How would their families and friends respond if they were married? Both were able to understand that though they had been together now almost 6 years, they were operating under the assumption that the relationship depended on a year-to-year renewal, founded on their unconscious belief that gay men were not really capable or entitled to a lifelong relationship. This assumption undermined Mr. E's right to expect more from Mr. D, and Mr. D's belief that he had a commitment that superseded the onset of illness.

With Mr. D's increasing fear that he would lose Mr. E and not be able to cope becoming more apparent, the couple separated for about 2 months. Mr. E told Mr. D that he didn't want pity or charity, and that if Mr. D couldn't love him—emotionally and sexually— then he felt he was better off relying on family and friends for support rather than on him. During the separation, the therapist continued to meet with both Mr. D and Mr. E, helping Mr. E to grieve not only the loss of the relationship but of his future as well. Although Mr. E remained firmly convinced that he still wanted and loved Mr. D, he was quite stubborn and felt that Mr. D had to "fish or cut bait."

Meanwhile, Mr. D attempted to date other men, but found himself comparing them all with Mr. E. Time and time again he would return to therapy bemoaning how other men were not able to make him feel as loved, needed, and happy as Mr. E had. At this point Mr. E's health had stabilized, although it remained delicate. Both men were wishing that the other would take the risk and swallow his pride. Gradually, both patients began to deal with the existential issues about love and how in all relationships one partner loses the other.

Sensing that time was running out and seeing the misery that both men were experiencing from being apart, the therapist took a very active role in encouraging each partner to admit to him that each really wanted the other back. The therapist pushed Mr. E to face the fact that time was not to be taken for granted and that he should decide what he wanted and make it known. With Mr. E's permission, Mr. D was informed that Mr. E wanted to reconnect with him, but, that as the vulnerable one, it would be up to Mr. D to make that move. The therapist pushed Mr. D to see how in contrast to his relationship with his father, he was not in fact destined to be helpless and destructive in his relationships. The therapist helped Mr. D confront his father with the anger he had about being called a sissy while growing up. Mr. D then asked the therapist if he would promise to be there for him when Mr. E died. Following that, therapy focused on working through Mr. D's feelings of being outlawed from his ostensibly supportive family and looking at what Mr. D meant when he asked if the therapist would "be there."

Mr. D called Mr. E and they moved back in together, continuing in couples treatment for several months and working on communicating their deepest fears and anxieties. Mr. E was able to let go of the need to have sex with Mr. D as a proof of his love, and Mr. D was able to make his commitment to Mr. E until the end. They became closer than ever, cutting through their fears and recognizing that they wanted to be with each other more than with anybody else they had ever met, that they were indeed a couple, and that they would be there for each other "till death do us part."

The therapist allowed them to determine the frequency of sessions, which they tapered down to once a month and then discontinued for several months, while they pursued their relationship in many of the same ways they had at the beginning, including a renewed, though rarely acted-upon, sexual connection. The therapist continued to hear from one or both members of the couple, receiving a card when they traveled, as they did when Mr. E's health permitted it. Neither doubted that the therapist would be there for either one or both of them, should the need arise.

Couples with dissimilar HIV statuses may find support in groups and social settings with others facing the same dilemmas. Often the seronegative partner believes that because he is not sick he has no rights within the relationship, feeling resentful when he cannot fight back against the HIV-positive partner for fear that he is being selfish or might precipitate a new health crisis. More difficult to work through is the wish of the seronegative partner that his partner would die and "get it over with soon." The guilt and shame of wanting to move on with one's life, of wanting to put an end to his partner's pain and the uncertainty about the future, can manifest itself in many ways, including withdrawal, increased substance use, and a lack of attention to the emotional needs of the seronegative partner. The therapist can help by normalizing the wide range of feelings and tremendous ambivalence the seronegative patient has about his partner.

When the consequences of HIV infection include a loss of cognitive function, and the couple is facing a process in which the infected partner's capacity will become increasingly diminished, many difficult issues arise in therapy as the couple attempts to both deny and cope. Neurocognitive impairment changes the qualitative nature of the relationship and puts an incredible burden on all involved. Nothing is so frightening to an individual as the loss of mental function, an experience that can engender powerful feelings within himself and within his partner. The issues of suicidal ideation and self-determination often surface again, threatening whatever sense had been made of this earlier by the couple.

Likewise, the therapist is faced with having to assess and adjust to the impact that the neurocognitive dysfunction has on the patient's ability to work in therapy (i.e., to process feelings and information). A dramatic change may occur in the dynamics within the couple in terms of issues of control and responsibility for the day-to-day decisions and the decisions looming in the near distance. Actions that are a physiological consequence of brain dysfunction may be interpreted by the healthier partner as being manipulative, uncaring, or caused by depression. Decreases in affect or lability of mood may be frightening to one or both of the partners. Denial of cognitive deficits by both may force the therapist into an uncomfortable position of having to ask very difficult questions, such as, Is he still driving? Have there been any unusual accidents at home? Is it possible for him to stay at home alone, without supervision? Is it time to find home health care? Is hospice care an option? Can the partner cope with the eventually disabling consequences of the progressive loss of function? If one or both members of a couple show signs of cognitive dysfunction, the therapist may need to refer them to other professionals for complete neurological evaluations. This may be experienced by the therapist as a limitation, as an acknowledgment of failure (i.e., the therapy could not protect the couple from this terrible process). For the therapist it means becoming comfortable with changing roles in the couple's life and with a changing quality to the therapeutic interaction. The later stages of HIV-related neurocognitive impairment precipitate profound sadness and emotional pain for all involved and provide the greatest challenge to the therapist to be professional, yet human and available.

Conclusions

Gay couples who seek therapy in this decade may not have an immediate or conscious appreciation for the impact of HIV infection on their relationship. In addition to gathering information and developing a formulation of the dynamics within the relationship, a therapist must assess sexual behavior within and outside the relationship, the use of controlled substances, and what is known about HIV status. Even if the HIV status is not known, the therapist must keep in mind how the fears and anxieties of being infected might be playing a role in the dynamics within the couple. When the status of one or both partners is known, the impact this information has on the couple and their social network must be ascertained. A psychoeducational approach might be useful at various times throughout the treatment, which requires great flexibility on the part of the therapist. The therapist must be aware that the members of a couple can collude with each other against the therapist when intolerable affects or ambivalences are raised to a conscious level.

HIV intrudes into the lives of gay couples at all points along the spectrum of concerns, from being at risk to dying from AIDS. No gay man, and hence no gay male couple, has been unaffected by the HIV epidemic. Therapists who work with these male couples are often confronted with changing dynamics within the couple and between members of the couple and the therapist. Aware of the lack of legal protections and the potential within medical and social institutions to undermine, ignore, or devalue the male couple as a legitimate entity, the therapist may serve as advocate, case manager, and surrogate family for the couple. The therapist must carefully enter into the private and complex relationship of two outlaws trying to make a place for themselves as a couple, fending off the assaults of stigma and a disease that may threaten the fabric of their lives. Amid the unremitting loss of gay men to HIV and the background of violence and prejudice towards gay people, the therapist must find a way to help the couple celebrate life and make sense of loving in the time of AIDS.

References

Blumstein P, Schwartz P: American Couples. New York, William Morrow, 1983

Carl D: Counseling Same Sex Couples. New York, WW Norton, 1990

Forstein M: Psychodynamic psychotherapy with gay male couples, in Contemporary Perspectives in Psychotherapy With Lesbians and Gay Men. Edited by Stein T, Cohen C. New York, Plenum, 1986

Mendola M: The Mendola Report: A New Look at Gay Couples in America. New York, Crown, 1980

McWhirter DP, Mattison AM: The Male Couple. Englewood Cliffs, NJ, Prentice Hall, 1984

Silverstein C: Man to Man—Gay Couples in America. New York, William Morrow, 1981

Stein T: Homosexuality and new family forms: issues in psychotherapy. Psychiatric Annals 18:12–20, 1988

Section III

Specific Treatment Populations

Chapter 15

African American Gay Men and HIV and AIDS: Therapeutic Challenges

Shani A. Dowd, L.C.S.W.

A ny discussion of the mental health of African American gay men must begin by acknowledging the particular social circumstances confronting all African Americans. African American gay men must not only master the normal developmental challenges but also cope with the effects of racism, poverty, violence, and lack of access to educational and economic resources. However, unlike their heterosexual counterparts, African American gay men must manage these developmental tasks with the additional burden of the homophobic responses of both the Anglo-American majority culture and the African American community.

The stresses inherent in living with human immunodeficiency virus (HIV) infection further challenge the flexibility and strength of the African American gay man's normal personality and defenses. The social sequelae of HIV infection may erode basic life supports and isolate these men from interpersonal support. High rates of substance abuse, victimization, and unemployment may make these issues important in the psychotherapy of some African American men.

In this chapter, I address these issues in the context of evaluation and treatment of HIV-positive African American gay men. I discuss practice models, as well as issues related to delivery of services and case management.

Cultural Context

African American men are presented with social and economic challenges that greatly impact their lives and make their day-to-day experiences different from those of other American men. African American men, regardless of their sexual orientation, are four times more likely than other American men to be raised in families with incomes below the poverty line, seven times more likely to die as the result of homicide, and three times more likely to be unemployed. Although African Americans make up only 12% of the population, they comprise 47% of all prisoners incarcerated and 28% of all deaths from acquired immunodeficiency syndrome (AIDS)–related illnesses (U.S. Department of Commerce 1990). These realities add a great deal of stress to the lives of African American men, influencing the kind of opportunities they experience and their perception of possible life choices.

Within the African American community, an African American boy may have both positive role models (e.g., father, neighbor, community leader) and other, somewhat more complicated role models (e.g., the street hustler, gangster, drug dealer). Although these less-than-ideal, aggressively heterosexual images are derogated by most of the African American community, for many African American adolescents they may embody personal power and an unwillingness to submit to domination by the larger non–African American culture and its supporting social structures.

Available models of gay men either are white and predominately middle class or are derogatory stereotypes of African American gay men. In the absence of positive African American models of healthy gay relationships, African American men must invent their own roles, develop a strong personal identity, and find ways to establish relationships with other African Americans.

African Americans place high value on positive relationships with other African Americans, and regard intimate relationships with those outside their culture with suspicion. Consequently, any African American man who has an intimate relationship with a non–African American is likely to experience criticism from family, friends, or other members of the community. Because these values are internalized throughout a lifetime, those gay African Americans for whom all or part of their intimate relationship experiences occurs in the largely white gay community will experience significant conflict in the process of reconciling the contrasting values and life-styles of both communities and in negotiating conflicting allegiances to the ethnic community and to the gay community (Morales 1990). Many African Americans tend to assign to non–African Americans the responsibility for events or attributes negatively valued by the African American community. It is not unusual to hear heterosexual African Americans describe homosexuality as originating with and "belonging" to non–African Americans and homosexual African Americans being described as not really African American (Fullilove 1989).

Because African Americans maintain close family bonds throughout their lifetime, have fairly frequent contact with kin, and use kinship networks as one of the most important resources for interpersonal and financial support, rejection by their family may have a devastating impact on them (Mays and Cochran 1987). African American gay men who are rejected by their families because of homophobia or fears related to HIV transmission may be much more profoundly isolated than their non–African American counterparts who experience similar rejection. African American gay men may not feel comfortable using resources available to non–African American gay men, and may not feel accepted in the larger, predominately non–African American gay community. Many report feeling quite isolated in largely white support groups for HIV-infected gay men unless there are other African Americans also present.

The combination of racism in the larger American community and homophobic attitudes within the African American community presents difficult choices for African American gay men. By openly identifying themselves as gay in the their own community, African American gay men risk rejection, isolation, or even physical assault by other African Americans. By concealing their gay identity, they continually risk disclosure, and struggle with an inner experience of devaluation and alienation. African American men are often quite open and casual in their denunciation of homosexuality, and among themselves routinely use pejorative labels of gay men to indicate undesirable personal characteristics, such as physical or sexual cowardice, weakness, or incompetence (Fullilove 1989).

Despite these attitudes, African Americans have maintained an ambivalent relationship with their gay and lesbian kin. On the one hand, there may be a certain degree of acceptance and even tacit approval: same-sex "friends" may be occasionally invited to family functions, and friends and family may collude to avoid addressing an individual's sexual orientation or openly expressing their feelings about the matter. On the other hand, there is little tolerance for discussion of homosexuality and little opportunity for open acknowledgment of an individual's sexual orientation (Sullivan 1990). Gays and lesbians tacitly agree not to speak of their sexual preference or of their relationships; silence is the price of acceptance (Dalton 1989).

In the face of these powerful messages, most African American gay men conceal their sexual orientation, and many split off their same-sex attractions and behavior from their sense of personal identity. Many marry and then have same-sex relationships outside of the marital relationship; such men may consider themselves bisexual, heterosexual, or homosexual. Others may not seek to establish enduring same-sex intimate relationships, and may rely on a series of relatively brief relationships or on anonymous sexual partners to meet their sexual needs, turning to friends for relational and intimacy needs. Still other gay African American men may establish long-term live-in relationships. Those who can establish a close and stable circle of African American gay friends experience less isolation, although they are rarely out to the larger African American community.

Adding to the complexities of possible relational patterns found among African American gay men is the cultural heterogeneity of the African American communities. In most such communities one finds both families who are beset by poverty and middle-class families with greater access to educational, economic, and social resources. Families may be only one generation away from the rural life of a sharecropper or may have been part of an urban life-style for several generations. Community standards of masculine identity and attitudes about homosexuality will be interpreted quite differently by a second-generation Trinidadian African American gay man growing up in New York City and an African American gay man growing up in a small town in North Carolina. The relational patterns adopted by individuals are creative resolutions of the conflicts engendered by the need to integrate to some degree a set of powerfully stigmatized self-images and to retain a sense of connection to significant community roles, expectations, and institutions.

The more visible African American gay men are more likely to be middle class, to be allied with the white gay community, and to form social networks that are racially integrated. This may lead to the assumption that African American gay men are more like their white gay counterparts than they are like the majority of African American men. African American gay men who come out in the public sense usually do so only after distancing themselves from the African American community. Some strongly identify with the gay community, but find themselves isolated as one of a few African American men in an essentially non–African American social environment. African American gay men report frequent experiences of racist behavior in gay bars and other predominantly white gay social settings (DeMarco 1983). Non–African American gay men may respond to gay African Americans out of stereotyped beliefs about African American men and their sexuality, and may only be willing to relate to them in narrow and highly sexualized roles. Other African American gay men remain closeted within the African American community and may socialize within that community through a network of men's social clubs and bars known to be meeting places for African American gay men but which are otherwise indistinguishable from straight clubs. The African American church has traditionally been an important social support for African American gay men, provided they maintain the pretense of heterosexuality. Few African American churches openly tolerate gay or lesbian members.

Gay African American Adolescents

Most gay African American adolescents are indistinguishable from their heterosexual peers in appearance and behavior. They may be involved in a variety of community activities and organizations, both positive and negative. Like male adolescents from other ethnic groups, African American youths experiment with both heterosexuality and homosexuality.

A significant problem for gay adolescents of all ethnic groups is the issue of reasonably safe access to other gay adolescents and to older gay role models. Although some adolescents may be befriended by older gay men who act as gay mentors, providing guidance and protection, other adolescents may be preyed upon by both gay and heterosexual men. Gay adolescents below the legal drinking age are often admitted to gay bars, where they may be exposed to drugs, heavy drinking, and sexual relationships with men much older than themselves. Adolescents may frequent well-known cruising areas, thereby placing themselves at increased risk for sexually transmitted diseases and violence.

Easy access to alcohol and other drugs during an important developmental period so complicated by conflicting value systems, economic oppression, racism, and homophobia, places an adolescent at extremely high risk for problems with substance abuse. In studies of the drinking behavior of African American men, it has been reported that heavy drinking may begin as early as age 12 or 13 (Robin et al. 1984). In 1988 Baker noted that, among African American men between the ages of 25 and 34, the rate of deaths caused by cirrhosis was 10 times as high as that for white men in the same age bracket. Because 15–25 years of heavy drinking are usually required to produce a severely cirrhotic liver, adolescence emerges as a critical time for both the initiation of problem-drinking patterns and for opportunities for intervention (Baker 1988).

Gay adolescents who are alienated from their families either because of their homosexuality or for other reasons may become homeless. Many homeless youths, both gay and straight, use drugs and alcohol to manage the stresses inherent in living in the streets. Drug and alcohol dependency can induce a youth to continue earning money in the streets, often through prostitution. Such a life-style greatly increases the likelihood of HIV infection and other sexually transmitted diseases. African American gay men who may have spent some part of their adolescence involved in prostitution or drug-related activities often avoid addressing these events in their lives.

Prevention of HIV Infection

African American men, regardless of their sexual orientation, use a wide network of interpersonal contacts for assistance and information, including the doctor's office, church, social clubs, and barbershops, and frequently turn to close male friends and relatives (Jones and Gray 1983). African American gay men who attempt to educate themselves about HIV infection and its prevention frequently encounter educational and economic barriers in finding such information. For example, African American gay men who are middle class and integrated into the predominantly white gay community are most likely to have had extended exposure to information presented in a wide variety of formats: printed materials, videos, television announcements, plays, movies, and lectures (AIDS Action Committee 1991). In contrast, African American gay men who are not part of the so-called gay community may have limited access to information, may receive nonspecific information (e.g., public service announcements), or may have literacy problems, which further limit their access to available information. Homophobic attitudes in the African American community often prevent access to detailed and specific information about sexual transmission of HIV, even in educational programs designed to reach African American men.

There is a wealth of specific information provided to African American drug users regarding the need for clean needles, but almost none available regarding risk reduction in oral or anal sex. As a result, African American gay men have been found to be less well informed about HIV infection, AIDS, and reducing their risk to these than African American drug users (Peterson and Marin 1988).

Young African American gay men may experiment with behavior that places them at increased risk for HIV infection at fairly young ages. A young man may not have access to appropriate information or may not perceive that the information has any relevance to his own behavior. Adolescents often use denial to manage anxiety and ambivalence, and so literally may not remember having engaged in certain behaviors. Many African American men who become symptomatic in their 20s may have been exposed to the disease in their early- to middle-teenage years. When we consider that most HIV prevention programs have been aimed at older teenagers and even then have been quite constrained in the material they present and the kind of language permitted, it is evident that our prevention and outreach efforts have not taken sufficient advantage of what we know about adolescent sexuality or behavior. In addition, young African American men may resist messages that are seen as intrusions by the institutions of the majority culture into the private realm of sexuality.

All health and mental health providers should receive in-service training on strategies for reducing the risk of HIV infection, have some knowledge of how the virus functions, and be reasonably knowledge-able about community resources and services (Peterson and Marin 1988). Such an approach enables providers to answer basic questions and provide sensitive referrals when appropriate. African American physicians in particular should be aware of their own avoidance of topics related to homosexuality, as many African American gay men will attempt to assess their physician's attitudes before asking openly for needed information. A physician's silence or failure to include questions about sexual orientation may serve as an unspoken warning to the patient not to discuss issues related to sexual orientation (Butts 1988). African American physicians may treat patients for years and never know they are gay or bisexual, thereby robbing the patient of an opportunity for education and counseling about risk reduction and early intervention.

Treatment Considerations

Cultural and Socioeconomic Issues

African American gay men struggle with the same anxiety, depression, fearfulness, and anger described by observers of white gay persons who are HIV infected. Nichols (1985), Ostrow et. al (1988), and Forstein (1984) have described some of the symptomatology com-monly presented by HIV-positive individuals seeking mental health services. African American gay men do not differ significantly in the symptoms they experience at different phases of illness, but bring to the therapeutic encounter a very different world view; different views about psychotherapeutic, psychological, and interpersonal strategies; and different ways of relating to the world and to other people. These differences can profoundly affect the success or failure of psychother-apy with African American men who are HIV positive.

Economics and a lack of health insurance are both factors that prevent African American men from seeking routine or preventive health care and that increase their reliance on emergency rooms (Neighbors 1988). Even when care is delivered in the physician's office or neighborhood health center, African American men are more likely to use health services for urgent requests, thus making education and counseling difficult.

The African American gay man who presents for psychotherapy may have developed a profound distrust of white individuals in an effort to protect himself against physical assault, slander, humiliation, and mistreatment (Grier and Cobbs 1980). Individuals and institutions identified with the majority American culture must prove themselves in his eyes. For most African American men to enter a majority-culture institution with trust, openness, and an eagerness to self-disclose would require so profound a denial of the African American experience that the very denial would be pathological in itself. An African American man must be convinced that he will be treated with respect and courtesy and that his needs will be taken seriously.

African American gay men live in a cultural milieu in which they can neither take for granted that others will behave towards them with common courtesy nor assume that even those whose task it is to be helpful can be trusted to do so. Negotiating such difficult interpersonal terrain requires the patient to maintain a high degree of vigilance and constrain expression of dependency needs until a certain level of safety is experienced. As a result, African Americans have raised to an art form the ability to be "cool": to not express one's true thoughts, needs, or opinions, and yet give the appearance of being fully engaged in the interaction. It is not at all uncommon for African American men to consult with a health or mental health provider and seem quite calm, collected, and generally in control. Such an initial presentation may be quite at odds with inner feelings of extreme conflict, overwhelming anxiety or depression, or fears of loss of control (Grier and Cobbs 1980). The ability to maintain one's "cool" may also be linked to a certain view of one's self in such a way that showing vulnerability, especially to a stranger, may represent an injury to self-esteem. Individuals may adopt interpersonal stances of autonomy and isolation as a defense against overwhelming fears of abandonment (Pinderhughes

1982). It is important that clinicians exercise patience in the initial evaluation of an African American gay man to avoid underestimating the degree of his distress. African American men may refer to their own distress with a self-deprecating humor that obscures the intensity of their pain, or use anger, belligerence, or derogation both to conceal their true distress and as an unconscious acting out of their own fears of encountering a hostile or indifferent reception. As illustrated in the following case example, African American gay patients may resist full participation in an evaluation process.

Case 1

Mr. A, a 46-year-old African American man, was referred by his internist for evaluation after he refused further treatment for AIDS-related illnesses. Mr. A had been evaluated by two different psychiatrists, both European Americans, within the previous 2 months. In both interviews, Mr. A had presented as a calm, intelligent, appropriately dressed man who seemed depressed, although he denied vegetative symptoms. On both occasions Mr. A reported sadness related to the death the year before of his lover of 10 years. He stated that he felt that he was handling things well, functioned in a reasonable way, and felt the quality of his life was good. He said that he wished no further treatment because he understood that treatment could prolong his life but could not save it. Mr. A denied suicidality and refused antidepressants. Both of the clinicians who interviewed Mr. A felt that they had made a good connection with him, and expressed some surprise that, despite outreach, he had not followed up in treatment.

Mr. A's third interview with a mental health practitioner was with an African American social worker. During that evaluation, Mr. A expressed relief at having an opportunity to talk with an African American clinician. He described extreme depression and a persistent and overwhelming wish to die and rejoin his lost lover. He reported loss of appetite, inability to rise out of bed in the mornings, and extreme tearfulness. In response to the social worker's inquiry, Mr. A reported that these symptoms had been present at the time of his first two evaluations, but that he distrusted the motives of the clinicians and did not feel comfortable in opening up to them. It is significant that Mr. A could name no behavior on the clinicians' part that led to his feeling; he described them both as kind, empathic, sensitive, and apparently knowledgeable. It was the fact of their being European American that made them untrustworthy. After several sessions of focusing on the experience of losing his lover, Mr. A accepted the social worker's recommendation that he begin antidepressant medication; following this, his depressive symptoms improved.

Internalized Anger

Few adult gay men or lesbians are free of internalized homophobia (Cabaj 1988), and early, negative images of the gay self may surface during times of psychological crises. An individual may have reached a comfortable resolution of earlier conflicts about homosexuality, but experience a reemergence of these issues under the stress of HIV-related concerns. These feelings are often accompanied by both guilt and shame and should be understood in the context of a reactivation of old conflicts occurring under stress. Gay patients will often express surprise at reexperiencing conflicts they had believed to be settled long ago, and may require assistance in working through such conflicts.

The management of anger in assessment and psychotherapy often becomes difficult for both patients and therapists. So many stereotypes present the image of the angry African American man as being in poor control of his impulses that both the therapist and the patient may find themselves reacting to internalized stereotypes (Jones and Gray 1983). Patients may suppress or deny their angry feelings, either in an effort to avoid seeing themselves in this stereotyped view or as a projection of fear of their own anger, including the feeling that the therapist could not tolerate the open expression of anger. Other patients may express their anger in a dramatic, confrontational, or threatening manner, thereby distancing others. Clinicians may project anger onto the patient or project their own conflicts regarding anger onto the patient. Because intense feelings of anger are a common response to the experience of living with HIV-related illnesses, it is critical that issues relating to the internalization or expression of anger be confronted and worked through in the treatment. Clinicians should use supervision to assist them in working through their own feelings and their unconscious stereotypes of African American men and their anger. Case 2 illustrates a patient's use of a demanding confrontational style as an attempt to ward off powerful feelings of shame.

Case 2

Mr. B, a 44-year-old African American gay man, presented as an emergency referral after several heated conversations with triage staff in which he demanded an appointment with a clinician who was an "expert on black men's issues." In the initial interview with an African American female therapist, he continued repeating this demand and, on being asked to elaborate, stated that he was not "one of those tame black men who'll take any old thing." He was finally able to say that he feared being misunderstood and that he felt like he wanted to kill someone. When the therapist offered an interpretation that he may have been feeling out of control and feared that the staff might see him as a berserk animal rather than as a man in intolerable pain, Mr. B began to cry and left the office. He returned almost immediately. He then cried openly and began to describe how difficult it was for him to disclose to anyone that he was gay and had recently discovered that he was HIV positive. In subsequent sessions, Mr. B revealed that he had not really feared his homicidal impulses, recognizing them as expressions of distress, but that he had feared that staff might have dismissed him as a "hysterical sissy" if he had come in crying openly.

Although Mr. B's presentation was much more dramatic than is typical, his dilemma of seeking help for himself while concealing his vulnerability is often seen in clinical practice with African American men. In the example of Mr. B we may also see the effects of his internalized homophobia, projected outward. Mr. B had reached a partial resolution of his conflicts around being gay, but under the stress of learning about his HIV status, early, negative images of gay men again surfaced, expressed in his fear of being seen as a sissy or as looking "too gay."

Countertransference Reactions

Countertransference reactions on the part of the clinicians working with African American gay men also contribute to problems in the psychotherapeutic relationship. Clinicians who are themselves gay may overidentify with the patient or project onto the patient their own fears or wishes (Dunkel and Hatfield 1986). When patients are racially different, clinicians may project onto the patients their own racial stereotypes, and may develop either extremely warm feelings toward a patient, grounded in positive stereotypes, or hostile feelings, grounded in negative stereotypes. Both types of responses create problems as they are not authentic responses to the individual but responses to what the clinician believes about an entire class of people.

Gay clinicians, regardless of ethnicity, who have struggled to come to terms with their own homosexuality and have become open about their gay identity may be intolerant of the African American gay patient who states that he is bisexual or even heterosexual. The African American gay patient may be seen as denying his "real" identity and may arouse in the clinician unconscious feelings of ambivalence around the clinician's own life choices. Therapists may have trouble understanding these self-labels as compromises between conflicting value systems and identifications. Non–African American gay clinicians may err by assuming that trust and rapport exist, based on a shared sexual orientation or life-style. Although this common bond may help ease an individual's anxiety, it probably has little impact on the awareness of the racial differences between the clinician and the patient. A premature assumption of intimacy may actually have the effect of causing the patient to retreat emotionally, as illustrated in Case 3.

Case 3

Mr. C, a 28-year-old African American gay man, consulted an openly gay European American clinician after experiencing several panic episodes that he related to the progression of his HIV status from being asymptomatic to symptomatic. He described the first interview as comfortable, but described increasing discomfort in the next two interviews. He described the therapist as "talking to me as if he had known me forever and knew all about me" and making many assumptions about a shared experience of being gay. Mr. C experienced resentment and anxiety in response to feeling as if his identity as an African American man was being rendered invisible. Mr. C accepted a fourth appointment but did not keep it and dropped out of treatment. Three months later, recurrent episodes of panic resulted in Mr. C's seeking care at a local hospital emergency room where he accepted a referral to a different clinician.

Ethnic minority clinicians are not exempt from troublesome countertransference reactions. African American heterosexual clinicians may have difficulty in accepting the gay or bisexual patient or may find that after years of receiving subtle messages enforcing a kind of silence around issues of sexual orientation, it is extremely difficult to comfortably discuss sexuality, relationships, or other areas directly related to sexual orientation. Some therapists will use denial, asserting that the gay patient is just like other heterosexual patients, and actively avoid any discussion of these issues. Ethnic minority clinicians may experience conflict between their roles as representatives of the majority culture institutions that may employ them and their membership in a disempowered ethnic community (Fernando 1988). These conflicting allegiances may be played out in the relationship between the therapist and the patient, and sometimes result in either a blurring of boundaries and limits of the therapeutic relationship or the therapist's inappropriate use of the power imbalances between patient and therapist to distance the patient in order to affirm his or her status or to control the patient's behavior. Case 4 illustrates the complex interplay of transferential and countertransferential responses.

Case 4

An African American heterosexual male psychiatrist sought consultation to assist him in his work with Mr. D, a 41-year-old African American bisexual man who had been diagnosed as being HIV positive a year earlier. Both the physician and the patient were interviewed. Mr. D was married and had an 8-year-old son. For most of his adult life he had had male lovers, although he maintained that his relationship with his wife was the "important one." He had disclosed his bisexuality to his therapist about 6 months before the consultation.

The psychiatrist felt that a reasonable amount of time had been spent in exploring the patient's sexual attractions to men and felt the patient was resisting moving on to the core issues of his fears of intimacy with women. The psychiatrist openly acknowledged that he had little experience in working with gay or bisexual men and reported that, although he found Mr. D quite likable and engaging, he also found himself feeling increasingly uncomfortable with what he saw as the patient's increasingly graphic and explicit descriptions of his sexual relationships with men. The psychiatrist noted that he had found many parallels among Mr. D's experiences as an African American man, and experienced a positive empathic connection in his work with him. At this point in the treatment, however, he wondered whether he should set firmer limits in the treatment or even offer to terminate treatment to test the patient's motivation.

Mr. D described feeling angry at his therapist for refusing to explore his sexual conflicts with him. He was struggling with profound guilt regarding the probability that his pattern of becoming intoxicated, picking up a stranger in a cruising area, and having unprotected sex with him was the route of his becoming infected with HIV. Mr. D had never reconciled his disdain for gay men with his own need for sexual contact with men. He strongly felt that receptive anal sex was for "real sissies," whom he disparaged, and had difficulty acknowledging that he enjoyed it, even when it emerged that receptive anal sex was a usual part of his sexual activities with men. Mr. D was not conscious of the ways in which his description of sex in his sessions was serving as a distancing strategy; he relentlessly described to the psychiatrist the details of his sexual encounters but avoided addressing any of his feelings about these experiences. Mr. D projected onto the psychiatrist his view of himself as a "weakling," describing him as somebody who "just couldn't handle it." Mr. D had not yet begun to acknowledge his growing wish to have the psychiatrist's respect or his wish to be close to and trust his therapist.

The psychiatrist responded with withdrawal and anger to the unconscious distancing of his patient and was uncomfortable with his growing positive feelings about Mr. D. Although he had correctly identified conflicts around intimacy as a core issue, the complexity of his own feelings toward Mr. D and the content of the sessions made it difficult for the psychiatrist to recognize this issue when it emerged in the transference or in Mr. D's attempts to address his conflicts around sexual intimacy with his male sexual partners. The role of Mr. D's use of alcohol to defend against these conflicts had not yet emerged as a treatment focus.

Models of Care

Traditional psychotherapeutic models of care tend to isolate the therapist from other caregivers and from the patient's psychosocial network. Generally, therapists tend not to become involved in the medical care of their patients and, except in the case of patients with disabling major mental illnesses, often have little contact with spouses, lovers, or family members. On the other hand, the traditional models of care among social workers are flexible enough to be ideal for caring for HIV-positive individuals. Social workers are more likely to feel comfortable in using a variety of treatment formats with an individual; family, couples, and individual treatment modalities may be combined with assistance in providing linkages to social services, medical care, and financial assistance.

In working with HIV-positive individuals, treatment typically begins with an assessment of the individual. When individuals are relatively healthy and asymptomatic, individual psychotherapy that takes place in the clinic or private office may be appropriate and sufficient. As the disease progresses, relationship issues may emerge that require some couples or family intervention. A willingness on the part of the clinician to provide an evaluation and assist in referral often greatly increases the African American man's willingness to comply with treatment recommendations. Receiving information, recommendations, and assistance from an individual known to the patient provides a psychological parallel to the ways in which African Americans traditionally use kinship and community networks.

Therapists working with HIV-positive African American gay men would do well to become reasonably knowledgeable about community networks and social services and to develop professional relationships with colleagues working in those areas. For therapists in private practice, the problems of loss of employment, reduced income, or loss of insurance are likely to become issues at some point, particularly given that African American men are more likely to be marginally employed or underemployed. Therapists who work in neighborhood health care networks often find that changing eligibility requirements interrupt treatment or limit treatment options.

HIV-positive patients generally must receive care from an increasing number of health care providers, particularly as their condition progresses from being asymptomatic to having frequent and often disabling opportunistic infections. Often the psychotherapist is in a position to observe important changes in the patient's physical or mental status. The therapist may have known the patient longer and have had more frequent opportunities to observe the patient than many of the specialists who see the patient intermittently or who have not known the patient well enough to see more gradual changes. Changes in gait, speech, cognition, or mood and affect are not always a result of stress. Clinicians should review the elements of the traditional neuropsychiatric mental status exam and be alert to subtle changes that are often overlooked (Tross and Hirsch 1988). Whenever possible, the therapist should seek the patient's permission to establish and maintain contact with key medical and social services providers as such communications often result in more comprehensive care and better coordination of treatment and services. This approach also greatly aids the caregiver by creating a team of providers who share the emotional burden of caring for very ill patients, thus mitigating the effects of stress on providers.

Summary

In addition to the predictable responses of an individual to the various stages of HIV infection, clinicians must be sensitive to the particular psychosocial issues confronting all African American men and African American gay men in particular. All health and mental health providers should receive in-service training in order to have a working knowledge of strategies for preventing HIV infection and of local resources to be able to make appropriate referrals for HIV-infected individuals.

Whenever possible, providers should be in contact with one another and share observations, information, and recommendations for treatment. Therapists should attempt to develop working relationships with professionals in other institutions and social service settings to facilitate the coordination of services and the flow of information between providers and through them to the patient.

Psychotherapists must use supervision and peer support to assist them in exploring their stereotypes of African American gay men and in managing the often complex transference and countertransference issues that are frequently encountered in psychotherapy with African American gay men. Currently very few data are available about African American gay men who live primarily within the African American community. Research initiatives in this area will no doubt be difficult, given the resistance of the African American community to discussing homosexuality, but such efforts are imperative if better prevention and intervention strategies are to be developed.

References

AIDS Action Committee: A Survey of AIDS-Related Knowledge, Attitudes and Behavior Among Gay and Bisexual Men in Greater Boston: A Report to Community Educators. Boston, MA, AIDS Action Committee, 1991

Baker FM: Afro-Americans, in Clinical Guidelines in Cross Cultural Mental Health. Edited by Comas-Diaz L, Griffiths EEH. New York, Wiley, 1988, pp 151–181

Butts JD: Sex, therapy, intimacy and the role of the black physician in the AIDS era. J Ntl Med Assoc 80:919–922, 1988

Cabaj RP: Gay and lesbian couples: lessons on human intimacy. Psychiatric Annals 18:21–25, 1988

Dalton HL: AIDS in black-face. Daedalus 118:205–227, 1989

DeMarco J: Gay racism, in Black Men/White Men: A Gay Anthology. Edited by Smith M. San Francisco, CA, Gay Sunshine Press, 1983, pp 109–118

Dunkel J, Hatfield S: Countertransference issues in working with persons with AIDS. Soc Work 31:114–117, 1986

Fernando S: Race and Culture in Psychiatry. London, Routledge, 1988

Forstein M: The psychosocial impact of the acquired immunodeficiency syndrome. Semin Oncol 11:77–82, 1984

Fullilove M: Social denial: a barrier to halting AIDS. MIRA: Multicultural Inquiry and Research on AIDS 3:5–6, 1989

Grier WH, Cobbs B: Black Rage. New York, Basic Books, 1980

Jones BE, Gray B: Black males and psychotherapy: theoretical issues. Am J Psychother 37:77–85, 1983

Mays VM, Cochran SD: Acquired immunodeficiency syndrome and black Americans: special psychosocial issues. Public Health Rep 102:224–231, 1987

Morales ES: Ethnic minority families and minority gays and lesbians, in Homosexuality and Family Relations. New York, Harrington Park Press, 1990, pp 217–239

Neighbors HW: The help-seeking behavior of black Americans. J Ntl Med Assoc 80:1009–1012, 1988

Nichols S: Psychosocial reactions of persons with the acquired immunodeficiency syndrome. Ann Intern Med 103:765–767, 1985

Ostrow D, Grant I, Atkinson H: Assessment and management of AIDS patient with neuropsychiatric disturbances. J Clin Psychiatry 49:14–22, 1988

Peterson JL, Marin G: Issues in the prevention of AIDS among black and Hispanic men. Am Psychol 43:871–877, 1988

Pinderhughes E: Family functioning of Afro-Americans. Soc Work 27:91–96, 1982

Robin LN, Murphy GE, Breckenridge MD: Drinking behavior of young Negro men. Quarterly Journal of Studies in Alcohol 19:657–684, 1984

Sullivan A: Gay life, gay death. New Republic, December 1990, pp 19–25

Tross S, Hirsch DA: Psychological distress and neuropsychological complications of HIV infection and AIDS. Am Psychol 43:929–934, 1988

U.S. Department of Commerce: Statistical Abstract of the United States: 1990 (110th Edition). Washington, DC, U.S. Department of Commerce, 1990

Chapter 16

Issues in the Psychosocial Care of Latino Gay Men With HIV Infection

José A. Parés-Avila, M.A.
Rubén Montano-López, M.A.

Listen: homesickness can also be a kind of consolation, a sweet sadness, a way of seeing things and even enjoying them. Our triumph is resisting. Our revenge is surviving.

Reinaldo Arenas
End of a Story[1]

Although the volume of literature on the psychosocial aspects of white gay men being human immunodeficiency virus (HIV) positive has grown tremendously, there are very few references to or writings

---

[1] From W. Leyland (ed.): *My Deep Dark Pain is Love: A Collection of Latin American Gay Fiction.* San Francisco, CA, Gay Sunshine Press, 1983. Copyright Estate of Reinaldo Arenas. Used with permission.

The authors gratefully acknowledge the helpful comments provided by Lourdes Argüelles and Carlos Vega-Matos, M.P.A. We dedicate this work to all our Latino/a gay brothers and lesbian sisters living with AIDS and we thank the many friends, patients, and colleagues who have shared their stories with us. They have taught us the importance of *la familia* as a key to surviving in this racist and homophobic society.

about Latino gay men (Carballo-Diéguez 1989; Ceballos-Capitaine et al. 1990; Kaminsky et al. 1990; Morales 1990; Parés-Avila 1989). Before addressing the specific issues surrounding psychosocial care of HIV-positive Latino men, we feel it is important to familiarize the reader with some basic sociodemographic and epidemiological data related to Latinos in the United States and the impact of the acquired immunodeficiency syndrome (AIDS) epidemic on this population. Although an in-depth discussion of this sort is beyond the scope of this chapter, we do intend to offer a common framework from which we may begin to examine the mental health needs of Latino gay men who have been affected by the AIDS epidemic.

Sociodemographic Data

Latinos[2] number approximately 20 million (or 7.25% of the population) in the United States (U.S. Census Bureau 1990). This figure does not include Puerto Ricans who reside on that island or the large number of undocumented Latinos who reside in the United States. It is estimated that 1 in 12 Americans is Latino, and that Latinos constitute the youngest and fastest growing subgroup in the United States (McKay 1988). In fact, it is estimated that by the year 2000 Latinos will be the largest ethnic minority group in this country (Spencer 1986).

Demographic and socioeconomic characteristics of the Latino population indicate that this group is in a highly disadvantaged position in American society. One such indicator is the educational attainment of the Latino population. Whereas over 75% of the United States adult population has obtained at least a high school diploma, only 50% of their Latino counterparts have done so (Institute for Puerto

---

[2] We have chosen the term *Latino* as the term that best reflects the sociopolitical circumstances of all peoples of Latin American origin or ancestry in the United States. The term *Hispanic* was adopted by the federal government in the 1970s and includes European peoples of Spanish origin, who are quite different from peoples of Latin American origin. Because this is not a settled controversy, the reader is referred to Hayes-Bautista and Chapa (1987) and Treviño (1987) for further discussion.

Rican Policy 1990). Moreover, only 8.4% of Latinos are college graduates compared to 20% of whites (McKay 1988). Educational attainment goes hand in hand with other socioeconomic indicators, such as unemployment, underemployment, and living in poverty. The unemployment rate of Latinos is twice as high as that for whites (Institute for Puerto Rican Policy 1990) and those who are employed tend to have low-wage, low-skill jobs (McKay 1988). Nearly 30% of the Latino population live below the poverty rate, compared with only 12% of non-Latinos (Institute for Puerto Rican Policy 1990).

It is important to acknowledge that the terms *Latino* or *Hispanic* are umbrella terms that refer to a highly heterogeneous group. Thus they do not reflect the diversity that exists among Latinos. According to the United States census figures (U.S. Bureau of the Census 1990), 63% of Latinos are of Mexican origin, 12% of Puerto Rican origin, 5% of Cuban origin, and 21% of another Latin American origin. Country of origin or ancestry carries an important historical and sociopolitical significance that greatly influences the demographic and other important characteristics of Latino subgroups. For example, the fact that Cubans tend to be older, be more highly educated, and have a higher income in comparison with the two other largest Latino subgroups in the United States (Mexicans and Puerto Ricans) is a reflection of the sociopolitical climate in the United States when many Cubans migrated following the Cuban Revolution of 1959.

Latinos and AIDS

Health statistics show that Latinos experienced morbidity and mortality greater than that of the general population even before the AIDS epidemic (Hahn and Castro 1989). As of June 1991, 28,831 cases of AIDS had been reported among Latinos (Centers for Disease Control 1991). This amount constitutes over 16% of the total number of AIDS cases and shows a twofold overrepresentation of Latinos in this epidemic in proportion to their representation in the United States population. It is important to know that HIV-positive people of color have a significantly shorter life expectancy than HIV-positive whites. This holds true even after introducing controls for initial diagnosis, date of diagnosis, risk group, and gender (Centers for Disease Control 1986). These striking findings suggest the possibility of differences in disease progression tied to ethnic origin (Ceballos-Capitaine et al. 1990). At this point it is unclear which psychological factors contribute to this rapid progression of the illness. However, we can speculate that Latinos, as a highly disempowered group, feel easily defeated by this diagnosis.

AIDS prevention efforts in Latino communities have focused primarily on needle sharing among intravenous drug users and have tended to overlook homosexual behavior as an equally important mode of transmission. In fact, 40% of AIDS cases in the Latino population are among gay and bisexual males and an additional 6% of the cases are among men who reported both intravenous drug use and homosexual behavior.

The cumulative incidence (CI; i.e., the number of cases per each 100,000 individuals in the United States) of AIDS among Latino gay and bisexual men is 32.1 compared with 19.9 for whites, and their relative risk (RR) is 1.6 times that of whites (Selik et al. 1989). When Selik et al. examined the birthplace of all Latinos diagnosed with AIDS in the United States, they found that foreign-born Latino gay and bisexual men have much higher CI and RR rates than those of United States–born Latinos; the only exception to that finding were Mexicans, who appeared similar to the reference group of non-Latino whites (see Table 16–1). The fact that foreign-born Latinos have a higher risk rate than United States–born Latinos probably means that,

Table 16–1. Cumulative incidence and relative risk rates of different Latino populations for contracting AIDS

Country of origin	Cumulative incidence rate	Relative risk rate
United States	21.7	1.1
Puerto Rico	45.9	2.3
Other Latin American countries	64.9	3.3
Cuba	97.2	4.9

Source. Selik et al. 1989.

although both groups of Latinos face structural barriers to AIDS prevention related to cultural and socioeconomic factors, foreign-born Latinos are the most likely to "fall through the cracks."

Although much more could be said about preventing the spread of HIV infection among Latino gay men, for the remainder of this chapter we focus on the issues that are germane to the psychosocial care of Latino gay men diagnosed with an HIV-related condition. The following sections should assist clinicians in identifying cultural issues relevant in the treatment of Latino gay men. They include a discussion of cultural beliefs and values, views of homosexuality within the Latino culture, and the identity development of Latino gay men as double minorities.

Cultural Beliefs and Values

For Latinos, as with any ethnic group, the patients' cultural context is considered to be a critical factor for the effective delivery of mental health services (Comas-Díaz 1985). Any discussion of Latino cultural issues, however, requires the use of generalizations that may be more appropriate for Latinos as a group rather than as individuals. Hence we must emphasize that our discussion in this chapter does indeed deal with generalizations, but that the accuracy of these generalizations may vary as a result of the acculturation process, individual personality differences, or subgroup variations (B. V. Marín, in press). With this in mind, the following segments are dedicated to the discussion of beliefs and values embraced by most Latinos that distinguish them from other broader ethnic groups.

Familismo and Family Dynamics

Latinos tend to place a strong emphasis on the importance of the family (Carballo-Diéguez 1989; Comas-Díaz 1988). The term *familismo* has been used to describe Latinos' tendency to view the family as a primary source of support (G. Marín 1989). This value emphasizes interdependence, affiliation, and cooperation. These characteristics are frequently interpreted as being reflective of an enmeshed rather than a disengaged family (Arce and Torres-Matrullo 1982). From this viewpoint, dynamics within the Latino family are characterized by overinvolvement, dependence, and discouragement of self-differenti- ation. Be that as it may, Latinos can usually rely on their families in times of crisis as well as during the small emergencies of day-to-day life: grandmothers frequently baby-sit their grandchildren; parents loan money to their adult children; and uncles take their nephews and nieces on field trips. These things are not only common, they are ex- pected. A strong sense of obligation is felt toward the family.

Latinos value their family ties; often these ties extend beyond the immediate family members to include even non–blood-related indi- viduals. One way in which this is achieved is through the system of *compadrazgo*, which refers to the close relationship that is established when a couple participates in the baptism of another couple's child. The couples will refer to each other as *compadres* and *comadres* (co- fathers and comothers) and will assume responsibility for the child's welfare if the biological parents die. At times, the coparent system need not be specifically around the actual baptism of a child but is established on the basis of *buena fe* ("good faith"). Regardless of how the coparent relationship is established, *compadres* traditionally con- sult with each other around family crises and are involved in the fam- ily decision-making process (Comas-Díaz 1989).

Gender Roles

The gender roles and social scripts ascribed to men and women in Latino cultures are traditionally rigid. This inflexibility could suggest that roles and scripts are straightforward and clear, when in actuality they are infinitely complex. The terms *machismo* and *marianismo* are commonly used when describing gender roles in Latino culture. *Ma- chismo* is a complex phenomenon that emphasizes male superiority and the need for the man to appear to be in charge. Although the term may connote a domineering male who is abrasive, possessive, and, at his worst, even abusive, *machismo*, in fact, includes a blend of cultural virtues such as courage, fearlessness, accountability, and leadership. At times, the *macho* may be overbearing and oppressive, but he is also considered the head and protector of his family who is responsible for the family's safety and well-being and the defender of its dignity and honor (Abad et al. 1974). How this ideology translates behaviorally will depend on a number of factors. De La Cancela (1986) suggested that Latino males' own experience of oppression, usually in the form of socioeconomic limitations, defines and molds how machismo becomes manifested in their interpersonal and family relationships. It should be noted that although the *machismo* code places men in a more empowered position than women, it also makes it harder for them to accept help or demonstrate vulnerability, as a *macho* should be self-sufficient and strong.

Marianismo is the female counterpart of *machismo*. It is based on the worship of Mary in the Catholic religion, who is both virgin and madonna. The term connotes the chaste and docile female who is dominated by the men in her life, and whose purpose is to bear children (preferably boys) and be forever self-sacrificing, initially in favor of her family (particularly her father), then her husband, and finally her children. The basis of such self-sacrifice is the *marianista* notion that women are spiritually superior to men and, hence, can endure all suffering inflicted on them by men. This spiritual superiority offers *marianista* women a way (albeit indirect) in which to enjoy greater power (Comas-Díaz 1988). Thus in spite of their outward submissiveness under the *marianista* code, women can be elevated to sanctity and assume indirect power through the sacred responsibilities of motherhood (Bernal and Flores-Ortiz 1984; Comas-Díaz 1988). This notion of the mother as saint is illustrated clearly in the common use of the phrase *mi santa madre* ("my holy mother") in reference to Latina mothers.

Interpersonal Relationships, Communication Styles, and Language

Interpersonal relationships and communication styles among Latinos are heavily influenced by a number of cultural values that are often misinterpreted by non-Latinos (Sluski 1985). Overall, it can be said that Latinos' interpersonal styles are characterized by their placing greater value on cooperation than on competition (Arce and Torres-Matrullo 1982). This is noted in the concept of *personalismo,* which refers to the tendency of Latinos to trust and cooperate with individuals who they know personally and to dislike impersonal and formal structures and institutions. Three other concepts dominate Latinos' social relations: *simpatía* refers to Latinos' preference for smooth social relations based on politeness and respect and the avoidance of confrontation and criticism; *respeto* is the special consideration and respect that should be shown to elder members in the family and authority figures within the community; and *confianza* refers to the notion of trust between individuals that is enhanced by *personalismo* and *simpatía* but which requires time to fully develop. In its absence, intimate topics are usually avoided. These values can be evidenced through a number of nonverbal gestures and cues. For example, silence and lack of eye contact, although frequently interpreted by non-Latinos as indications of withdrawal, are commonly indications of respect and courtesy.

Other important considerations in examining Latinos' interpersonal styles include their notion of time and the personal distance they establish in their interactions. Latinos are known for their flexible understanding of punctuality and their aversion to a hurried pace, especially vis-à-vis their emphasis on warm social relations (G. Marín 1987). An emphasis on saving time versus being cordial is viewed as rudeness and not necessarily as efficiency. Personal space among Latinos is usually closer than among whites. In addition, Latinos tend to touch more frequently than whites. Handshaking, hugging, knee- and backslapping, rib nudging, and cheek kissing are frequently observed among Latinos.

Regarding language, Spanish is standard in Latin American countries, with the exception of Brazil, the Guyanas, and other Caribbean nations. However, although Spanish is a unifying force among Latinos, it has been modified by other languages in different countries (e.g., by indigenous influences in Mexico and other Central and South American countries, and by the language of the Yoruba and other African peoples in Puerto Rico, Cuba, the Dominican Republic, and other Caribbean regions of Latin America [Bernal and Flores-Ortiz 1984]). The particular blend of indigenous African and European influences varies from country to country; it accounts, in part, for the richness and diversity that Spanish has achieved in the Americas and the Caribbean. It is in the United States that the different accents, nuances, and linguistic regionalisms intersect. In spite of the English-only initiatives in many states and jurisdictions across the United States, it is the fourth largest Spanish-speaking country in the Americas. It is estimated that between 30% and 60% of Latinos in the United States speak only Spanish or prefer to speak Spanish at home (U.S. Bureau of the Census 1983).

Religion and Folk Beliefs

Although Catholicism is the predominant religion among Latinos, religious diversity is noted in the significant presence of Protestants, Pentecostals, and Jehovah's Witnesses, as well as followers of other evangelical and fundamentalist faiths throughout Latin America. Regardless of their particular religious affiliation, Latinos place a high value on spiritual matters (Comas-Díaz 1985). Furthermore, Latinos seek both spiritual and social support through the church, which frequently serves as a substitute for or complement to the extended family.

Concomitant to their religiousness, many Latinos believe in folk healing, which is practiced in a variety of ways among different Latino subgroups. One folk healing system, *Curanderism,* is more common among Latinos originally from countries with stronger indigenous influences, such as Mexico. The *curanderos* use prayers, massages, and herbs to cure physical, spiritual, and emotional ailments. Their healing abilities are considered a gift from God (Maduro 1983). *Santería* is a belief system common among Cubans and other people from the Caribbean. It combines Yoruban deities introduced by African slaves with the Catholic saints, and blends pagan and Catholic beliefs and rituals. Through its practice, the believer seeks divine intervention by way of prayer, the use of amulets and charms, and devotion to a particular saint or deity.

Espiritismo is a belief system common among Puerto Ricans and other Latinos that has been described by its major proponent, Allan Kardec, as "the science that deals with the nature, origin and destiny of the spirits, and with their relationship with the material world" (Machuca 1982). *Espiritismo* postulates that the spirits of the dead, whether of religious or "common" individuals, manifest themselves to and intervene with the living. Through the practice of this belief system, the *espiritista*, who is deemed to possess *facultades* (mediumistic faculties), has *la misión* of helping others with their dilemmas in love and interpersonal affairs, as well as in their physical and mental health problems. This is achieved through communications and negotiations with the intervening spirit or spirits.

Awareness of religious and folk healing practices among Latinos is extremely important to a clinician attempting to work with this group (Abad et al. 1974). The culturally sensitive clinician respects the manner in which Latinos meet their spiritual needs, whether that is through an affiliation with the more formal religions or an adherence to some form of a folk-healing belief system.

Homosexuality and Latino Culture

To date, there is a dearth of empirical data on homosexual behavior among Latino men in the literature on homosexuality in the United States (Amaro et al. 1989). For example, the most comprehensive data set on homosexuality in the United States (Bell and Weinberg 1978) did not include Latinos. Most of the literature available on male homosexuality among Latinos comes from anthropological field studies conducted in Mexico and other Latin American countries (e.g., see Carrier 1976, 1985). Many of these studies have described what is known as the *gender-defined organization of homosexuality* in which sexual behavior mirrors heterosexual norms (i.e., one partner is passive and the other is active). In sexual exchanges or relationships, only the passive partner identifies himself as homosexual whereas the active partner identifies himself as heterosexual and leads an otherwise heterosexual life-style. Thus the active partner is neither labeled nor stigmatized because what becomes stigmatized is the cross-gender behavior (i.e., being the receptive partner). This interpretation is questionable because there is no evidence that the active homosexual role is accepted among Latinos. Rather, the active partner's identification with a heterosexual life-style despite his bisexual behavior may reflect the active partner's mechanism for coping with homophobia in his community of origin.

The conclusions reached in these anthropological studies should be read with caution. Speculations about the influence of Latino culture on homosexual behavior and a gay life-style need to integrate other aspects of the life of Latino men in the United States. Although cultural values, beliefs, and attitudes play an important role, the depiction of homosexuality in Latin America does not apply entirely to Latino men who were either born and raised in the United States or who migrated to the United States after spending their formative years in their countries of origin.

The impact the dominant Caucasian culture has on the attitudes, beliefs, and behaviors of Latino gay men in the United States raises a number of relevant questions for researchers and clinicians. Some of these questions have been explored by Carrier and Magaña (1991) in their ethnographic fieldwork conducted with Mexican-born and Mexican American gay men in Orange County, California. They found that the sexual behavior of Mexican male immigrants can be modified through contact with the Caucasian culture. However, many men continue to show behaviors patterned after their prior experiences in Mexico. These researchers concluded that such selective acculturation varies according to where the adolescent socialization took place. More variability was observed among Mexican American males. Once again, adolescent socialization seemed to determine choice of partners (i.e., whether Mexican or Caucasian) and sexual behavior. In another study in which focus groups were conducted with Latino gay men, Sabogal and Otero-Sabogal (1990) explored the role of acculturation on gay life-style. The group of Latino gay men from San Francisco they studied acknowledged that their sexual behavior was more conservative when they were in their countries of origin.

It is important to note that all of these data come from Mexico or California where most Latino gay men are of Mexican origin or ancestry. We should be cautious in generalizing these findings to all Latino gay men, and should assume that less traditional Latino men may not fit the gender-defined dichotomy of homosexuality. Important differences exist between men of Caribbean origin (e.g., Puerto Ricans, Cubans, Dominicans) and men of Mexican, Central American, and South American origin or ancestry. Although these differences have not been studied systematically, we can deduce from clinical and anecdotal data

that Latino men of Caribbean origin do not necessarily fit the dichot-
omous model. For example, although the gay community in Puerto
Rico does not have the level of political organization seen in urban gay
communities across the United States, the availability of outlets for
gay socialization there (e.g., bars, discos) has resulted in more diverse
social and sexual relationships that go beyond the traditional roles
described in the literature. This is one example in which a Puerto
Rican–born gay man may be significantly different from a gay man
raised in a more conservative Latin American country.

Issues of Identity Development in Latino Gay Men

Clinicians working with Latino gay men must also consider the impact the oppression these men face as ethnic and sexual minorities has
on their identity development. We are fortunate to have a growing
body of literature by several gay and lesbian scholars of color based
on their clinical experience and theoretical thinking on the topic (de
Monteflores 1986; Espín 1984, 1987; Gock 1986; Morales 1983).

Latino gay men face the developmental task of integrating and
embracing aspects of the self that are stigmatized by the dominant
culture as well as by the culture of their communities of origin. They
must deal with coming out or remaining closeted within a homophobic Latino community that is caught up in its own struggle for preser-
vation in a racist and class-conscious society. For some, the natural
choice is to seek refuge and gain acceptance within the gay community. However, they quickly find themselves "between a rock and a
hard place" when they realize that the racism and classism seen in
society at large permeate the values and attitudes of the mainstream
gay community. Others may choose to lead a more closeted gay life-
style in order to protect their ties to their families and the Latino community. Such is the choice of many Latino gay men who give priority
to investing their energy and talents in causes that affect the Latino
community at large. These men may have a more marginal relationship with the Caucasian gay community through participation in its
social structures (e.g., going to gay bars) but limited participation in

its political structures. These men are perceived by the Caucasian gay community as being "too closeted" for the advancement of gay civil rights. Thus Latino gay men constantly face an array of difficult dilemmas and choices. In the social and interpersonal arenas, they have to choose or go back and forth between opposing cultures in order to satisfy their needs for friendships, love, nurturance, and intimacy. In the political arena, Latino rights and gay civil rights pull the Latino gay man from opposite sides. Morales (1983) has called this issue the *conflict of allegiance*. He described the perceived choice as one between the gay community as a source for satisfying one's need for intimacy or an ethnic community as a source of emotional and cultural grounding.

Because an in-depth discussion of the theoretical aspects of identity development is beyond the scope of this chapter, we refer the reader to the work of two Latina lesbian scholars and clinicians: Espín (1987) and de Monteflores (1986). In her work, Espín integrated and looked at the parallels between Atkinson's model of minority identity development and Cass's model of homosexual identity development (see Espín 1987). Both of these models look at the integration of negative aspects of the self. However, Atkinson's model refers to an *ascribed label* (e.g., being different from the dominant culture because of one's race and ethnicity) whereas Cass's takes into consideration a *chosen label* (e.g., choosing by the act of coming out to the self).

Regardless of whether the labels are ascribed or chosen, both of these models propose a series of developmental stages that may not necessarily be linear. In the initial stages, individuals take on traits and values from the dominant group (a practice call *passing*), and their attitude toward themselves and their reference group may be one of depreciation. De Monteflores (1986) stated that individuals in this stage of assimilation use passing as the main coping device. Feelings of self-betrayal may accompany this stage. The next stages involve resistance and rejection of the dominant culture, and may involve intense feelings of separatism and the establishment of strict psychological and possibly geographic boundaries (e.g., ghettoization). The later stages involve a more integrated sense of self through which one can value one's own culture and survive in the dominant culture without paying the price of denying any of the stigmatized aspects of the self. There is a greater ability to recognize sameness and difference, and the attitude toward the dominant group is one of selective appreciation (de Monteflores 1986; Espín 1987). Gock (1986) argued that the resolution of these developmental tasks is fluid and never totally complete. An awareness and understanding of these issues of identity development are critical for effective delivery of mental health services to Latino gay men affected by HIV, who serve as a double minority.

Implications for Assessment and Treatment

In this section we provide the reader with guidelines and suggestions that may be useful in providing competent and sensitive care to Latino gay men. Making assumptions solely on the patient's ethnicity may constitute insensitivity on the clinician's part. The challenge presented to the clinician is to bring into his or her practice a set of skills that would establish an atmosphere of cultural sensitivity as well as a gay-affirmative stance.

When initiating work with a Latino gay patient, standard assessment procedures should be used in gathering data. However, there are several critical areas that must be explored in order to ensure the gathering of a thorough psychosocial and developmental history that may result in accurate formulation and treatment planning.

Country of Origin

A first consideration is the patient's country of origin. In the case of foreign-born Latinos (including Puerto Ricans born on that island), there is a need to explore the patient's migration history: When did the patient move to the United States? Where did he move to? Who else moved with or before him? Who has moved since? What connections has he maintained with family and friends that stayed behind? In the case of Latinos born in the United States, a similar migration history should be collected regarding the patient's family, and should include a determination of how many generations ago the move occurred. Furthermore, the clinician should explore the patient's experiences of being a minority in the United States (e.g., incidents of discrimination or racism).

Language

Assessment of language use and dominance is another critical area. When the Latino patient is seen by a monolingual Caucasian therapist and the patient is fluent in English, this area is frequently overlooked. The therapist should find out whether the patient's language is predominantly English or Spanish, or whether he is bilingual. Even for patients whose dominant language is English, it is important to determine what language is spoken at home and through what language the patient was schooled (i.e., through a bilingual or an English-only program). The therapist should be aware that the predominantly Spanish-speaking or bilingual patient speaking English may invest more energy in expressing himself correctly, thereby giving precedence to the cognitive aspect of communications over the affective component of his language. This may have the effect of his demeanor appearing to be more constricted or flat.

It is important to note that researchers (see Crespo González EI: "It Loses Something in the Translation: The Communication of Emotions Among Puerto Ricans Living in the United States." Unpublished doctoral dissertation, New York, Adelphi University, 1990) have found that Caucasian therapists evaluating and treating bilingual patients tend to "overpathologize" and even misdiagnose. Furthermore, in Crespo González's study, in which bilingual Puerto Ricans were administered projective testing in Spanish and English, it was found that found that both languages serve different sociocultural and emotional functions. Even when a patient uses English on a daily basis to communicate with his friends, coworkers, or partner, Spanish may still be his "emotional language." In the context of bilingual psychotherapy (i.e., when both the therapist and the patient are bilingual), clinicians have found that bilingualism becomes part of the defensive structure. The patient may discuss certain emotionally charged topics in his nondominant language as a way of gaining some emotional distance. At other times, however, the patient may choose the dominant language in order to gain access to meaningful memories or experiences. In the context of therapy with an English-speaking therapist, these issues represent a hindrance to which the clinician must be sensitive. A technique that the English-speaking therapist may use is to allow the patient to think out loud in his dominant (emotional) language in order to facilitate his access to and organization of meaningful material.

Available Support System

Another area to consider during assessment is the patient's natural support system. The availability of such support will be crucial in helping the patient cope with his HIV diagnosis. The type and quality of the patient's interpersonal relationships will also assist the clinician in understanding the patient's stage of development with regard to his identity as a Latino and as a gay man. An assessment of the patient's social network should include a list of friends and acquaintances and their ethnic background and sexual orientation. If the patient has a group of heterosexual friends, it will be important to find out to whom he has come out.

The current state of the patient's relationship with his family is particularly important. In this regard, both family meetings and genograms are useful assessment and therapeutic techniques that should be considered. Particularly when it is not possible to interview family members because of their geographic or emotional distance, use of a genogram (multigenerational maps of the extended family) is highly recommended in gaining an understanding of the family dynamics and relations. Furthermore, the clinician should assess whether the patient has attributed family status to non–blood-related individuals. This is frequently done by Latino gay men when they create a "chosen" family with their Latino gay and lesbian friends. If such is the case, the therapist should treat them accordingly and include this *familia* in the assessment and therapeutic process.

Finally, gathering a history of intimate relationships is also crucial. If the patient is currently in a relationship, it is important to explore whether his lover is Latino or non-Latino. If he is in a relationship with a non-Latino man, the clinician should assess how the partners deal with their cultural differences, and how these differences are played out in the couple's dynamics. In its entirety, the social network data will be useful in anticipating potential transference issues that may emerge in a therapeutic relationship. How the patient deals with homophobia and racism will be seen in the patient's interpersonal relationships and his choice of friends and partners. Some patients may give priority to ethnicity and have a predominantly Latino social network regardless of sexual orientation. Others may have a predominantly gay social network regardless of ethnicity. Still others will have more of a mix. In each case the composition of the patient's social network will offer the therapist interesting data regarding the patient's sexual and ethnic identity development and how he deals with stressors therein.

Patient-Therapist Dynamics

Another source of valuable information is the dynamics that result from the similarities and differences in the patient-therapist match. Patients who knowingly or unknowingly follow what is suggested in the literature regarding the benefits of shared cultural experiences between patients and their therapists (Isay 1991; Liljestrand et al. 1978; Rochlin 1981) will seek out a therapist who is as similar to themselves as possible. Accordingly, a Latino gay male may feel inclined to initiate therapy with a Latino gay therapist. Patients who seek out therapy through mental health clinics, hospital outpatient departments, or health maintenance organizations may lack freedom of choice in the assignment of a therapist. In either case, given the scarcity of Latino gay clinicians, patients are most likely to find themselves matched with a non-Latino heterosexual therapist. With some luck and resourcefulness the patient may find a heterosexual Latino therapist or a non-Latino gay or lesbian therapist. However it may have resulted, the match should be explored in the assessment process as it may illustrate meaningful psychosocial issues. If the patient had freedom of choice with regard to the match, the therapist should explore what considerations in terms of sexual orientation and ethnicity led to his choice. If the match was left to chance or limited resources, the therapist must explore how the patient feels about his choice (or lack of), what difficulties he may be experiencing, and what concerns he may have.

The resulting match will also have significant transference and countertransference implications. Whenever the therapeutic dyad is discordant in terms of sexual orientation, ethnicity, or both, the therapist must explore the implications of the discordance and seek out ways of increasing his or her sensitivity to gay and ethnic minority issues. Furthermore, therapists must be particularly sensitive to power differentials in the therapeutic relationship when the match is discordant along the lines of both ethnicity and sexual orientation. Then, more than ever, the therapist must find ways to deal with cultural differences by acknowledging and exploring the differences, and be flexible and open-minded in the management of these differences.

In addition to the issues discussed above, gender and social class may be equally critical and need to be addressed in the patient-therapist match.

Practical Application of Principles Discussed Above

The following case example and discussion highlight many of the issues discussed throughout this chapter.

Case Example

Mr. A, a 29-year-old Latino gay male of Puerto Rican origin, was diagnosed as having AIDS 6 months before seeking psychotherapy. He was born and raised in a small, rural Puerto Rican town within an intact family of five siblings. He moved to a large urban area in Puerto Rico to attend college, where he met his first lover, Mr. B. They both moved to the northeastern United States shortly after graduating from college.

Mr. A came out when he was 19 but did not tell anybody in his family in part because of comments his mother had made that, "If I ever found out a son of mine was queer, I would set myself on fire." In spite of not coming out directly to his family, Mr. A felt that they knew about his sexual orientation. Surprisingly, Mr. A described his mother as very *entendida* (accepting). When this was explored further, Mr. A explained that his mother always treated Mr. B as part of the family and would scold her son if he attended a family function without him. Furthermore, she had cried when Mr. A told her that his "roommate" had moved out, asking, "Who's going to take care of you?"

Mr. A broke up with Mr. B 3 years after their move to the United States. Following that he dated a number of men but did not establish a stable relationship. His ensuing partners were primarily Caucasian men. Mr. A did not know he was HIV positive until his first hospital admission for treatment of Pneumocystis carinii pneumonia. Initially, he did not tell anybody about his illness except for his ex-lover, Mr. B. Mr. A sought therapy after his third hospital admission. He had just lost his job as a bilingual school teacher and felt very depressed. His mother had been taking care of him since his last hospital admission and wanted him to return with her to Puerto Rico. His ex-lover, Mr. B, felt he should stay in the United States because the treatment was better there and Mr. A's friends would take care of him.

The central issues that brought Mr. A to therapy seemed to be his depression about remaining in the United States versus returning to Puerto Rico with his family, a decision precipitated by his deteriorated health and the loss of his job. His ambivalence illustrates many cultural issues of which therapists should be aware. First and foremost is the Latino's strong sense of family loyalty. Mr. A felt compelled to be with his family during this difficult time. However, he also felt compelled to stay away so that he would not have to face his family. He may have been struggling with intense feelings of *vergüenza* (shame) and *culpa* (guilt), which may have been related to his Catholic upbringing and the homophobic nature of his social context during his formative years. It was imperative that the therapist explore with Mr. A what his priorities were in this regard, while simultaneously serving as a reality check for Mr. A in terms of the advantages of remaining in the United States and receiving better medical treatment and social welfare benefits.

Some of the questions that needed to be addressed include the following: How important was it to Mr. A to be with his family during his illness? How would the family respond to his diagnosis? What were his particular fears in returning? Could the possibly *machista* father assume his protective role with an HIV-infected son? What family or social network had Mr. A formed in the United States? Could he rely on these individuals to the same extent as he could on his family? In order to better deal with these questions, meetings with Mr. A's mother as well as with his ex-lover were considered useful. Mr. B appeared to be an important figure in Mr. A's social support network and also might have been a key member of Mr. A's chosen family. These interviews would offer crucial information and would also have important therapeutic implications. In many instances, establishing direct and cordial contact with family members of Latino patients is highly recommended. By emphasizing *simpatia* and *personalismo* during these contacts, the therapist helps the family change its view of him or her as an outsider, and may minimize any tendencies of external sabotaging.

Another important treatment issue with significant cultural underpinnings is the family members' level of knowledge regarding Mr. A's sexual orientation and their attitudes toward homosexuality. Some therapists might have felt apprehensive regarding the dramatic level of homophobia conveyed by Mr. A's mother. However, as always, her comments had to be interpreted within a cultural context. The use of melodrama and hyperboles is not uncommon among Latinos. Furthermore, the mother's comments needed to be closely reexamined. It is important to note that she said, "If I ever found out a son of mine was queer. . . . " rather than "If a son of mine were queer. . . . " At first glance, the comment is simply outrageously homophobic. However, given her familial treatment of the Mr. B, the message may be interpreted as, "I know you're gay, but let's not talk about it." Indeed, this seemed to be Mr. A's interpretation given that he described his mother as *entendida,* a term that conveys acceptance and knowledge or understanding. Thus both mother and son seemed to be following cultural norms regarding the avoidance of confrontation and the maintenance of smooth social relations. This avoidance may be difficult for the non-Latino therapist to understand and he or she may have felt tempted to suggest that Mr. A be more direct with his family. However, to make a major issue of this could have proven injurious to Mr. A and the therapeutic process. Extreme caution would be in order.

An obvious issue to be dealt with in Mr. A's treatment, as in the treatment of all HIV-infected individuals, was his concept of death and dying. Although each individual has his or her own ideas in this regard, the topic is so culturally charged that there may be some general considerations that are specific to Latinos as a group. Perhaps the most weighty consideration here is the value Latinos place on spiritual matters. Although Mr. A was raised in a Catholic family, it was not clear how prominent Catholicism was in his upbringing nor whether he continued to practice it. It should be noted that many Latinos return to the church (or turn to it for the first time) when confronted with a life-threatening illness. Given the central role church and religion tend to play in the lives of many Latinos (regardless of their particular affiliation), it is imperative that this aspect of their lives be explored with them and that the therapist assess the manner in which their spiritual needs are being met.

In addition to organized or traditional religious affiliations, Mr. A might have had his needs met through less orthodox faith approaches such as *Curanderismo, Santeria,* or *Espiritismo.* Being Puerto Rican, the latter two were most likely. However, because these beliefs are considered taboo by the non-Latino culture, Mr. A might have hesitated in presenting them to the therapist, particularly if he or she was a non-Latino. This obstacle could be overcome by the therapist by his or her posing a direct question about Mr. A's beliefs in a nonjudgmental and culturally sensitive manner. Even if Mr. A's religious or folk healing beliefs seemed foreign to his therapist, she or he had to respect and validate them as long as they did not interfere with appropriate health care choices. Moreover, it is extremely helpful for therapists to appreciate the usefulness of these practices as coping mechanisms for events that are perceived as uncontrollable or external in nature.

A final consideration in the management of Mr. A's case concerns supervision and case consultation. Particularly if the therapist is of a different ethnic background or belongs to a non–Puerto Rican Latino subgroup, she or he should seek out advisory services from a supervisor or colleague who is culturally similar to the patient (in the case of Mr. A, preferably a Puerto Rican or other Latino from the Caribbean). Such consultation would help the therapist be more cognizant of his or her own biases and insensitivities. It would also help the therapist interpret Mr. A's cultural reality more accurately and be more aware of how clinical interventions may affect this reality. Thus, ideally, these consultations would increase the therapist's ability to treat a specific

Latino subgroup in a respectful, noncondescending, and culturally sensitive manner.

References

Abad V, Ramos J, Boyce E: A model for the delivery of mental health services to Spanish-speaking minorities. Am J Orthopsychiatry 44:584–595, 1974

Amaro H, Montano-López R, Parés-Avila JA: Sexual and contraceptive knowledge, attitudes, and practices among Hispanics: implications for AIDS prevention. Paper commissioned by the National Institute on Drug Abuse, 1989

Arce AA, Torres-Matrullo C: Application of cognitive behavioral techniques in the treatment of Hispanic patients. Psychiatr Q 54:230–236, 1982

Bell AP, Weinberg MS: Homosexualities: A Study of Diversity Among Men and Women. New York, Simon & Schuster, 1978

Bernal G, Flores-Ortiz Y: Latino families: sociohistorical perspectives and cultural issues, in Nueva Epoca. Edited by Cordero T. San Francisco, CA, BASSTA, 1984, pp 4–9

Carballo-Diéguez A: Hispanic culture, gay male culture, and AIDS: counseling implications. Journal of Counseling and Development 68:26–30, 1989

Carrier JM: Cultural factors affecting urban Mexican male homosexual behavior. Arch Sex Behav 5:103–124, 1976

Carrier JM: Mexican male bisexuality, in Bisexualities: Theory and Research. Edited by Klein F, Wolf TJ. New York, Haworth, 1985, pp 75–85

Carrier JM, Magaña JR: Use of ethnosexual data on men of Mexican origin for HIV/AIDS prevention programs. Journal of Sex Research 28:189–202, 1991

Ceballos-Capitaine A, Szapocznik J, Blaney NT, et al: Ethnicity, emotional distress, stress-related disruption, and coping among HIV seropositive gay males. Hispanic Journal of Behavioral Sciences 12:135–152, 1990

Centers for Disease Control: Acquired immunodeficiency syndrome (AIDS) among blacks and Hispanics. Morb Mortal Wkly Rep 35:655–666, 1986

Centers for Disease Control: HIV/AIDS Surveillance Report. Atlanta, GA, U.S. Department of Health and Human Services, 1991

Comas-Díaz L: Culturally relevant issues and treatment implications for Hispanics, in Crossing Cultures in Mental Health. Edited by Koslow DR, Salett E. Washington, DC, SIETAR International, 1985, pp 31–48

Comas-Diaz L: Mainland Puerto Rican women: a sociocultural approach. Journal of Consulting and Community Psychology 16:21–31, 1988

De La Cancela V: A critical analysis of Puerto Rican machismo: implications for clinical practice. Psychotherapy 23:291–296, 1986

de Monteflores C: Notes on the management of difference, in Contemporary Perspectives on Psychotherapy With Lesbians and Gay Men. Edited by Stein TS, Cohen CJ. New York, Plenum, 1986, pp 73–101

Espín OM: Cultural and historical influences on sexuality in Hispanic/Latin women: implications for psychotherapy, in Towards a New Politics of Sexuality. Edited by Vance C. London, Routledge & Kegan Paul, 1984

Espín OM: Issues of identity in the psychology of Latina lesbians, in Lesbian Psychologies: Explorations and Challenges. Edited by the Boston Lesbian Psychologies Collective. Urbana, IL, University of Illinois Press, 1987, pp 35–55

Gock TS: Issues in gay affirmative psychotherapy with ethnically/culturally diverse populations. Paper presented at the 94th annual meeting of the American Psychological Association, Washington, DC, August 1986

Hahn RA, Castro KG: The health and health care status of Latino populations in the U.S.: a brief review, in Latinos and AIDS: A National Strategy Symposium. Edited by Martínez-Maza O, Shin DM, Banks HE. Los Angeles, CA, University of California Press, 1989, pp 1–7

Hayes-Bautista DE, Chapa J: Latino terminology: Conceptual bases for standardized terminology. Am J Public Health 77:61–68, 1987

Institute for Puerto Rican Policy: Puerto Ricans and other Latinos in the United States. Datanote on the Puerto Rican Community 8:1–2, 1990

Isay RA: The homosexual analyst: clinical considerations. Psychoanal Study Child 46:199–216, 1991

Kaminsky S, Kurtines W, Hervis OO, et al: Life enhancement counseling with HIV-infected Hispanic gay males. Hispanic Journal of Behavioral Sciences 12:177–195, 1990

Liljestrand P, Gerling E, Saliba PA: The effect of social sex-role stereotypes and sexual orientation on psychotherapeutic outcomes. J Homosex 3/4:361–372, 1978

Machuca J: ¿Qué es el espiritismo? (What is espiritismo?), 2nd Edition. Santurce, PR, Casa de las Almas, 1982, pp 1–20

Maduro R: Curanderismo and Latino views of disease. West J Med 139:868–874, 1983

Marín BV: Hispanic culture: implications for AIDS prevention, in Sexuality and Disease: Metaphors, Perceptions and Behavior in the AIDS Era. Edited by Boswell J, Hexter R, Reinisch J. New York, Oxford University Press (in press)

Marín G: Attributions for tardiness among Chilean and United States students. Journal of Social Psychology 127:69–75, 1987

Marín G: AIDS prevention among Hispanics: needs, risk behaviors, and cultural values. Public Health Rep 104:411–415, 1989

McKay EG: Changing Hispanic Demographics. Washington, DC, Policy Analysis Center, National Council of La Raza, 1988

Morales ES: Third world gays and lesbians: a process of multiple identities. Paper presented at the 91st annual meeting of the American Psychological Association, Anaheim, CA, August 1983

Morales ES: HIV infection and Hispanic gay and bisexual men. Hispanic Journal of Behavioral Sciences 12:212–222, 1990

Parés-Avila JA: Mental health, in Latinos and AIDS: A National Strategy Symposium. Edited by Martínez-Maza O, Shin DM, Banks HE. Los Angeles, CA, University of California Press, 1989, pp 21–41

Rochlin M: Sexual orientation of the therapist and therapeutic effectiveness with gay clients. J Homosex 7:21–29, 1981

Sabogal F, Otero-Sabogal R: Latin Sexuality, AIDS, and Drug Use, in Gay Males, I.V. Drug Users, and Heterosexual Males: A Focus Group Approach. San Francisco, CA, Center for AIDS Prevention Studies, University of California, 1990

Selik RM, Castro KG, Pappaioanou M, et al: Birthplace and the risk of AIDS among Hispanics in the United States. Am J Public Health 77:69–72, 1989

Sluski C: The Latin lover revisited, in Ethnicity and Family Therapy. Edited by McGoldrick M, Pearce JK, Giordano J. New York, Guilford, 1985, pp 492–498

Spencer G: Projections of the Hispanic population: 1983 to 2080. Current Population Estimates and Projections, Series P-25, No 995. Washington, DC, U. S. Bureau of the Census, 1986

Treviño FM: Standardized terminology for Hispanic populations. Am J Public Health 77:69–72, 1987

U.S. Bureau of the Census: 1980 Census of the United States: Population and Housing. Washington, DC, U.S. Government Printing Office, 1983

U.S. Bureau of the Census: The Hispanic Population in the United States: March 1989. Current Population Reports, Series P-20, No 444. Washington, DC, U.S. Government Printing Office, 1990

Chapter 17

Negotiating HIV Infection in Rural America: Breaking Through the Isolation

Jane K. O'Rourke, L.M.S.W.
Perry S. Sutherland, A.C.S.W.

D uring the second decade of the acquired immunodeficiency syndrome (AIDS) epidemic, gay men in rural communities increasingly faced the devastation that had been endured by gay men mainly in urban epicenters. Demand for services for human immunodeficiency virus (HIV)–positive patients in these rural areas has increased whereas the supply has fallen short. For example, in our community in rural New England, an HIV-positive gay man must contend with complex social and delivery-of-care issues in addition to coping with the medical manifestations of the HIV-related illnesses. Urban areas have the advantage of having vocal community leaders, broad-based media coverage, skilled and informed mental health practitioners, aggressive tertiary care hospitals, and politically savvy gay and lesbian health advocates to create sophisticated responses to the spread of HIV (Drucker 1992; Eberle 1992; Nieto 1989). This is rarely true for rural America and is not our experience in Maine.

In this chapter we explore some of the complex issues surrounding treatment of HIV-infected patients from the informed perspective of two clinical social work practitioners in rural Maine. Our social work practice settings contrast significantly, and the differences determine the nature of our work. One (J. O'Rourke) works in the AIDS

Consultation Service, a medical setting offering psychosocial assessment, information, and referral services; the other (P. Sutherland) works in a community-based mental health counseling center with a wide variety of treatment modalities, including long-term therapy. Both of us provide services to gay men who are HIV infected or diagnosed with AIDS. Despite the differences between our settings, our work shares salient themes vis-à-vis treating HIV-positive gay men in rural settings. Social isolation, fear of unwanted disclosure, and lack of information and transportation are common issues in rural areas (Rounds 1988).

Men seek the comprehensive services of the AIDS Consultation Service at all points on the continuum of the HIV-related illness process. They are referred by their primary care provider, from any community throughout Maine, to be seen by an infectious disease physician, a nurse practitioner, and a clinical social worker for a full consultation and recommendations. This decentralized interdisciplinary approach to patient care offers a useful holistic perspective for understanding more than the limited set of presenting symptoms (Eberle 1992). The focus of the psychosocial assessment is the whole person and all aspects of his health. The AIDS Consultation Service team approach incorporates a complete understanding of the person when offering treatment recommendations, recognizing both mind and body have an impact on each other.

Implications of Being Gay and HIV Positive in Rural New England

Demographics

Eberle (1992) described the late 1980s as the "second wave" of the AIDS epidemic, noting that it included the increased spread of the epidemic to semirural and rural areas. Between 1988 and 1989, newly reported AIDS cases in rural America increased by more than 30%, compared with 8% in the entire country.

The prevalence of HIV infection in Maine, New Hampshire, and Vermont is relatively low compared with that in urban areas of the northeastern United States, and is distributed fairly evenly across these areas. As of 1993, 373 patients had been reported to have AIDS in Maine and 180 of those had died. This number does not reflect the number of patients who were diagnosed in other states and then migrated to Maine (Rumley et al. 1991). To include this group would increase the number by 30%. Half of the diagnosed cases are now from nonurban areas of the state. Little is understood about the epidemiology of the 2,800 people who are estimated to be HIV positive.

Social Stigma

One might hypothesize that in Maine, as in most rural areas, so little gay culture is visible that disclosure of gay identity could be stigmatizing and lead to social isolation and little support (Andersen and Civic 1989; Cleveland and Davenport 1989; Dhooper and Royse 1989; Hudson and Donovan 1989; Nieto 1989; Rounds 1988). Given the underground nature of the rural gay culture, roadside rest areas and truck stops have often become a rural alternative to gay bars. Certain locations are identified and become the outlet for sexual expression.

The majority of the HIV-positive people assessed at the hospital-based AIDS Consultation Service are Caucasian gay men who are sexually active with male partners. This reflects the statewide statistic that 81% of adults and adolescents diagnosed with AIDS in Maine since the beginning of the epidemic are identified as homosexual or bisexual males. However, not all of these men necessarily think of themselves as gay. This disassociation from the gay culture is not unique to men who live in rural areas.

The most profound common theme among rural men who have sex with other men is social isolation. Rounds (1988) described the unavoidable double bind in which rural gays are trapped: In order to avoid stigma, ostracism, and violence, they must hide their sexual orientation and fit into the traditional family unit. This often leads to an internalization of dystonic negative messages toward their own sexuality. The indigenous traditional values of rural conservatism combined with the lack of privacy create a tempest of intolerance and discrimination—often giving way to self-loathing, substance abuse, or flight (Andersen and Civic 1989; Cleveland and Davenport 1989; Dhooper and Royse 1989; Hudson and Donovan 1989; Nieto 1989; Rounds 1988; Rounds et al. 1991).

Some gay men live their entire lives in Maine. Some manage to find support and community discreetly, whereas those who come out pay the price of being excluded or exploited. Only a few gay men overcome these obstacles and assert their rights (Dhooper and Royse 1989). One common scenario for many gay men is that they leave rural Maine early in their lives to find sanctuary in the anonymity of major cities where they hope to pursue a life-style free from judgment. For many, their hope dissolves as a series of lovers and friends pass away and they ultimately become sick themselves and need the love and support of the family they left behind. This creates a potential crisis for all involved: family members learn about the returning gay man's sexual orientation at the same time as they learn about his sero-positivity, and the gay man is returning at a time when he is both emotionally and physically vulnerable. Neither family members nor the gay man may be up to the task of negotiating this assault on their lives (Andersen and Civic 1989; Hudson and Donovan 1989; Peabody 1987). An HIV-positive gay man's reunion with his family can be an emotional setup with disastrous consequences (Andersen and Civic 1989; see also Chapter 13 on gay men returning home to die).

Social and Delivery-of-Care Issues

Educational opportunities about homosexuality or the AIDS epidemic are not readily available in rural settings. For example, the information families receive is often filtered by the narrowly defined moral ethics of the local and regional media. Community centers such as churches or places of employment offer no frame of reference from which family members can comprehend their loved one's experience and, in fact, actually may be sources of misinformation.

Confidentiality is much more challenging in smaller communities than in larger urban areas (Cleveland and Davenport 1989; Neito 1989). It is not uncommon for the local Social Security clerk to be a neighbor or family friend (Hudson and Donovan 1989). Fear of disclosure keeps many men and their families from seeking the comfort

and support of others as well as the resources to which they are entitled. Many discuss their condition only with their medical team and
have no other outlet. One poignant story recently recounted at an
AIDS conference by a minister from a neighboring rural state centered
on nine separate families in her community, each of which had a HIV-
positive loved one. The minister shared her desperate frustration that
each family felt completely alone because they had no idea that the
other families were experiencing the same crisis.

Lack of transportation to medical appointments, let alone to psychotherapy or to support groups, can be a considerable hindrance to
care and support for rural gay men. There is no public transportation
in outlying rural areas and very little in the more densely populated
areas. As these men experience the unyielding loss of control in all
spheres of their life, including their body and environment, the simple
task of traveling to and from an appointment becomes a daunting obstacle. This challenge siphons their energy away from the real business
of taking care of themselves and diverts their life force into logistical
negotiations.

Gay men with HIV-related illnesses may become completely dependent, losing all previous autonomy. When asking for assistance,
they often feel compelled to lie about their condition. Often they tell
people they have cancer. Many families are also more comfortable
using this explanation. The secret veils the family in a cloak of deceit
and mutual distrust at a time when truth and openness could not be
more important (Rounds et al. 1991). This process also parallels the
secrecy and self-loathing that may have been experienced by the family as a result of the patient's sexual orientation (Andersen and Civic
1989).

All of these factors may contribute to an existential crisis in the
life of the HIV-positive gay man living in a rural community. He may
be reeling from the accumulated losses of friends and lovers, and he
may have given up his independence and authentic public self in the
face of a deteriorating, debilitating illness. He may have limited access
to others who might identify with either his sexuality or his diagnosis
as he contends with significant issues of life and death (Drucker 1992;
Shelby 1992).

Psychotherapy can be an important resource for HIV-positive gay men but access to the few experienced practitioners in rural New England is limited. The issues of social isolation, breach of confidentiality, limited community understanding, and restricted transportation options can combine to prevent the rural gay man from receiving the support and help he deserves (Human and Wasem 1991).

Treatment Issues

The following two case examples reflect a variety of clinical concerns unique to serving HIV-infected gay men in rural Maine. Rural factors impinge on the efficacy of treatment in both cases. The first case demonstrates how the patient's previous experiences of being abused and socially isolated were only reinforced by the separateness imposed on him by his rural constraints. Not only did he have to face a life-threatening and demoralizing illness with only limited access to his primary support (his partner), but also, because of his painful family history, he was not able to trust in himself or others. It was only within the therapeutic relationship that he could find consistent hope for a relatedness beyond the limited opportunity available from his family or rural environment. The therapist supported the patient's strengths and generated a treatment plan that included cognitive and psychodynamic interventions.

The second case illustrates a reasonably successful negotiation of rural barriers despite the intensity of the patient's symptoms. The therapist reached out to him in his home and together they created a treatment plan focusing on the impact of HIV-related illnesses, the availability of support, and unresolved life issues. Although this man was physically isolated from his friends, he was able use his inner strength to create positive change and to teach others about living with HIV-related illness. Again, the thoughtful use of both cognitive and psychodynamic paradigms provided an evenhanded approach to working with this gay man, diagnosed with AIDS and living in a rural setting. The following case example illustrates the struggle with isolation and the use of the therapeutic relationship as an important connection.

Case 1

Mr. A, a 25-year-old gay man, was referred to the counseling center by his case manager from a regional AIDS service organization. Mr. A's 27-year-old ex-lover of 3 years had died of AIDS 8 months prior to Mr. A's contact with the center. His ability to grieve this loss was impaired in part because of his own HIV-positive status, as well as because of the deaths of several friends from AIDS-related illnesses and the ongoing illnesses of others.

Mr. A reported feeling very depressed, with components of loneliness, hopelessness, insignificance, and a persistent "sinking" feeling. These feelings had been predominant for most of his life, as had feelings of anxiety and fear. Mr. A reported that he had previously received psychotherapeutic treatment for 5 years with a clinical psychologist, adding that he had been in counseling off and on for most of his life. He had been treated with several antidepressants, but had experienced no consistent relief from his symptoms. The center's consulting psychiatrist rendered the diagnosis of dysthymia, primary type, early onset.

Mr. A was the fifth of seven children, the fourth boy, growing up in a small Maine city. He had a very turbulent childhood and identified himself as the black sheep of his family. He experienced both intrafamilial and extrafamilial sexual abuse between the ages of 10 and 14. Mr. A reported having a marginal relationship with his family, with little trust in his parents or siblings, and reported having no interest in involving them in his treatment. He saw himself as having been mistreated by both his family and society, and experienced strong feelings of resentment toward both.

When Mr. A came out in junior high school, he experienced severe harassment from other students and had to be escorted to and from school by the local police. Although he clearly experienced significant ongoing trauma from his childhood and adolescence, his life began to settle down by age 18 when he left his family to venture out on his own. He was, however, diagnosed as being HIV positive a few months after his 18th birthday.

At the time of intake, Mr. A resided in a very small township located approximately 1 hour from medical and mental health services. He lived with his current partner in this small town, where residents tended to "know too much of each other's business." Because he was disabled as a result of the physical manifestations of his illness, Mr. A applied for general assistance funding from the town office. As he appeared to be physically healthy, the town clerk did not believe that general assistance was truly needed. Instead, Mr. A was encouraged to search for employment. Mr. A was compelled to bring his case worker to a second meeting with the town clerk in an effort to explain the dynamics of his illness. After convincing information was provided to the clerk, Mr. A was granted general assistance support from the town.

Mr. A had previously attended a support group for HIV-positive individuals in a city 45 miles away, but found the group somewhat exclusive. He was not asked to join the others for coffee after group meetings ended, which reignited feelings of rejection that stemmed from his childhood and adolescence. Instead of sharing with the group these feelings of rejection, he discontinued group attendance and isolated himself from available community supports.

As his depression deepened, Mr. A began to sleep 12 to 14 hours per day, having little reason to either rise out of bed or leave his home. He was encouraged to seek volunteer or support group activities in the nearby city, which he agreed to consider. Because he and his partner shared a car, Mr. A would have to leave home when his partner left for work at 6:00 A.M. in order to have transportation for the day. He would then have to remain in the city for the day or travel from home in the afternoon to pick up his partner from work. His lack of transportation supported his resistance to establishing a more positive network of support. To complicate matters, Mr. A had a history of cruising for anonymous sexual contacts. Having access to transportation raised his anxiety about his sexual obsessiveness, as he was unsure that he could set limits on his sexual desires.

The treatment goals for Mr. A's therapy focused on 1) examining the sources of and decreasing the occurrence of anxiety, 2) identifying and enhancing those things in his life that elicited feelings of happiness and comfort, 3) using the therapeutic setting to talk about feelings related to being HIV seropositive, and 4) clarifying issues from his past that continued to affect his daily functioning.

Eventually Mr. A developed a severe bronchial infection, which left him feeling very tired and restless and contributed to his already disrupted sleep pattern. When he felt physically sick, Mr. A tended to become quite verbose and obsessive in his thinking. His physical isolation left him alone at home, which added to his feelings of abandonment and rejection. Although he had friends who were willing to visit, he would not call them, as he did not feel deserving of their attention. Mr. A also expressed increased concern about his lethargy and weight gain. He also questioned the impact of his ongoing cannabis use on his emotional well-being. Acknowledging that his cannabis use was problematic at times, he considered the possibility of admitting himself to a substance abuse rehabilitation program. However, his physical isolation again contributed to his decision to forgo substance abuse treatment, as available services were far from his home. His concern about substance use diminished as he began to focus more on current and historical feelings of depression.

As treatment progressed, Mr. A began to speak about a decline in both the frequency of and pleasure received from the couple's sexual relations. His partner had reportedly become more detached, and plans were made to provide couples therapy. Because of his partner's schedule and transportation conflicts, conjoint sessions were difficult to arrange and as a result were postponed.

Mr. A was a young man with a long history of being mistreated by others. He seemed to have never had the chance to get back on his feet following his childhood trauma. At too young an age he had to deal with the new trauma of HIV-related illness. His decision to live in a rural setting complicated both his ability and his willingness to establish a positive network of support. The rural setting of his home played an important role in contributing to his ongoing isolation and feelings of depression. He did, however, appear to be motivated to engage in treatment, and was hopeful that therapy would help to lift his depression. Case 2 describes a man with more ego strengths than Mr. A who also struggled with the trauma of his illness. By using the treatment relationship to deal with his feelings, he was able to stay engaged with resources around him.

Case 2

Mr. B, an artist, was first diagnosed with Pneumocystis carinii pneumonia at age 20. He referred himself to psychotherapeutic treatment 2 years later after a period of emotional turmoil. He had symptoms of anxiety, depression, and suicidal ideation, as well as visual hallucinations. Mr. B had been hospitalized shortly before beginning psychotherapy because of an intestinal parasitic infection, which continued to cause significant pain and discomfort throughout the period of treatment. He had begun a course of antiviral medication (zidovudine [AZT]), which had to be administered every 4 hours.

Mr. B agreed to weekly psychotherapy sessions, making his way on his own to the office for the first 2 months. However, because of progressive neuromuscular deterioration in his legs, he became unable to walk significant distances. Subsequent psychotherapy was provided in Mr. B's home.

Mr. B was the oldest of two sons, born in a very small Maine city. His family home in a small village was approximately 45 minutes away from available medical services. He reported that his family provided him with a happy and nurturing home environment during childhood. There was no history of substance abuse or other remarkable family dysfunction. Family members were aware of both his sexual orientation and his AIDS diagnosis.

Initially, Mr. B revealed tremendous feelings of anger and resentment toward his illness, his family and friends, and the medical and social service systems available to him. He perceived that his physical condition was rapidly deteriorating and was worried about the beginning of possible neurological impairment. Mr. B was upset that he had "seen" a former roommate of his, who had died of AIDS 6 months prior to the commencement of therapy, walk across the room while Mr. B was resting on the couch in his apartment. His hallucination made him worry that he might be "going crazy." He also expressed strong feelings of frustration and ambivalence toward his primary physician, who, at that time, was one of two infectious disease specialists in the area who were knowledgeable about HIV.

Mr. B's therapy focused on 1) identifying and expressing his feelings related to his AIDS diagnosis and ongoing physical deterioration, 2) identifying those individuals in his support network who could be counted on for support as his illness progressed, and 3) identifying and discussing those issues that remained unresolved during his lifetime, with a focus toward resolution.

Mr. B's anger and hostility fluctuated as treatment progressed. He experienced difficulty becoming dependent on friends, family, and the social welfare system. At times he felt guilty that he was "burdening" his family and friends. The necessity of depending on others for transportation to appointments and to social gatherings became very frustrating to this highly independent young man.

Although he had had several significant romantic relationships during his early adulthood, one of Mr. B's primary concerns was that he was currently single. His physical isolation limited his possibilities of meeting potential partners. However, Mr. B became active in HIV education efforts, joined the board of directors of a regional AIDS organization, and attended both domestic and international conferences. Through these social activities, he dated and became involved for brief periods in satisfying romantic relationships.

During the early years of Mr. B's illness, his access to social services was limited. Frequently he would not qualify for services because of agencies' ignorance about HIV or the lack of HIV-related policies given by service providers. Mr. B's initial response was to become angry with the social service system. As treatment continued, he became more assertive and effective in responding to such challenges and educating service providers. His efforts resulted in landmark changes in policy and service delivery throughout the state's social service system.

Eventually Mr. B stopped taking AZT because the every-4-hour doses interfered with his sleep and because he believed the medication was not making a difference in his health status. He reported impairment in short-term memory, with disorientation at times, and a continuation of hypnagogic auditory and visual hallucinations, which remained disturbing to him. Four months after discontinuing AZT, Mr. B began to tire of the battle with his HIV-related illnesses. He became tearful and discouraged. Neurological symptoms continued to limit his daily functioning. He became extremely angry during one therapy session and picked up his wheelchair and threw it across his apartment. He eloquently expressed his anger and resentment toward the virus, his illness, and the losses that he had experienced.

Mr. B's family, especially his mother, had been very supportive of him during his illness. However, the family's denial of his prognosis was remarkable. When AIDS was discussed, he recalled his mother seeing his illness as a "temporary problem," which invalidated Mr. B's struggle to deal with his mortality. In therapy, he began to talk about issues of spirituality, which he had never addressed before. He had also resisted dealing with funeral arrangements, as well as preparing a will and power of attorney, all of which he began to consider and plan. As Mr. B's decompensation became more visible, he began to address more substantially the issues of grief, dying, and death, which seemed difficult and frightening for him. He was a very proud young man who had difficulty asking for support. By venting in therapy, he was freed from some of his feeling of burdening others. Furthermore, he was able to validate his right to express anger and discomfort without labeling himself as a hypochondriac. His decision to focus on the reality of his terminal diagnosis enabled him to integrate his death. With greater acceptance of his illness as his physical condition worsened, he began to invest more time in his art work, as well as participate in AIDS education presentations to area schools and organizations.

After almost a year in treatment, I informed Mr. B of my intention to leave the agency for a placement overseas. Both of us discussed our feelings about termination as well as my recommendation for him to continue his therapeutic work. As I arranged for a case transfer, we both recognized and accepted the reality that he might die during my absence.

I returned from my overseas commitment after 9 months to find Mr. B more active and in better health than when I left. He resided very near his parents, who had become much more involved in his day-to-day care. He was also receiving support from a regional visiting nurse service. Although he was physically isolated in his rural environment, he broke through the isolation by continually reaching out to his support network of family and friends, as well as by providing media interviews and educational presentations up to the time of his death.

Summary of Case Examples

These case examples highlight some of the different challenges that face HIV-positive gay men in rural America. Both Mr. A and Mr. B had problems of depression and isolation. However, their needs and treatment goals contrasted substantially. Mr. A used the opportunity to see the therapist in his office as a way to extricate himself from what felt to be a stifling environment that made him recall his earlier experiences of trauma and abuse in his childhood home and community. The convergence of substance abuse with medical and psychiatric issues complicated his isolation and created significant barriers to effective treatment.

In contrast, Mr. B's isolation was more the interactive result of the debilitating progression of his illness combined with his rural environment. The therapist bridged some of the patient's isolation by providing treatment in Mr. B's home and by strengthening Mr. B's ongoing relationships. The case of Mr. B demonstrates the possibility of more effectively using available supports and developing new ones despite significant physical isolation. Through his supportive friends and his own proactive manner, Mr. B was able to overcome barriers in his rural environment.

In both cases, treatment goals included breaking through rural isolation by connecting the patient with existing resources and actively developing new resources. Mr. A had not crossed the threshold from being HIV positive to having AIDS and his treatment had to incorporate living with a chronic terminal illness in a small community that offered minimal support. Although Mr. B's family was fully aware of his diagnosis, they tended to discount its seriousness. This became one of the central themes of Mr. B's therapeutic work, as we looked at death and considered how to live with the family's denial.

Conclusions

Being HIV infected in rural America is a challenge not only for the gay man but for the therapists who work with him as well. The patient must deal with his isolation and negotiate a network that is supportive despite limited institutional support. The treatment goals in therapy with an HIV-positive gay man must include a thorough psychosocial assessment. The therapy must be conducted in terms of his pre–HIV infection character and family history in addition to an awareness about the attitudes and resources in his rural community. Issues of confidentiality and limited resources must be managed. The therapist must be flexible and improvise to meet the patient's needs.

The countryside can be a very unprivate place despite its wide expanse. Because patient and therapist may become outcasts in their own communities if the nature of their work together is known, the therapist often must take extreme measures to preserve the confidentiality of their relationship. The therapist's vigilance about boundaries can isolate the therapist in the work. Furthermore, in rural HIV work therapists often witness injustices and have to contend with inadequate service systems. Because the work can be frustrating, isolating, and demoralizing for the therapist, support for the therapist is critical. Consultation and support can be regularly obtained from a variety of sources: local colleagues, a network of colleagues who live and work throughout a large region but who meet for monthly peer supervision, or conferences at nearby urban centers. Because the majority of providers travel to cities for initial and continuing education, the urban training centers must become familiar with the different demands of rural HIV work.

Contending with a possibly homophobic, AIDS-phobic rural community with limited resources complicates the life of an HIV-infected gay man. The therapist's task is to offer an opening out of his rural isolation that may have exacerbated his shame. In the therapeutic relationship, the therapist creates a safer holding environment that may enable him to further break out of his social isolation as he takes on the challenges of integrating his life.

References

Andersen H, Civic D: Psychosocial issues in rural AIDS care. Human Services in the Rural Environment 13:11–16, 1989

Cleveland PH, Davenport J: AIDS: a growing problem for rural communities. Human Services in the Rural Environment 13:23–29, 1989

Dhooper SS, Royse DD: Rural attitudes about AIDS: a statewide survey. Human Services in the Rural Environment 13:17–22, 1989

Drucker A: HIV-related challenges for the rural therapist. Focus: A Guide to AIDS Research and Counseling 7:5–6, 1992

Eberle S: Beyond the urban epidemic. Focus: A Guide to AIDS Research and Counseling 7:1–4, 1992

Hudson CJ, Donovan TC: Two cases of acquired immune deficiency syndrome encountered in rural mental health outpatient facilities. Human Services in the Rural Environment 13:39–41, 1989

Human J, Wasem C: Mental health in the rural U.S. Am Psychol 3:232–239, 1991

Nieto DS: AIDS and the rural family: some systems considerations and intervention implications for the human service practitioner. Human Services in the Rural Environment 13:34–38, 1989

Peabody B: The screaming room: a mother's journal of her son's struggle with AIDS. New York, Avon Books, 1987

Rounds K: AIDS in rural areas: challenges to providing care. Journal of Social Work 33:257–261, 1988

Rounds K, Galinsky MJ, Stevens LS: Linking people with AIDS in rural communities: the telephone group. Journal of Social Work 36:13–18, 1991

Rumley RL, Shappley NC, Waivers LE, et al: HIV migration to rural America. AIDS 5:1373–1378, 1991

Shelby RD: If a Partner Has AIDS: Guide to Clinical Intervention for Relationships in Crisis. New York, Harrington Park Press, 1992

Chapter 18

Trauma Revisited: HIV and AIDS in Gay Male Survivors of Early Sexual Abuse

Robert A. Burnham, Jr., Ph.D.

In this chapter, I examine how the psychological and somatic dimensions of earlier sexual traumatization are closely intertwined with the psychophysiological sequelae of human immunodeficiency virus (HIV)–related illness in adult gay male survivors of such trauma. I explore this interaction within the context of five stages along the full spectrum of HIV illness: 1) unsafe sexual behavior, 2) HIV testing, 3) severe immunosuppression and the development of opportunistic infections, 4) growing dependency on providers and the experiencing of intrusive medical procedures, and 5) the process of dying. Throughout the chapter I emphasize identifying and exploring the ways in which the occurrence of sexual traumatization in childhood can be concealed behind the more immediate trauma associated with HIV-related illness and acquired immunodeficiency syndrome (AIDS). Identification of earlier traumatization provides an indispensable key to understanding the deeply personal meaning of the later HIV-related trauma.

Introduction

Several studies confirm that earlier traumatic experiences predispose adults to developing posttraumatic sequelae in reaction to later trauma (Burgess and Holstrom 1979; Helzer et al. 1987; Hendin et al.

1983). When this occurs, various isolated fragments of the original trauma may be reexperienced as ideomotor or ideosensory activity (i.e., *body memories*), visual flashbacks, nightmares, behavioral reenactments, or hypermnesias (Brett and Ostroff 1985; Putnam et al. 1986; Rossi 1986; Rossi and Cheek 1988; van der Kolk 1987, 1988). Memories of earlier traumatization are almost always fragmented, as children characteristically both react to trauma and store traumatic memories by means of ideosensory and ideomotor activity (Pynoos and Eth 1985; Rossi 1986; Rossi and Cheek 1988). Children are much more likely to remember the sensory qualities rather than the context of events transpired (Jacobs and Nadel 1985; Squire 1987). Because traumatic events lack the contextual (spatial and temporal) referents of other types of events that occur during childhood, adults later find that they did not symbolically represent the traumatic events in a manner required for ready retrieval (van der Kolk 1988).

Adults appear to retrieve memories of earlier traumatization in much the same fashion as they originally stored them as children—that is, somatically, with little or no cognitive representation. For adults, it is a profoundly regressive experience to be besieged by generalized somatic and affective states but to be unable to contextualize these reactions. Hyperarousal and emotional flooding do not permit traumatized adults to gauge the relative danger of perceived threats (Strian and Klicpera 1978 [in van der Kolk 1988]), fostering instead immediate action in an attempt to reduce the impact of intense sensation and emotion. Traumatized adults may attempt to inhibit hyperarousal and flooding through emotional distancing, numbing, and other dissociative phenomena; chemical dissociation by means of drug and alcohol abuse; and through dissociation via sexually addictive behavior. The danger and persistence of these responses are frequently compelling enough to distract the clinician from assessing their traumatic etiology (van der Kolk 1988).

Unsafe Sex:
The Sexual Partner as Perpetrator

As soon as HIV was isolated and its modes of transmission identified, educational campaigns were launched by AIDS education specialists, gay community leaders, and health service providers to inform the gay male population of the risks of unsafe sex and to promote safer sex procedures. Despite these efforts, some men persistently engaged in unsafe sexual behavior, disregarding what they knew to be true about the virus and its transmission; others engaged in unsafe sex intermittently, and still others appeared to resume practicing unsafe sex after initially adopting safer procedures for a period of time.

It is misleading to assume that the underlying motivation for practicing unsafe sexual behavior is simply the unconscious desire for self-annihilation (see Chapters 20 and 21). In many if not most cases, the gay male survivor of earlier trauma who practices unsafe sex operates with the basic paradoxical motivation of surviving in an atmosphere of perceived danger. For the survivor, any type of sexual contact, particularly contact that is not self-initiated, carries the potential of setting in motion a somatosensory process of retrieving earlier memories of sexual traumatization. The process of accessing these earlier memory fragments eclipses the survivor's mature cognitive capacity to mediate sensation and emotion, and regresses him to an infantile, trauma-induced mode of internal experience characterized either by hyperarousal and flooding or by severe dissociation. Once regressed, it is not uncommon for the survivor to experience complete paralysis in the face of what is perceived to be extreme danger, mirroring the vulnerability once experienced at the hands of a perpetrator. As a child, it would have been dangerous to refuse the sexual advances of an adult who threatened violence, even death, as a consequence of noncompliance. The child's survival depended on compliance with the perpetrator's wishes. As an adult, the child's paralysis in the face of threatened violence is reexperienced as the inconceivability of halting the inevitable progression of unsafe sexual behavior for the same reason—that is, survival depends on compliance with the wishes of the sexual partner.

The loss of judgment evident in initiating unsafe sexual contact and the paralysis of the will to act seen in accepting another's unsafe sexual advances may both be amplified by the dissociation that frequently accompanies the retrieval of traumatic memories. *Dissociative phenomena* are psychological defensive strategies for escaping the somatic and affective realities of trauma that occur when a perpetrator blocks by force or the threat of violence the actual bodily escape of the victim. Trauma survivors characterize the experience of dissociation as leaving the body or leaving the scene, reflecting both the element of escape and a reduction in the intensity of sensation and emotion experienced. It is particularly difficult to monitor the safety of sexual behavior and to disengage from behavior that is life threatening when the intensity of all somatic and affective experience has been sharply lowered or completely extinguished. Not only does the survivor describe having left his body while engaged sexually, he may further develop amnesia for the entire sexual encounter. Drug and alcohol use exacerbate dissociation, clouding judgment and paralyzing the individual's will to act.

In a certain proportion of gay male survivors, persistent unsafe sexual behavior appears to be a compulsive reexposure to events that either reenact the original trauma or duplicate certain aspects of it. This phenomenon has been variously described as behavioral reenactment, fixation on the trauma, or addiction to the trauma (van der Kolk 1987; van der Kolk et al. 1985). It takes the form of re-creating one's own victimization (Pattison and Kahan 1983) or of identifying with the aggressor by perpetrating abuse on others as a manifestation of the same type of abuse once directed against the self (Burgess et al. 1987). In the initial stages of treatment, victims-turned-perpetrators who compulsively use unsafe sexual behavior to reenact their trauma with others vehemently rationalize their own behavior and denigrate others for not behaving similarly. In these cases, identification with the aggressor appears to have become a philosophy of living, and the philosophy as well as the behavior it engenders must be maintained rigidly or the individual risks intensely reexperiencing the affective and physiological correlates of his own trauma. The following case example illustrates many of the dissociative phenomena described in this section.

Case 1

Mr. A was in weekly individual psychotherapy for 3 months when he reported that he had sought anonymous sexual contact in a park located in an area well known for its high frequency of violent crimes committed against gay men. After being in the park only a short time, a man whom he found attractive approached him and, with no words spoken, the two initiated sexual contact. A short time later, still silent, the man initiated anal intercourse, with Mr. A in the receptive role. This continued until the man withdrew from Mr. A and hurriedly began to dress himself. Startled, as though having suddenly awakened from a dream, Mr. A examined his rectal area with his hand and found to his great astonishment that it was wet. As the other man was leaving, Mr. A asked in shocked disbelief, "You came inside me?"

As he reported this encounter, Mr. A exhibited the same shocked disbelief in the office as he had felt in the park. Presumably experiencing the same dissociative state as he related the incident that he had experienced after his sexual encounter, Mr. A's sense of self appeared to be in eclipse, for it had not yet occurred to him that he shared any responsibility whatsoever for this incident of unsafe sexual behavior. We used this dissociative state in therapy as a naturally occurring bridge back to an earlier, similarly dangerous sexual encounter, in which a much younger Mr. A was also dissociated from his body and completely paralyzed. It was this younger Mr. A who was accessed during the sexual encounter in the park. His adult sense of self had been driven from his body in a very real sense by the danger of the violation in progress.

Mr. A's passive participation in unsafe sexual behavior is illustrative of two distinct modes of remembering earlier traumatic events commonly used by trauma patients: 1) behavioral remembering or reenactment, represented by Mr. A's search for a type of sexual contact that mirrored his earlier sexual abuse, and 2) somatosensory remembering, exemplified by the rapid and dramatic loss of ideosensory responsiveness or the profound dissociation Mr. A manifested.

Testing Seropositive or Seronegative: HIV as Perpetrator

In this section I discuss three distinct approaches to the challenge of HIV testing, each one having been clinically presented by gay male survivors of childhood trauma. These different scenarios demonstrate the extraordinary potential of HIV testing to trigger posttraumatic sequelae.

Avoiding HIV testing altogether, believing oneself to be seropositive, without a history of high-risk sexual behavior.   Most trauma survivors are internally fragmented to some degree; their internal experience is chaotic because one or more memory fragments were frozen in time and split off from consciousness at the moment the individual was in grave danger. Each of these fragments contains the vivid details of specific traumatic events that were experienced immediately prior to the act of splitting off from consciousness. The break with consciousness appears to occur because the level of danger to the self has risen to an intolerable degree. In the case of earlier sexual traumatization, the danger that has become intolerable typically takes one of the following forms: 1) a directly or indirectly stated or nonverbally implied threat to kill the victim should he disclose the abuse; 2) the somatic experience of suffocation, of being "crushed" or "broken open" or "ripped apart," resulting from being pinned underneath the full weight of an adult's body or of having been violated; or 3) the overwhelming fear of decompensating in the presence of danger that is too massive to bear.

Although memory fragments do effectively break away from consciousness, this does not mean that they remain completely repressed. Each fragment continuously replays the traumatic events experienced just prior to the splitting of consciousness, but in as somatically heightened and cognitively unmediated a form as they were originally experienced. What a survivor eventually recalls to have been a directly stated threat against his life is first experienced only as the persistent threat of immediate anger. For example, the crushing and suffocating weight of an obese uncle's full body weight on the abused child's chest is first experienced only somatically as the recurring feeling of suffocation because of a lack of air.

The anticipatory anxiety of testing seropositive triggers memory fragments of the earlier trauma and brings them partially to consciousness. These fragments are retrieved in the forms in which they were originally stored (i.e., as somatic or affective memory fragments), and they are usually experienced as intense sensations or emotions that occur without reference to their original context. Once these fragments have been accessed, many survivors fail to discriminate between the perceived future and the past trauma. They react to the prospect of testing seropositive as they reacted to the earlier sexual abuse. They may experience debilitating fear, overwhelming dread, a sense of extreme danger resulting from the certainty that disaster is imminent, and a developing paralysis commensurate with the sense of encroaching danger. The earlier sexual abuse has scripted a role for the prospect of testing seropositive to play: the role of imminent disaster. The virus is clearly in the role of perpetrator. It is important to approach a survivor who manifests these reactions to HIV testing as gently and respectfully as one would approach a young child who has just experienced severe trauma. This precludes intervening educationally, as so often happens, as though the reason the gay survivor avoids testing is because he lacks information.

Avoiding HIV testing altogether, believing oneself to be seropositive, with a history of and possibly ongoing high-risk sexual behavior. The prospective trauma of testing seropositive evokes the same type of fragments of earlier trauma for survivors in this category as those just described, with one important difference. Survivors in this category appear to blame themselves most severely for having become infected with HIV. They frequently excoriate themselves for their past sexual behavior and easily adopt the perspective that their contraction of the virus was justly deserved. Although they may morally judge themselves and others who share similar histories, the moral tone of their negative self-labeling reveals a deep and abiding confusion between the experiences of the self as perpetrator and the self as victim.

This confusion functions as a medium through which the survivor indirectly remembers the shame that followed his earlier sexual humiliation. In many cases it is a medium through which the survivor symbolically recalls the dialogue following the traumatic incident in which his experience was disclosed to someone in a position of trust. Having exposed the abuse, the survivor was then blamed for its occurrence, attacked for constructing lies about the perpetrator, or labeled "crazy" for misperceiving reality. Once this second-order abuse occurred and its memory was split off from consciousness, the survivor was effectively turned against himself by having been cast simulta-neously as perpetrator and victim. From this point in time, the sec-ond-order abuse is reenacted in one part of the survivor's self turning against another part.

It is common for survivors in this category to fear that they will impulsively suicide or decompensate in response to a seropositive test result. It is important that the clinician assess the potentially traumatic underpinnings of this fear. Patients who have experienced the second-order abuse described above are more likely to frame HIV testing as a referendum on their status as perpetrators or victims, with a seropos-itive result confirming their status as perpetrators. These survivors are at an especially high risk for suicide and other less lethal self-destruc-tive behavior from the point in time at which they begin to consider taking the test. The level of danger to these survivors decreases as soon as the traumatic underpinnings of their fears are raised for exploration and memories of the second-order abuse in particular begin to surface.

Rushing into HIV testing with no apparent anxiety, believing oneself to be—or seeking to be—seropositive, with a history of and ongoing high-risk sexual behavior.   After testing seropositive, it is not un-common for survivors in this category to react with a sense of great calm. Paradoxically, they often describe feeling as though they have just won, not lost, a great battle. Unlike survivors in the previous cat-egory, these survivors appear to have constructed seropositivity as confirmation that they are in fact victims, not perpetrators. Before these survivors have brought memories of earlier trauma to con-sciousness, a period in time that usually coincides with the behavior of seeking to become infected, HIV infection appears to function as a symbolic embodiment of the traumatized state, a condition marked by one or more of the following characteristics: 1) a vaguely defined yet unmistakably experienced internal sense of feeling broken or defec-tive, 2) a sense of shame or of having been humiliated, and 3) a sense of guilt or of having done something bad or wrong. Until these survi-vors can identify having been specifically traumatized, these general-ized feelings, which are affective memory fragments, carry the full burden of remembering the earlier sexual trauma.

Remembering trauma indirectly through the prism of generalized affective states without concrete experiential referents on which to base the sense of one's own personal history leads the survivor inevitably to feel ungrounded, unmoored, or unreal. HIV is experienced by survivors in this category as the previously missing factor that grounds them in a reality that makes sense to them internally. HIV externalizes, concretizes, and legitimizes the vaguely defined yet unmistakably experienced traumatized state these survivors have experienced since childhood. Upon confirmation of their seropositive status, these survivors frequently mobilize their internal resources and live life more fully because HIV has mirrored their internal sense of themselves as no person or circumstance had done before.

Immunosuppression and Opportunistic Infections: The Body as Perpetrator

As an HIV-infected gay man progresses along the spectrum of HIV infection, his body's immune response is incrementally suppressed, leaving him with a corresponding increase in vulnerability to opportunistic infection. The appearance of immunosuppressive symptomatology confronts the gay trauma survivor with a heightened sense of bodily vulnerability to the unpredictable onslaught of multiple infectious agents. The prospective (or ongoing) trauma of facing serious infection with only diminishing resources with which to combat it has a tremendous potential for evoking the affective and physiological correlates of the earlier traumatization. Immunosuppressive symptomatology frequently appears to evoke memory fragments of second-order abuse (i.e., the retraumatization that occurs when the survivor is blamed, further humiliated, or disqualified after having disclosed the original trauma to a trusted individual) through two distinct experiences of bodily vulnerability: 1) when the body is experienced as the enemy that turns and attacks the self, or 2) when the body fails to defend or protect the self from the combined assault of HIV and various infectious agents. The somatic and affective memory fragments of the *original trauma* may be retriggered when, having experienced the body's diminishing capacity to provide protection from illness, the survivor waits in fear for opportunistic infection to strike.

Experiencing Immunosuppression as a Reenactment of Second-Order Abuse

The Body as the Enemy

Trauma survivors differ in their capacity to experience *bodily safety,* defined variously as a sense of having control over another's access to one's body, as the experience of feeling a protective space surrounding one's body, or as a boundary that demarcates one's body as a distinct entity. Almost all survivors have experienced bodily sensations associated with the somatic retrieval of earlier traumatization, most of which are unpleasant and frightening. Long before acquiring the ability to assimilate the trauma cognitively, these survivors experienced their bodies as a source of pain rather than pleasure, as a source of an unfocused yet imminent danger rather than a shield that provided safe repose. These experiences account for the greatly augmented capacity of survivors to dissociate from their bodies. Once they have dissociated, the body is no longer experienced as connected to the self, but rather is split off and regarded as the "other." To this extent, most trauma survivors have experienced standing in opposition to their own bodies.

A smaller group of survivors adds to this experience the profound confusion they feel from simultaneously experiencing themselves as victims and as perpetrators, a phenomenon that stems from second-order trauma. When a recently lowered T cell count or newly manifested symptomatology that confirms the occurrence of further immunosuppression triggers memory fragments of second-order abuse, these survivors may present in treatment as having lost the will to fight, surrendering completely to the inevitability of succumbing to infection. Paradoxically, this may occur early in the course of HIV infection, when their T cell count remains above 500 and the types of opportunistic infections encountered are, relatively speaking, benign. From the time these survivors tested seropositive to their present position along the HIV spectrum, they may have conceptualized themselves as struggling to live with HIV as fully as possible and may have been judged by others to have done so with dignity and hope. However, when these survivors experience themselves surrendering completely to the early signs of immunosuppression, they must confront head-on the reality that what they had initially understood to be living in the face of HIV was in actuality either denying that they had contracted the virus or dismissing the potential of HIV to impact their lives negatively.

The most effective way to assess the potentially traumatic etiology of this denial is to facilitate the patient's exploration of recent changes in his relationship with his body. Once the early signs of immunosuppression have appeared, the trauma patient with a history of second-order abuse may express anger toward or hatred of his body, the sheer intensity of which the clinician could reasonably assume would be reserved for a perpetrator.

One survivor under these circumstances described his body as a "toxic waste dump poisoning the underground water supply" on which he depended to live. When the patient was asked whether he was referring to his body or to HIV, he immediately dissociated and began to reexperience, only somatically at first, having been beaten by his father after disclosing that his paternal uncle had sexually molested him. Another patient verbally assaulted his body for "having lied to and tricked" him and for having given him a "false sense of safety and comfort" by feeling well after having tested seropositive, thereby reassuring him that HIV infection would have only a minimal impact upon him. When this reaction to his body was explored over several sessions, this patient began to regress to an earlier period in which he felt "crazy" and then "mind fucked," as he put it, as though someone were attempting to drive him crazy systematically. After a great deal of work piecing together memory fragments, he eventually recalled a conversation he initiated with his mother in which he told her of his father's ongoing sexual abuse of him. His mother responded by reprimanding him for "having disgusting thoughts," and threatened to bring him before their parish priest whom she stated somewhat darkly "would certainly know how to deal with you" if the boy disclosed his "dirty thoughts" to anyone else. In the case of both these patients, memory fragments of second-order abuse had been stored primarily in the survivors' relationship with their own bodies, and these fragments began to be retrieved, somewhat mystifyingly at first, when the initial somatic effects of immunosuppression were manifested.

The Body That Fails to Protect From the Enemy

When, as just described, the body is experienced as an enemy to the self, the survivor is remembering the consequences of a particular type of second-order trauma (i.e., the confusion from experiencing the self as perpetrator and victim simultaneously, resulting from having been blamed for the original trauma). When, however, in response to further immunosuppression, the body is experienced not as an enemy to the self but as failing to protect the self from an unwanted intrusion, the survivor may be remembering a different type of second-order trauma. Instead of blaming the victim, the trusted individual to whom the original trauma was disclosed may have shirked his or her responsibility as a parental figure to provide safety for the child. In some cases, the parental figure may have regressed on hearing of the child's trauma and may have begun to access the memory fragments of his or her own earlier traumatization. The parental figure may then have attempted to reverse roles and parentify the child while the child was in the process of disclosing his own trauma, effectively communicating to the young survivor that he did not have a safe parental figure on whom he could lean for support. Under these circumstances the child may have felt that he had to toughen up enough to become a safe enough parental figure on whom his parent could lean for support.

When new evidence of further immunosuppression or the development of an opportunistic infection triggers memory fragments of this type of second-order trauma, the survivor may present himself in treatment as completely absorbed by the final stages of AIDS. He may visualize himself in the future as increasingly debilitated with no one to care for him as his dependency on others necessarily increases. The more absorbed he becomes in his projected future, the more deprived, neglected, and abandoned he feels in the present. The survivor in this predicament typically has intermittent difficulties with object constancy; when his projection of his earlier trauma into the future heightens feelings of deprivation and neglect in the present, the survivor may intermittently be unable to internalize another's love and care for him. When this happens, the survivor is at a greatly increased risk for suicide.

The most effective way to assess the potentially traumatic etiology of the survivor's projection of himself into the final stages of AIDS is to facilitate his exploration of recent changes in his relationship with his body. The patient who is remembering earlier sexual traumatization within the larger context of neglect reacts to the early signs of immunosuppression by feeling abandoned by his body, as illustrated in the following case example.

Case 2

Mr. B, a survivor of sexual abuse, stated in treatment that he used to feel "supported" by his body, that he used to feel that his body made it possible for him to exist as a person. Now he felt that the opposite was true, that his body endangered his continued existence. He felt that now it was necessary for him to care for his body in the way that his body was supposed to take care of him. When Mr. B was asked how his body was supposed to take care of him, he became agitated and then angry. He refused to speak for a long period of time, after which he grew sullen. He began to cry and, with a mixture of sadness and anger in his voice, described an incident that he said had "popped" into his mind during his long period of silence. He described a private conversation with his father during which he disclosed that he had been sexually abused by his uncle at regular intervals over a period of several years. After hearing this disclosure, Mr. B's father burst into tears and told Mr. B that he too had been sexually assaulted by his brother (Mr. B's uncle) since childhood and was still being assaulted by him.

It appeared from Mr. B's description that his father was attempting to join him in complaining about their common perpetrator. At this point in the session, Mr. B described feeling utterly hopeless and suicidal. He began to sob uncontrollably as he further described how as a child he had never felt secure any time he was in a vulnerable position vis-à-vis an adult. Before the memory of this incident had "popped" into his awareness, he had been indirectly remembering the incident by using two distinct yet related mechanisms: 1) he underwent a change in his relationship to his body from feeling supported by it to feeling abandoned by it, and 2) he projected himself into the final stages of his illness in which he felt abandoned by others at a time when he would be most dependent on their care. Both of these were affective memory fragments of second-order trauma that were evoked by new evidence of further immunosuppression.

When Immunosuppression and Opportunistic Infection Retrigger the Original Trauma

Sometimes the physical symptoms associated with immunosuppression (e.g., fatigue, dizziness, night sweats, skin rashes) or those related to opportunistic infections that occur first along the spectrum of HIV-related illness (e.g., upper respiratory symptoms associated with candidiasis, hairy leukoplakia in the mouth) occur in the same general areas of the body where the somatic memory fragments of earlier sexual trauma are experienced. These memory fragments usually take the form of sensations that have been previously experienced without reference to their original traumatic context, but they may also be body memories that have been accessed for the first time by the occurrence of HIV-related changes in the same or related body parts. At other times affective states associated with immunosuppression and infection access the affective memory fragments of earlier sexual trauma. When this happens, the affective bridge between HIV and earlier sexual traumatization appears to be the experience of bodily vulnerability to the uncertain yet anticipated attack of opportunistic agents, an experience that leaves one feeling broken and in need of healing.

Survivors for whom new evidence of immunosuppression and infection evokes the somatic and affective memory fragments of the original sexual trauma may present in therapy as preoccupied with the prospect of serious infection, which they anticipate with great trepidation. They appear agitated and morbidly afraid of infection. The most effective way to assess the potentially traumatic underpinnings of this fear is to facilitate exploration of the patients' physical and emotional reactions to the prospect of serious infection. It is important to note, however, that a traumatic history is not the only reason one would react strongly to, for example, a recently lowered T cell count, particularly when the new count places one within a range that is associated with increased vulnerability to infection. What appears to differentiate a trauma survivor under these circumstances is 1) the morbidity of his fear of infection, and 2) the fact that his fear appears to increase rather than subside over time as the therapist focuses more sharply on its underlying causes. In fact, as the following case example makes clear, the closer the focus of therapy is to the traumatic etiology underlying the fear of infection, the greater the degree of agitation and fear the patient experiences.

Case 3

Mr. C, a patient who had previously manifested candidiasis and hairy leukoplakia, had just received a T cell count that registered a 130-point drop over that of the previous 3 months. He immediately developed a sleep disturbance. He described habitually awakening in the middle of the night in a state of terror, assessing his body, one part after another, for the signs of developing infection. As he did this, he affectively alternated between the terror of discovering the signs of developing infection and the wish that he might discover them soon so that he might bring out into the open whatever danger was lurking. As Mr. C described his associations to the terror of imminent yet uncertain danger, his agitation increased to the point where he described feeling as though the only way he could experience relief would be to jump out of his skin. With a great deal of encouragement to breathe through and stay with these experiences, Mr. C eventually remembered how often he had lain awake at night when he was young anticipating the following sequence of events: hearing his father's footsteps as he arrived home intoxicated; hearing his father verbally assault his mother and then physically beat her into submission; hearing his father begin to break through the door to his bedroom, which he had previously barricaded shut; and then remembering only the sounds his father made as he sexually abused him. Mr. C's morbid fear of the prospect of serious infection mirrored his earlier experience of lying awake at night anticipating the trauma that was sure to come. The morbid fear itself was an affective memory fragment of the earlier sexual trauma that was evoked by his own understandably strong reaction to his recently lowered T cell count.

Intrusive Medical Procedures:
The Health Service Provider as Perpetrator

As the gay trauma survivor progresses further along the HIV spectrum, is diagnosed with AIDS, and develops increasingly serious opportunistic infections, his deteriorating medical condition renders him steadily more dependent on the services of health care providers in order to survive. He may experience episodes during which this dependency snatches away the privacy and independence that came with self-care. He may also be required to undergo painfully intrusive medical procedures for diagnosis and treatment.

As the trauma survivor grows more dependent on health care providers, who of necessity must have intimate access to his body, he may revisit traumatic earlier relationships with the adults who were charged with providing him with parental sustenance. When this mirroring does occur, the affective bridge that associates parental care to health care is comprised chiefly of two components: 1) the survivor's affective response to the issue of dependency, which frequently consists of feeling trapped in a dangerous relationship, outside of which the child is too young to survive and within which he is too endangered to feel safe; and 2) the survivor's affective response to the issue of intrusion, which often involves feeling violated by a procedure that the he must accept in order to survive that is performed by an individual with whom the survivor shares a healing relationship. In this section I explore issues of dependency and intrusion as they relate to the experience of trauma survivors in the later stages of HIV infection.

Dependency

As a group, trauma survivors react so uniformly negatively to the prospect of becoming dependent on another person that their friendships and intimate relationships inevitably experience strain. The recognition of growing dependency between partners, both or one of whom may be a survivor of earlier trauma, typically evokes regressive experiences on the part of the survivor(s) that are characterized by some or all of the following phenomena: 1) feeling young and vulnerable; 2) feeling trapped and looking for a way to escape the relationship; 3) experiencing panic attacks or generalized anxiety states; 4) fearing physical or emotional attack by the partner who had not experienced trauma; 5) developing somatic complaints; the causes for which seem difficult to understand; 6) developing visual flashbacks; and 7) experiencing strong and in some cases explosive rage toward the partner who had not experienced trauma.

The experience of feeling dependent appears to function as one of the fastest tracks back to the time of the survivor's original trauma, and, once back in time, the survivor reexperiences the sensations and emotions associated with the earlier abuse. The dependency evokes such intensely regressive experiences because it captures the essence of the child's vulnerability to abuse; children by their nature cannot exist independently from their adult parental caretakers, so they are forced to endure episodic abuse for the sole purpose of survival. Survivors experience dependency as an essential component of earlier sexual trauma, especially when it occurs within the context of the extended family, for they see dependency as the condition that more than any other force actually blocked their escape from relationships in which they were traumatized.

One of the most devastating ways in which HIV-related illnesses retraumatize survivors is by returning them to a state in which they are dependent on the care and assistance of others in order to meet their survival needs. Health care providers are in the sensitive, sometimes delicate position of providing life-sustaining care to survivors with AIDS. In their professional capacity, they often elicit the projections of the trauma-related memory fragments that are accessed by the survivor's "enforced" return to a dependent state of living. More often than not, survivors have little or no cognizance of their feelings toward providers, so these feelings are indirectly expressed through their behavior in the professional relationship. Some of the more common examples of this type of behavior are as follows:

1. Resistance to following the doctor's or nurse's treatment protocol. This may take the form of resisting therapy with particular drugs, resisting specific modes of delivering drugs to the body (e.g., refusing all drugs administered intravenously), or tampering with the prescribed dosages of medications.
2. Resistance to accepting the doctor's or nurse's advice on making life-style changes for the purpose of increasing longevity (e.g., changes in diet, exercise, sleep patterns, safer sex procedures, exposure to the sun, meditation) or accepting advice regarding alternative treatments (e.g., acupuncture, massage).

3. Avoiding necessary services or specific providers for extended periods of time.

This type of behavior toward providers simultaneously expresses and conceals the survivor's feelings toward the individual(s) who sexually abused him as a child. The survivor adopts this indirect method of expressing his feelings in order to avoid permanently endangering the lifeline that exists between the provider, who has taken over the role of the perpetrator in that the patient must depend on him or her, and himself. When speaking to the survivor about his resistance or avoidance it is helpful to keep two things in mind: 1) it is crucial not to confront the survivor head-on, interpret his behavior in an especially clinical fashion, or in any way usurp his sense of control; and 2) it is more effective to highlight whatever the clinician can glean about the affective qualities of the survivor's resistance, and to assist the patient in associating to this material to help him gain access to the original trauma in as nonintrusive a manner as possible. The rule of thumb here is to conceptualize the survivor's modes of resisting medical treatment as attempts on his part to resist the advances of the original perpetrator. When these attempts are respected, and the survivor does not have to fight a simultaneous battle with the clinician on a second front, he will move quite naturally toward exploring his reactions to his providers as soon as he feels safe enough to do so.

Intrusive Procedures

It is not difficult to understand why trauma survivors as a group experience terror in anticipation of intrusive medical procedures and rage in their aftermath. Bodily intrusion is a violation of the social and personal injunctions against 1) having internal or some other type of extraordinary access to another's body, and 2) exercising control over another's body. It was precisely these injunctions against bodily intrusion that were violated by the perpetrators of the original trauma.

The survivor will be overly sensitized to possible bodily intrusion by the provider. First, it is crucial that the provider understand what is likely to be evoked in the survivor by requiring him to be naked before a provider. The survivor feels more embarrassment and shame than a nonsurvivor feels in this situation; he also experiences terror in anticipation of nakedness and humiliation after being naked. To cope with his reactions, the survivor must understand why, how, how much, how long, and when to become naked before it is time to do so. Second, should the survivor be hospitalized, it is helpful for him to know the provider is actively protective of the patient's physical privacy during rounds or joint conferences with the patient. To be on display physically without prior consent will always be powerfully evocative of earlier sexual trauma. Third, it is absolutely necessary to explain the details of suggested intrusive procedures by answering the questions why, when, how, and how long before attempting to secure the survivor's permission to proceed. When permission to proceed with a procedure is given before the details of it are known, the patient will feel trapped in the procedure once it has begun. When bodily intrusion is added to the feeling of entrapment, the provider has unwittingly assembled the most important pieces of a traumatic reenactment.

It is all too common for providers-in-training in the hospital setting to violate survivors with AIDS in many of the ways just cataloged. When this occurs, patients typically react with some form of direct or indirect rage, and a mental health consultant may be requested to help the patient understand and cope with his reaction. If the patient has a preexisting psychotherapy relationship with a clinician, his therapist may be called in to help at this point. When the patient reacts to medical intrusion by some form of directly expressed rage, he usually does so by yelling, screaming, blocking and refusing access to his body, tampering with his intravenous apparatus, or insulting providers in a deeply personal way. Indirect rage in response to medical intrusion usually takes the form of a lack of cooperation of any type, suspiciousness with the offending provider or with all providers, and splitting providers into two groups: those who are all good and those who are all bad. Once the problem of medical intrusion has been identified by the consultant, it is important not only to help the patient understand the violation at hand and the earlier memories it may have unleashed, but also to equip the offending provider(s) with more sophisticated skills for approaching and treating trauma patients.

Most survivors experienced sexual violation at a formative time in their personal development, when boundaries were by definition much more fluid or diffuse. Boundaries take shape over time as a direct consequence of the respect and care extended to survivors and their bodies by the adults in charge. A major consequence of sexual violation at an early age is the boundary disturbance that afflicts most survivors throughout their life. In some cases, boundaries do not appear to exist at all. In others they appear rigid and inflexible. In still others they are brittle, appearing stiff but easily chipped away. In general, as adults, survivors tend to mismanage the task of negotiating physical and emotional boundaries by either demanding too much distance to facilitate the smooth exchange of intimacy, or allowing too much closeness to fortify the sense of self and maintain personal safety and comfort. As a result, survivors tend to alternate between feeling isolated and feeling violated.

Boundary disturbances severely impact the capacity of survivors to negotiate issues of personal safety and comfort with providers. In anticipating an office visit with a physician, a home visit by a nurse, or a physically intrusive diagnostic or therapeutic procedure, it is likely that the survivor will experience the loss of his adult interactional skills as he begins to regress. In this traumatized state, he will be highly sensitized to possible emotional and physical intrusion by the provider. To minimize the resulting emotional intrusion, it is first of all necessary for the provider to offer the survivor as much control as possible over the specific manner in which the procedures are to be performed. Second, it is important that the provider acknowledge and negotiate social and personal boundaries before examining a survivor or initiating an intrusive procedure. From the survivor's point of view, the situation has already proceeded out of control if the provider waits for him to negotiate boundaries or assumes that his silence means his acceptance of what is occurring at the moment or is about to occur. Third, the provider must understand that the patient's level of personal safety increases as the provider demonstrates vigilance in protecting the survivor's emotional and social privacy.

The Torture of Dying

One of the most harrowing issues raised for gay trauma survivors by the process dying from AIDS-related illnesses is the extreme degree to which the illnesses, in their final stages, wrestle control over virtually every aspect of living away from the self. The high degree of affective resonance generated by such a lack of control results from multiple interlocking levels of trauma that are triggered simultaneously by the circumstances of dying from these illnesses. The most readily apparent trauma is the assault of the illnesses themselves. AIDS-related illnesses prove traumatic for everyone they touch, but particularly for the young. They prematurely age young gay men, wasting their bodies and minds, leaving them gaunt and only a shadow of their former selves. AIDS patients in the later stages of dying have described the horror of alternating between the fear of losing control over one's mind and the fear of remaining sane.

Less immediately apparent yet still evoked by the assault of illness is the stigmatization gay men have experienced stemming from their sexual orientation. Gay men instinctively know the traumatic consequences of having trusted individuals, in many cases family members and close friends, control whether or not their most basic desires are fulfilled. This trauma is amplified by the stigmatization that is specifically targeted at AIDS patients. (For an extended discussion of this double stigmatization, see Chapters 1 and 22.) Less apparent still is the evocation of childhood sexual trauma, memory fragments of which are accessed during the process of dying from AIDS-related illnesses. At this level of trauma, loss of control over any bodily function or any other aspect of living rapidly overwhelms the survivor with searing flashes of terror and dread. Although these emotions may be experienced by the AIDS patient as expressions of the most readily apparent trauma (i.e., the assault of the illness itself), they may also appear to reflect a much earlier encounter with terror and dread at the hands of a perpetrator. In this final section of the chapter, I focus on how the gradual erosion of the survivor's control over his own life that is brought about by the dying process evokes memory fragments of earlier sexual abuse.

As every individual negotiates the specific tasks associated with each stage of human development, he or she must learn how not only to take control of certain aspects of living but also to surrender control over other dimensions of life. Some developmental theorists have argued that the issue of surrendering or sharing control is ultimately the most important developmental skill to master because of the central roles surrendering and sharing play in the development of intimate human relationships. Surrendering and sharing have also been described as the most difficult skills to develop because their mastery requires emergence from the narcissistic preoccupations of childhood. On a different level, the experience of losing control is a fundamental component of all developmental change because developmental turning points are times in life when, on one hand, previously mastered skills no longer suffice to meet changing needs and responsibilities and, on the other hand, the new skills required to cope effectively with change have not yet been developed.

As a group, survivors of earlier sexual trauma demonstrate extraordinary difficulty in responsibly surrendering or sharing control because, as children, their fledgling sense of personal control over their own bodies was violently overridden by deliberate sexual violation. Thereafter, any experience that raises the specter of losing control, regardless of its context, tends to evoke in affective and somatic terms the prospect of rape. When an AIDS patient initially grapples with the idea that he may be dying, he begins a process of developmental change that perhaps more than any other will require that he share and ultimately surrender control before he is able to make sense of and come to terms with what is happening to him. The difficult process of discerning 1) whether one is in the final stages of AIDS, and then 2) whether to fight the loss of control, to share control, or to surrender control, is rarely experienced by the survivor as a process of initiating developmental change. Instead, the experience is almost always shaped by the affectively and somatically determined sequelae of abuse. The survivor often reacts in one of three ways: 1) he may immediately surrender complete control at the first sign that the process of dying may have begun, essentially replicating the earlier experience of paralysis at the hands of a perpetrator; 2) he may refuse to share or surrender control to anyone under any circumstances, sometimes continuing in this vein until he takes his own life in a final manifestation of retaining complete control (in this instance the survivor will do anything to avoid reexperiencing the terror associated with the earlier traumatic loss of control); or 3) he may attack those who would most likely share or take over control as it becomes necessary, symbolically rebuffing the advances of an earlier perpetrator, one to whom he was previously forced to surrender.

Frequently, the trauma survivor with AIDS who begins to confront the proximity of death appears to be stuck in an endless rage of tremendous ferocity. Even when the survivor appears to target his rage solely at the issue of dying, it may simultaneously be covertly directed at other targets. At the deepest level, this rage is often an affective memory fragment of earlier abuse, and as such it is directed at the original perpetrator. This fact may be partially obscured by the survivor's preoccupation with overwhelming regret that he may be blocked from achieving many of his personal goals in life because of the likelihood of premature death.

For example, one patient who had survived sexual abuse in childhood experienced tremendous regret that death would rob him of the chance to develop an intimate relationship with another man. When he was encouraged to explore his regret, his rage at death emerged. When he was encouraged not to escape this feeling, his rage gradually began to be directed against himself for having lived a life characterized by distance and disconnection in his relationships. At this point in the process, his body and affect began simultaneously to explode with a dizzying mix of sensations and emotions. He began to feel enraged with the man who sexually abused him as a child for having rendered him "just a shell of a person," one who was ill equipped to sustain intimate relationships.

In general, the rage that is experienced at the prospect of dying from AIDS-related illnesses, but which actually has its deepest roots in earlier sexual traumatization, is characterized first by its propensity to be intractable (i.e., it completely envelops the survivor and does not allow him to progress through the subsequent stages of coping with the proximity of death), and second by its high degree of toxicity (i.e., it has a poisonous effect on the survivor's relationships).

In the final stages of AIDS, survivors may be extraordinarily preoccupied with suicide, particularly during the time of their initial confrontation with the prospect of dying. The reasons they cite for wanting to take their own lives may be deeply rooted in childhood abuse. Examples include 1) the survivor who experienced the virus as "stalking" him, with the growing certainty as death approached that the virus would ultimately overwhelm him; and 2) the survivor who experienced the increasing proximity of death as more and more dangerous, such that his only route to safety appeared to be the option of taking his own life. When the connection is made by the survivor between the affective experience of losing control to advancing death and the affective ramifications of having lost control over the access granted to one's body, it sometimes emerges that the wish to commit suicide is itself an affective memory fragment of earlier trauma. In this instance, the survivor, without recognizing it, revives the wish to die that he experienced as a child. There are many circumstances in which a traumatized child may have wished to die, but three occur most often: 1) when the abuse that was being perpetrated felt too massive to endure, 2) when the perpetrator threatened to kill the survivor, or 3) when the survivor feared that he would die as a direct result of the sexual abuse in progress (e.g., being unable to breathe under the full weight of an adult's body). When it is possible to recontextualize suicidal impulses, the process of dying from AIDS-related illnesses may no longer be required to function as the primary medium through which the survivor gains access to his memories of childhood trauma. No longer confounded with earlier abuse, the process of dying may, in some cases, resume the course originally charted by Kubler-Ross (1969); that is, after denial and rage have been experienced, it is possible for the survivor to move through the additional states of bargaining and despair before achieving acceptance of death.

Summary

Many survivors of childhood sexual abuse initially report tremendous difficulty remembering the original events that traumatized them. The characterization of their common experience as amnesia, however, is based on an understanding of memory as it functions under normal circumstances and is not altogether accurate. These same patients continually replay their psychophysiological responses to childhood trauma as though the original danger never subsided (Kardiner 1941), reinforcing the idea that they have never, even for a moment, ceased to remember earlier trauma. The moment of extreme terror that comprised the core of a traumatic episode appears to have been encoded by an alternative form of memory that freezes the psychophysiological correlates of terror (Herman 1992). These somatic and affective responses are experienced by trauma survivors as reactions in search of a context because they exist without a comprehensible narrative to explain them.

The lives of people who were sexually abused as children are quite often characterized by a heroic search for narrative events that would explain their traumatic responses to ordinary as well as unusual occurrences. For the most part, this search is conducted neither consciously nor linearly (deductively), but rather in a loosely associative fashion, in a manner similar to that used by a child. When an unremarkable occurrence serves as a disguised reminder of childhood trauma and triggers a traumatic response, the survivor unknowingly reacts to the triggering occurrence, as well as to the people and circumstances associated with it, as he previously responded to the original abuse. It would not be unusual for him to respond to any of the specific components of the triggering occurrence as though the abuse were being perpetrated by the original abuser at that moment. This is the way in which the survivor most often makes sense of his recurring traumatic psychophysiological responses.

For gay men who have been sexually abused, the psychological sequelae of AIDS-related illnesses may serve to trigger somatic and affective responses associated with earlier sexual abuse. The process by which the survivor unconsciously associates his experience of AIDS-related illnesses with childhood trauma must be fully appreciated by the clinician for all that it reveals about the original abuse rather than be disqualified as a distortion of present-day events. When this process is understood to be the patient's naturally occurring mode of remembering childhood trauma, and it is positively framed for the patient as such, it may then serve as the basis for identifying and ultimately piecing together the isolated memory fragments of the original trauma.

References

Brett EA, Ostroff R: Imagery and posttraumatic stress disorder: an overview. Am J Psychiatry 142:417–424, 1985

Burgess AW, Holstrom E: Adaptive strategies in recovery from rape. Am J Psychiatry 136:1278–1282, 1979

Burgess AW, Hartman CR, McCormack A: Abuseu to abuser: antecedents of socially deviant behavior. Am J Psychiatry 144:1431–1436, 1987

Helzer JE, Robins LN, McEvoy L: Post-traumatic stress disorder in the general population. N Engl J Med 26:1630–1634, 1987

Hendin H, Pollinger Haas A, Singer P: The influence of precombat personality on post-traumatic stress disorders. Compr Psychiatry 24:530–534, 1983

Herman JL: Trauma and Recovery: The Aftermath of Violence—From Domestic Abuse to Political Terror. New York, Basic Books, 1992

Jacobs WJ, Nadel L: Stress-induced recovery of fears and phobias. Psychol Rev 92:512–531, 1985

Kardiner A: The Traumatic Neuroses of War. New York, P. Hoeber, 1941

Kubler-Ross E: On Death and Dying. New York, MacMillan, 1969

Pattison EM, Kahan J: The deliberate self-harm syndrome. Am J Psychiatry 140:867–872, 1983

Putnam FW, Guroff JJ, Silberman EK: The clinical phenomenology of multiple personality disorder. J Clin Psychiatry 47:285–293, 1986

Pynoos RS, Eth S: Developmental perspectives on psychic trauma in childhood, in Trauma and Its Wake. Edited by Figley CR. New York, Brunner/Mazel, 1985

Rossi EL: The Psychobiology of Mind-Body Healing: New Concepts of Therapeutic Hypnosis. New York, WW Norton, 1986

Rossi EL, Cheek DB: Mind-Body Therapy: Methods of Ideodynamic Healing in Hypnosis. New York, WW Norton, 1988

Squire LR: Memory and the Brain. New York, Oxford University Press, 1987

van der Kolk BA: Psychological Trauma. Washington, DC, American Psychiatric Press, 1987

van der Kolk BA: The trauma spectrum: the interaction of biological and social events in the genesis of the trauma response. J of Traumatic Stress 1:273–290, 1988

van der Kolk, BA Greenberg MS, Boyd H, et al: Inescapable shock, neurotransmitters, and addiction to trauma: towards a psychobiology of post-traumatic stress. Biol Psychiatry 20:314–325, 1985

Chapter 19

HIV and Substance Abuse in the Gay Male Community

Robert P. Cabaj, M.D.

A s this entire book makes clear, the human immunodeficiency virus (HIV) has had a profound impact on the gay community and on all therapists working with gay men. In addition, it has been evident for many years that gay men are at a particularly high risk for substance abuse. Although the link between HIV and intravenous (IV) drug use involving shared needles is obvious, there is also an important association between the spread of HIV and the use of all other substances of abuse, including alcohol. HIV and substance abuse in the gay population combine to create a difficult challenge in providing preventive and mental health interventions for gay men.

Homosexual Behavior, Substance Abuse, and HIV Infection

Link Between Substance Abuse and HIV Infection Among Gay Men

Men who have sex with men continue to be the largest at-risk group for current and new cases of HIV infection and acquired immunodeficiency syndrome (AIDS) in the United States; they accounted for 57% of all adult AIDS cases in the United States at the end

405

of December 1992 (Centers for Disease Control [CDC] 1993). Although most clinicians and researchers attribute the spread of HIV in this population to certain high-risk, unsafe sexual practices, the role of IV drug use is also significant. The same CDC report (1993) noted that an additional 6% of all adult cases of AIDS occurred in IV drug uses who were also gay or bisexual, meaning that 63% of all AIDS cases involve men who have sex with men. Those who claim their IV drug use to be their only risk factor comprise 23% of the total cases. All the CDC data need to be viewed critically, however, as many men in the IV drug use–only category may also have sex with men but fail to report this additional risk category for a variety of reasons—internalized homophobia and denial, fear of negative reactions from health care providers, cultural and ethnic variables, or fear of the reaction of friends and family who do not know they are gay or bisexual. In turn, many gay and bisexual men do not report IV drug use for similar reasons—fear of the negative reaction of friends and family, fear of rejection by health care providers, and the denial that accompanies substance abuse.

Sharing HIV-contaminated needles clearly increases the risk of spreading the infection. There is a more subtle, but extremely important, link between the spread of HIV infection and the use of alcohol, noninjected drugs of abuse, or abused prescribed medicines, all of which alter judgment and allow disinhibition in sexual behaviors. In several reviews of gay men and safer sex practices (Leigh 1990; Stall 1988; Stall et al. 1986), it was found that the great majority of men who were knowledgeable about safer sex failed to practice it while under the influence of some substance, whether it was alcohol or another drug. In addition, some high-risk sexual activities that certain gay men enjoy, such as sadomasochistic interactions or activities, such as *fisting* (insertion of fingers, hand, or forearm into the anus and rectum of a partner), are often performed with the use of drugs such as amyl nitrite (i.e., "poppers"), alcohol, and marijuana in order to reduce inhibitions and induce physical relaxation (Cabaj 1985; Goode and Troiden 1979; Lange et al. 1988; Smith et al. 1982). Judgment is clearly suspended or altered during even the moderate, let alone heavy, use of alcohol and other substances, often leading to the failure to follow safer sex guidelines. Furthermore, there is some evidence that most abused substances alter the immune system, which may well compromise the system's initial reaction to HIV exposure (MacGregor 1988).

With the widespread use of such substances by gay men, substance use and abuse are definite cofactors in the spread of HIV through sexual practices and may well be the primary cofactors in the continuing spread of HIV in the gay population.

Extent of Substance Abuse Within the Gay Community

Most studies and the experiences of most clinicians working with gay men and lesbians estimate an incidence of chemical dependencies among these patients at approximately 30% (with ranges between 28% and 35%) versus between 10% and 12% for the general population (Beatty 1983; Diamond and Wilsnack 1978; Fifield et al. 1975; Lesbian and Gay Substance Abuse Planning Group 1991; Lewis et al. 1982; Lohrenz et al. 1978; Morales and Graves 1983; Saghir and Robins 1973; Weinberg and Williams 1974). Most of these studies have been criticized for various reasons: poor control conditions, poor populations samples (many subjects were gathered at gay and lesbian bars), and failure to have uniform definitions of substance abuse or of homosexuality itself. The Lesbian and Gay Substance Abuse Planning Group of San Francisco (1991) did the most recent and thorough review, but also depended in part on self-report surveys. Nonetheless, it is very striking how uniform the results have been among various socioeconomic groups, in urban or rural settings, in the United States or other countries. Alcohol abuse or addiction was the primary focus of most studies. No specific studies of IV drug use and the gay population are currently available, although the CDC monthly *AIDS-HIV Surveillance Reports* clearly indicate a subgroup of IV drug–using gay and bisexual men (Centers for Disease Control 1993). The number of gay men who abuse substances is far greater than the number of HIV-infected men. The actual number of HIV-infected gay men who abuse substances is not known, but extrapolation from the above data implies that the likelihood of an HIV-infected gay man being a substance user or abuser is high.

Predispositions for Substance Abuse

In working with gay men who have substance abuse problems and who are affected by HIV directly or indirectly, it is useful to understand why there is such a high incidence of substance abuse in the gay population. The etiology is likely multifactorial, involving genetic, biochemical, biological, cultural, environmental, and psychological factors.

Genetic, biochemical, and biological factors.   New research continues to support the genetic, biological, and biochemical components of the substance abuse disorders. There is growing evidence that homosexual orientation may also have genetic, biological, and biochemical components (Bailey and Benishay 1993; Bailey and Pillard 1991; Pillard 1988; Pillard and Weinrich 1986; Pillard et al. 1982). Some of the studies of familial patterns (Pillard 1988; Pillard et al. 1982) have indicated that gay men have a greater than normal chance of having an alcoholic father. It is possible that the genetic materials for sexual orientation and substance abuse are chromosomally linked. However, although the results of several studies indicate that male and female homosexuality are different and have different familial patterns (Bailey and Benishay 1993; Bailey and Pillard 1991; Bell and Weinberg 1978; Bell et al. 1981; Pillard 1988), the rates of substance abuse are the same for gay men and lesbian women.

Social factors.   Although gay men and lesbians may not have a greater genetic predisposition for substance abuse than their heterosexual counterparts, they may have a greater expression of whatever genetic predisposition exists because of the combination of societal, cultural, environmental, and psychological factors that impact them. Most societies or cultures that are in turmoil or undergoing social change have higher rates of alcoholism (Cassel 1976; Vaillant 1983). The gay population certainly faces continuous stress and turmoil stemming from societal homophobia and legal prohibitions, and, over the last several years, from the effects of HIV infection.

Legal prohibitions and the failure of society to accept or even acknowledge gay men lead to limited social outlets for them, which are usually bars, private homes, or clubs where alcohol and other drugs play a prominent role. These sites are still the primary social environments available, although the number and type of alternative sites are increasing.

By following the early development and progression through the life cycle of most gay men, the link with substance use and gay identity formation may become clear. Gay men need to negotiate three steps that heterosexual men do not: 1) recognizing and accepting that they have a homosexual orientation that leads them to desire having their affectional and sexual needs met primarily by someone of the same sex; 2) negotiating a process of self-identity and self-recognition as a gay man, different from that of heterosexual males, known as *coming out*; and 3) confronting widespread and insidious dislike, hatred, and fear of gay men and homosexual activity and feelings, known as *homophobia*. Difficulties in progressing through these steps may help to explain their psychological predisposition to abusing substances.

Familial factors.   The Swiss psychoanalyst Miller (1981) described how parents form—and deform—the emotional lives of their talented or "different" children. Parental reactions shape a child's expression of needs and longings; parents reward what is familiar and acceptable to them and discourage or ignore behavior or needs they do not value or understand. Harm occurs when a parent is too depressed, preoccupied, influenced by drugs or alcohol, or narcissistic to respond to the actual needs and wants of the child. Children eventually learn to behave the way parents expect in order to receive rewards, and hide or deny the longings or needs that are not rewarded.

For the gay child, that awareness of being different, of having affectional and sexual longings that are different from the others around him, is usually evident quite early in life, especially in men. Male children who will grow up to be gay may require or desire a closer and more intimate relationship with their father or other males. This is not encouraged or even understood in our society (Isay 1989). The child hides his needs and longings, putting on a false front and creating a false self because these true needs are often rejected or described as wrong or bad. Dissociation and denial become major defenses in coping with internal feelings. Rejection and criticism lead to pain, denial, isolation, and fear, as demonstrated in the following case example.

Case 1

Mr. A, who sought help in maintaining sobriety after sustaining a job loss, seemed primarily concerned that his employer had discovered that he was gay and HIV positive and only secondarily concerned about his job situation. He was able to use both therapy and support groups to stay sober, but revealed a deep depression that required medication. In discussing his life, he recalled knowing he was different at age 4, even labeling himself as clearly gay at that age. However, he came out fully to himself and others as a gay man only at age 38, following years of social isolation. He remembered being a very active, friendly young child, and one who was in awe of his father's male friends until one day when his father saw him looking intensely at one of the older men and said to never do that again. He then withdrew and avoided all sexual activity in adolescence and early adulthood. He had been drinking heavily since high school.

The psychology of being different and learning to live in a society that does not readily accept differences shape the sexual identity development as the gay child emerges from childhood and during the latency period (de Monteflores 1986). In latency, children with gay feelings, especially boys with gender-atypical behavior, may fear other children and become more isolated. In adolescence, the gay sexual feelings emerge with great urgency, but with little or no context or permission for expressing them. Conformity is encouraged, which further supports denial and suppression of gay feelings, as adolescents often reject and isolate those who are different. As a result, the gay adolescent further develops dissociation and splitting off of affect and behavior.

Seeking Refuge in Mind-Altering Substances

Substance use relieves distress, can provide a source of acceptance, and, more importantly, mirrors the "comforting" dissociation developed in childhood. Alcohol and other drugs cause dissociation from feelings and anxiety, mimicking the emotional state many gay men had to develop in childhood to survive. The symptom-relieving aspects of this dissociative state help one fight the effects of homophobia; it can allow "forbidden" behavior, allow social comfort in bars or other unfamiliar social settings, and provide comfort just by its very nature. Some gay men cannot imagine socializing without alcohol or other mood-altering substances. Many men had their first homosexual sexual experiences while drinking or being drunk. This connection between the pleasure and release of substance use and the pleasure and release of sex is a powerful behavioral link that is difficult to change or "unlink" later in life. Furthermore, endogenous endorphins, which are associated with pleasure and euphoric effects, are released by both sexual activity and some of the drugs of abuse, possibly adding a physiological component that strengthens the link between sex and substance use, especially for gay men who may be depressed from the effects of homophobia.

The easy availability of alcohol and drugs at gay bars or parties encourages the use of substances early in the coming out and gay socialization process. The substance use helps many HIV-infected gay men brace themselves for rejection by family, friends, or partners that may be attendant with their coming out as a gay man, as HIV-infected, or as both. Many gay men persist in a powerful and destructive self-hatred, especially if they are HIV infected. The use of mood-altering substances both temporarily relieves this self-loathing and then reinforces it during the drug-withdrawal period. It allows denial and even "blackouts" around sexual behavior, allowing some HIV-infected men to not disclose or discuss their HIV status, such as in the following example.

Case 2

Mr. B was raised in the South and was told that gay men were evil and were disciples of the devil; they were also objects of ridicule and even violent attacks in his community. Mr. B became aware of his gay feelings in high school but denied them to himself. He prayed to be allowed to be straight. He began to have gay sex in college, but only when intoxicated. He would go through a period of disgust and self-punishment after every contact, increasing his drinking to help blot out the shame, then having gay sex again after drinking enough. The cycle continued until he was referred for treatment by his employer, who was concerned about his drinking on the job.

Finally, the internal state that accompanies internalized homophobia and that which occurs in active substance abuse itself are very similar—the *dual oppression* of homophobia and abuse (Finnegan and McNally 1987). The following traits are seen in both states: denial; fear, anxiety, and paranoia; anger and rage; guilt; self-pity; depression, with helplessness, hopelessness, and powerlessness; self-deception and development of a false self; passivity and a feeling of being a victim; inferiority and low self-esteem; self-loathing; isolation, alienation, and feeling alone, misunderstood, or unique; and fragmentation and confusion. These parallel intrapsychic experiences often make it very difficult for an HIV-infected gay man who cannot grapple with his sexual orientation to deal with either his substance abuse or his HIV-related care.

Treatment Issues With HIV-Positive, Substance-Abusing Gay Men

Because of the many factors that make gay men vulnerable to substance abuse, intervention treatment and recovery may be difficult for them, especially when HIV plays a role.

Finding Gay-Affirmative Recovery Programs

A brief list of the treatment issues facing HIV-positive gay men in recovery includes the following: clean, sober, and safer sex; clean and sober socializing; employment problems, such as being out as a gay man at work or dealing with the loss of a job because of HIV status; family issues, including the family's acceptance of the patient's sexual orientation and HIV status, and the family's support during the recovery process; couple and relationship concerns; confidentiality and record keeping, especially regarding reporting of a patient's sexual orientation and HIV status in his medical records; custody of children; continuing and worsening medical problems; and legal problems. Living clean and sober and gay may be extremely difficult. Once gay men are clean and sober, they will need to face living in a homophobic society without the help of mind-altering substances. Gay-sensitive individual and possibly group psychotherapy in addition to gay-sensitive substance abuse recovery work may be necessary for many gay patients in early recovery. Discussions about sexual orientation and awareness of the impact of HIV are absolutely necessary in all detoxification and rehabilitation programs. All gay men in early recovery need help in looking at internalized homophobia and in finding ways to accept sexual orientation, as in the following example.

Case 3

Mr. C had been to several recovery programs and managed to stay clean from drugs and alcohol for 6 months. He enjoyed being clean and sober but was also unhappy. He had learned he was HIV positive several years earlier and seemed to have always known he was gay, but was not really out to anyone. In the substance abuse treatment programs, he had discussed neither his sexual orientation nor his HIV status. He had never been asked about these matters. In treatment he stated he believed he deserved to be infected with HIV because he was gay. On his next relapse, he agreed to go to a gay-affirmative treatment program—one that was not only gay sensitive but one that advocated that a recovering gay individual needed to accept being gay in order to have a successful recovery. Mr. C completed the program and had been sober for more than 1 year at last contact.

Twelve-step recovery programs and philosophies are the mainstays of recovery. However, there may be no gay-sensitive or HIV-aware therapists or counselors in the recovering patients' communities. Alcoholics Anonymous (AA), although open to all with broad accepting tenants (Kus 1987), is only a group of people at any individual meeting, people who may reflect the perceptions and prejudices of the local community and not be open to, or accepting of, openly gay or HIV-positive members. In addition, some of the suggestions and guidelines of AA and Narcotics Anonymous (NA) and most treatment programs may be harder for some gay men, especially those who are HIV positive, to follow. Giving up or avoiding old friends, especially fellow substance users, may be difficult when the gay man has limited contacts who relate to him as a gay man or accept him as an HIV-positive individual; such isolation may lead to relapse. Staying away from bars or parties, which are often gay men's only social outlets, may be difficult, so special help on how not to drink or use drugs in such settings may be necessary. The selection of a sponsor in groups such as AA or NA may be difficult both because of potential homophobic concerns or potential sexual tensions and feelings between a gay sponsor and a new gay member. Finally, many gay men mistakenly link AA and religion. Because religious institutions in general have been hostile and rejecting of gay men, there may be resistance to trying AA or NA out of a misguided fear of encountering a similar hostility, as in the following example:

Case 4

Mr. D used both intravenous amphetamines and alcohol. He sought help in dealing with the emotional impact of learning that he was HIV positive. Mr. D acknowledged that his drug and alcohol use were out of control and that he knew he was addicted. He had tried both NA and AA and felt that they were "like cults." Mr. D did not want to hear others discuss his HIV status, and he reported wanting to use drugs more after he went to a meeting. In addition, when he went to a gay AA meeting, he felt it was nothing but a "pickup place," just like a gay bar. Eventually he found a gay men's support group that did not insist on total sobriety where he was able to discuss being both gay and HIV infected. He finally was able to use AA and NA when he saw he could go to gain what he needed from the meetings and ignore what was not helpful.

In addition, some treatment centers and programs may be too frightened to work with HIV-positive individuals, in spite of clear CDC risk-reduction guidelines and the American Society of Addiction Medicine guidelines for facilities treating such patients (American Society of Addiction Medicine 1991). Furthermore, counselors in these programs may resist talking about safer sex because they find such talk uncomfortable (Cabaj 1989). Some counselors may view discussions about safer sex and other prevention issues as detracting from recovery issues. A substance-abusing gay man who is HIV positive—

whether he is actively using substances or in recovery—faces many difficult clinical issues. These may include suicidality, potential or increasing dementia, negotiating safer sex, and legal issues regarding wills and powers of attorney (Cabaj 1989; Flavin et al. 1986; Ostrow et al. 1989, 1990). Finding a treatment setting that will accept a gay, clean, and sober HIV-positive individual may be very difficult (Cabaj 1989). There is great resistance to acknowledging homosexuality, let alone being open to HIV concerns, in many inpatient and community treatment programs (Hellman et al. 1989)

Clinicians and counselors must be aware of their own personal attitudes regarding homosexuality and HIV-related conditions. If a health care provider is homophobic or fears AIDS and cannot find help in working out these attitudes with a supportive colleague or supervisor, patients would be better off being referred to another staff member for help (Cabaj 1988). HIV-positive gay men facing recovery from substance abuse should not have to fight homophobia in a health care system to receive quality care.

There is a growing body of literature on working with gay men with substance abuse (Cabaj 1992; Finnegan and McNally 1987; Gorsiorek 1985; Hart 1991; Ziebold and Mongeon 1985). Most areas now have gay and lesbian health centers or mental health collectives, and almost all have a strong focus on recovery and substance abuse treatment. There are national organizations, some with referral services, to help therapists meet the needs of their gay and lesbian patients or to help gay men and lesbians find gay-sensitive care: the National Association of Lesbian and Gay Alcoholism Professionals, the National Gay and Lesbian Health Foundation, the Association of Gay and Lesbian Psychiatrists, the American Association of Physicians for Human Rights, the Association of Lesbian and Gay Psychologists, and the National Task Force of Gay and Lesbian Social Workers, to name a few. Many communities now have gay and lesbian AA, NA, and Al-Anon meetings, as well as supportive meetings for HIV-positive individuals, such as Positively Sober groups.

However, some gay men in recovery from substance abuse may not have come out about their sexual orientation or HIV status or may not feel comfortable in meetings specifically targeted to HIV-positive gay men. This is especially likely if looking at and attempting to accept and integrate sexual orientation were not part of their earlier recovery interventions. Groups similar to AA have formed to meet the needs of these gay men, such as Alcoholics Together, and many big cities sponsor "roundups" (large 3-day weekend gatherings focused on AA, NA, lectures, workshops, HIV information and support, and drug- and alcohol-free socializing) for such people.

Deciding to Be Tested While in Recovery

Being tested for HIV status poses special challenges for the gay man who abuses substances. If not in recovery, the active abuser is not likely to consider testing, as denial is the cornerstone of substance abuse. The abuser who believes he will test positive may see the result as his justification for continuing to use substances as it is too late to affect his health by any behavior change. To the abuser who wants to continue using, even a negative test may be interpreted as evidence that his existing behavior does not put him at risk for HIV infection. In either case, the active substance abuser may not benefit from the pretest counseling. If in recovery, his stress and anxiety before being tested and after receiving the results may lead to relapse. Patients in early recovery are often urged to do almost nothing except focus on recovery—not to form new relationships, move, change jobs, and so on. Seeking information about HIV status shifts their focus and may lead to withdrawal of support of sponsors, counselors, or clean and sober friends, and possibly to an outright relapse.

The Need to Develop a Different Social Network

The patient's loss of his original network of friends and supporters cannot be underemphasized as a potential problem. The gay man who enters sobriety will usually need a new social environment, one that does not have a primary focus on bars and parties. Friends who continue to drink or use drugs may not be able to understand the need for remaining clean and sober and may insist, as either a social connection or as a way of denying their own abuse problem, that the newly sober gay man return to using drugs or alcohol. The death of gay men from AIDS-related conditions may weaken the support network for clean and sober men, and lead to the almost continuous bereavement among gay men.

Issues Related to Special Subgroups

Some special subsets of the gay community, such as the leather set or men into sadomasochism, may use drugs and alcohol as part of the very nature of the subculture, such as beer busts or drugs to relax the muscles of the body for fisting or anal intercourse. Such gay men will need special help in learning how to remain part of the subculture and yet remain clean and sober, or in finding new groups to belong to or new ways to have sex.

Young gay men must deal with both substance abuse and HIV concerns to a greater extent than their heterosexual counterparts. The developmental steps previously described most often occur in adolescence, making gay youths especially vulnerable to substance use and abuse. The ego-dystonic phase may be a very uncomfortable one for a young man; this uncomfortableness may foster the use of substances for relief. A young gay man may seek sex as a way of being accepted, thus possibly making him vulnerable to exploitation by older men. If he is alcohol- or drug-dependent, the young gay male with financial limitations may turn to sex in exchange for drugs (or for money to buy drugs) and be at an extremely high risk for HIV infection. These youths' turmoil and sexual confusion are worsened by substance use. No real acceptance or understanding will be possible if the young male abuses substances.

People of color who are gay or who are dealing with early awareness of a homosexual sexual orientation may be even more at risk for substance abuse because of the cultural norms and pressures of their particular group and background, as well as because of the societal and psychological forces faced by all gay men. Providers will need to be sensitive not only about gay issues and recovery concerns, but also to patients' particular ethnic and cultural concerns. As an example, many African American or Latino gay men may describe themselves as bisexual, even if they are sexual exclusively with men, and may resist help if the provider insists on approaching them as gay men with a focus on gay treatment interventions.

Issues Related to
Treatment-Resistant Patients

Although most HIV-positive gay men make great efforts not to put others at risk, behavior becomes unpredictable under the influence of alcohol or drugs. As mentioned above, men who fail to follow guidelines do so when drinking or using drugs. The IV drug user may clean his needle on first use, but once high may not bother. The urgency to become high with quick-acting injectable drugs such as speed or cocaine often leads to users' bypassing clean needle techniques.

Many clinicians have learned that the 12-step, one-day-at-a-time relapse prevention model helps patients not return to the use of substances or, if they do relapse or "slip," not punish themselves but instead return more quickly to a clean and sober state. The same model is now being used to look at the relapse into high-risk behaviors—a one-day-at-a-time approach with no punishment or excessive guilt if there is a "relapse," allowing, it is hoped, a quick return to less risky behavior (Silven 1993).

Trying to help a gay man deal with his HIV or AIDS status and deal with recovery at the same time can be very difficult. Denial needs to be confronted in both areas. Many men feel that they will die anyway, so they wonder why they should bother with recovery. Some will say they want to party until the end. Efforts to instill a fear of medical illness or dire consequences of what could happen if alcohol or drugs are continued to be abused usually do little good. Instead, the clinician should ally with the patient and focus on trying to help him have as much control as possible over the course of his HIV illness. Pointing out that use of substances clouds judgment and leads to failure to follow through on needed medical and social treatment may be helpful and actually can be an incentive to enter recovery. The substance-abusing patient can have the fullest possible choices of what will happen to him and what he will do for himself if he becomes and stays clean and sober.

Learning about his HIV status may be the chance for a gay man to explore his substance use or abuse, admit he has a problem with drugs or alcohol, and become motivated to begin recovery, such as happened in the following case example.

Case 5

Mr. E was involved in a long-term relationship and believed it was monogamous. He and his lover did not practice safer sex, but felt they were not at risk. On a whim, they went to be tested together. Both were found to be HIV positive. Mr. E became profoundly upset, left his lover, and sought help. He acknowledged that he had been shooting IV speed (amphetamines) for years, sometimes using shared needles, but had never discussed this with anyone as safer sex was all anyone ever talked to him about when he mentioned being gay. Following discovery of his HIV status, Mr. E decided that he wanted to stop his drug use so he could maximize his life and try to do all the things he had not yet had time to do. He felt his HIV status put a clear time frame on his life and future.

Suicidality in HIV-Positive, Substance-Abusing Gay Men

Suicidal thinking is common in the substance abuser, especially as the illness of drug addiction has progressed. As noted in Chapter 5, suicidal ideation as well as suicidal behavior and even suicide attempts are problems for HIV-positive individuals. People are more likely to act on impulses if intoxicated.

Structuring Effective Therapeutic Interventions

Every medical and emotional setback in an HIV-positive man—a drop in T cell count, an allergic reaction to medications, news of another friend being diagnosed with AIDS, the death of a friend, rejection by a friend or family member—may be the excuse for him to break his recovery and drink or use drugs. A very solid and individual treatment plan and recovery program, therefore, are necessary for the HIV-positive gay man. The ideal treatment plan would focus on group treatment, both psychotherapeutic and recovery oriented. A group of HIV-positive men in recovery can help each other deal with the many setbacks and challenges to recovery that they face.

The stance of the therapist in individual therapy is also crucial. Rather than being aloof, purely psychodynamically focused, or strictly therapeutically neutral, the optimal role of the individual therapist is often, especially in early recovery, a solid and consistent presence through which support, guidance, information, and advice on how to negotiate the many social service, governmental, and medical systems an HIV-positive individual will have to face are offered.

Because a patient in early recovery will usually be affected by the "wet-brain syndrome" (i.e., mild cognitive impairment secondary to alcohol and drug use and the withdrawal from the substances), he will not always fully comprehend what is happening or make the best and clearest decisions. If he has a concurrent HIV-related dementia, special clinical interventions will be needed (see Chapter 6).

If the HIV-positive gay man in recovery is already in psychotherapy, the focus of therapy may have to shift to looking at his internalized homophobia and his tendency to use defense mechanisms such as dissociation, isolation, and denial. Psychotherapy will not treat or "cure" his substance abuse, but may enhance and support recovery. Psychodynamic psychotherapy is not recommended in early recovery if the patient is not already in therapy as it may often open areas too painful to handle without the old escapes provided by substances. Psychodynamic psychotherapy at too early a point in recovery may lead to relapse into substance abuse, and in addition may be ineffective because of the patient's mild dementia from substance withdrawal (Vaillant 1983). The following case example illustrates the importance of concentrating on the substance abuse treatment before any substantive insight-oriented work can be done in psychotherapy.

Case 6

Mr. F had been in therapy for years. He was a heavy, frequent drinker and had originally sought help years before for the drinking problems. Over the years of therapy, he had explored the meaning of his homosexuality and his relationships with his mother, father, siblings, and a series of short-term boyfriends. He had continued his drinking throughout the entire therapy. After learning he was HIV positive, Mr. F sought therapy again to help cope with the stress concerning his new status and with his increased drinking. The treatment focused on his first becoming sober. Mr. F tried to constantly return to psychodynamic issues, denying the need to become sober. Finally, he agreed to enter a treatment program and was able to stop his alcohol use completely, returning to therapy only for support around his HIV concerns.

Clinician Burnout

Burnout, the biggest challenge facing clinicians working with HIV-positive individuals, is compounded by work with substance abusers. The persistent denial of many substance abusers frustrates providers and makes them wish to give up trying to intervene. The defenses most substance abusers have developed as a result of their substance abuse—projection, denial, manipulation, avoidance, isolation, or dissociation—are challenging to work with on a continual basis.

It is easy to buy into a patient's denial and frustration and develop an attitude of "why bother." The clinician who does not recognize that relapse is part of the nature of the illness of substance abuse may feel personally offended or guilty if an HIV-positive patient relapses. The clinician may develop the fervent hope that the patient's living clean and sober will stave off the effects of his HIV infection, as many patients hope, and feel betrayed and hurt if the illness progresses.

It is also quite easy to overidentify with a patient, especially if the patient and provider share some demographic traits or are at similar positions in life, training, or professional growth. This close identification can be a very useful, empathic tool, but it can also lead to a blurring of therapeutic boundaries or a failure to see the patient as he really is, resulting in missed medical and psychiatric interventions (Cabaj 1991).

Burnout prevention is best done through group supports. The provider may need to seek a support group whose members are knowledgeable about recovery and substance abuse, as many clinicians do not understand the illness-recovery model and how it provides hope and a viable treatment plan for substance abusers. Each individual provider must recognize his or her limits as to the number of such clinical situations that he or she can handle and must set firm limits. Each provider will need to have his or her own social support system available and a reasonable emotional balance.

Summary

If the clinician recognizes that the HIV-positive gay man also has the illness of substance abuse, that illness needs to be addressed at each visit in an attempt to break through the denial, thereby "planting the seed" for recovery. Stubborn or harsh confrontation is not necessary. Mental health and medical care should not be cut off if the patient refuses to enter recovery. An altered form of a full-scale intervention can be helpful—listing the symptoms and evidence that the clinician sees to support the diagnosis of substance abuse, and the probable problems ahead if something is not done to treat it.

Many HIV-infected gay men who abuse substances have used their HIV infection as the inspiration to begin recovery; the infection represents the "bottom" that is hit before experiencing total legal, social, medical, and work-related failures. Even if they progress to AIDS and face dying and death issues, many HIV-infected gay men report that being in recovery made the journey much easier and allowed them to make peace with themselves, deal with internalized homophobia, and open up to and accept the help, love, and support of families, friends, and providers.

References

American Society for Addiction Medicine: Guidelines for Facilities Treating Chemically Dependent Patients at Risk for AIDS or Infected with HIV. Washington, DC, American Society for Addiction Medicine, 1991

Bailey JM, Benishay DS: Familial aggregation of female sexual orientation. Am J Psychiatry 150:272–277, 1993

Bailey JM, Pillard RC: A genetic study of male sexual orientation. Arch Gen Psychiatry 48:1089–1096, 1991

Beatty R: Alcoholism and adult gay male populations of Pennsylvania. Unpublished Master's thesis. University Park, PA, Pennsylvania State University, 1983

Bell AP, Weinberg MS: Homosexualities: A Study of Diversities Among Men and Women. New York, Simon & Schuster, 1978

Bell AP, Weinberg MS, Hammersmith SK: Sexual Preference: Its Development in Men and Women. Bloomington, IN, Indiana University Press, 1981

Cabaj RP: Working with male homosexual patients, I: GI problems in homosexual men. Practical Gastroenterology 9:7–12, 1985

Cabaj RP: Homosexuality and neurosis: considerations for psychotherapy. J Homosex 15:13–23, 1988

Cabaj RP: AIDS and chemical dependency: special issues and treatment barriers for gay and bisexual men. J Psychoactive Drugs 21:387–393, 1989

Cabaj RP: Overidentification with a patient, in Gays, Lesbians, and Their Therapists: Studies in Psychotherapy. Edited by Silverstein C. New York, WW Norton, 1991, pp 31–39

Cabaj RP: Substance abuse in the gay and lesbian community, in Substance Abuse: A Comprehensive Textbook, 2nd Edition. Edited by Lowenson JH, Ruiz P, Millman RB. Baltimore, MD, Williams & Wilkins, 1992, pp 852–860

Cassel J: The contributions of the social environment to host resistance. Am J Epidemiol 104:107–123, 1976

Centers for Disease Control: U.S. AIDS cases reported through December 1992. HIV/AIDS Surveillance Report, Year-End Edition, February 1993, pp 1–23

de Monteflores C: Notes on the management of difference, in Contemporary Perspectives on Psychotherapy With Lesbians and Gay Men. Edited by Stein TS, Cohen CC. New York, Plenum, 1986, pp 73–101

Diamond DL, Wilsnack SC: Alcohol abuse among lesbians: a descriptive study. J Homosex 4:123–142, 1978

Fifield L, de Crescenzo TA, Latham JD: Alcoholism and the gay community. Summary of On My Way to Nowhere: Alienated, Isolated, Drunk: An Analysis of Gay Alcohol Abuse and Evaluation of Alcoholism Rehabilitation Services for Los Angeles County. Los Angeles, CA, Los Angeles Gay Community Services Center, 1975

Finnegan DG, McNally EB: Dual Identities: Counseling Chemically Dependent Gay Men and Lesbians. Center City, MN, Hazelden, 1987

Flavin DK, Franklin JD, Frances RJ: The acquired immune deficiency syndrome (AIDS) and suicidal behavior in alcohol-dependent homosexual men. Am J Psychiatry 143:1440–1442, 1986

Goode E, Troiden RR: Amyl nitrite use among homosexual men. Am J Psychiatry 136:1067–1069, 1979

Gorsiorek JC (ed): A Guide to Psychotherapy With Gay and Lesbian Clients. New York, Harrington Park Press, 1985

Hart JE (ed): Substance Abuse Treatment: Considerations for Lesbians and Gay Men, Vol 2. The Mobile AIDS Resource Team Series. Boston, MA, The Mobile AIDS Resource Team, 1991

Hellman RE, Stanton M, Lee J, et al: Treatment of homosexual alcoholics in government-funded agencies: provider training and attitudes. Hosp Community Psychiatry 40:1163–1168, 1989

Isay RA: Being Homosexual: Gay Men and Their Development. New York, Farrar, Straus & Giroux, 1989

Kus RJ: Alcoholics Anonymous and gay American men. J Homosex 14:253–276, 1987

Lange WR, Haetzen CA, Hickey JE: Nitrites inhalants: patterns of abuse in Baltimore and Washington, DC. Am J Drug Alcohol Abuse 14:29–39, 1988

Leigh B: The relationship of substance use during sex to high risk sexual behavior. Journal of Sex Research 27:199–213, 1990

Lesbian and Gay Substance Abuse Planning Group: San Francisco Lesbian, Gay and Bisexual Substance Abuse Needs Assessment, Vols 1 and 2. Executive Summary; Appendices A, B, C. Prepared by EMT Associates, Sacramento, CA, 1991

Lewis CE, Saghir MT, Robins E: Drinking patterns in homosexual and heterosexual women. J Clin Psychiatry 43:277–279, 1982

Lohrenz L, Connelly J, Coyne L, et al: Alcohol problems in several midwestern homosexual communities. J Stud Alcohol 39:1959–1963, 1978

MacGregor RR: Alcohol and drugs as co-factors for AIDS, in AIDS and Substance Abuse. Edited by Siegel L. New York, Harrington Park Press, 1988, pp 47–71

Miller A: The Drama of the Gifted Child. New York, Basic Books, 1981

Morales ES, Graves MA: Substance Abuse: Patterns and Barriers to Treatment for Gay Men and Lesbians in San Francisco. San Francisco, CA, San Francisco Prevention Resources Center, 1983

Ostrow DG, Monjan A, Joseph J: HIV-related symptoms and psychological functioning in a cohort of homosexual men. Am J Psychiatry 146(6):737–742, 1989

Ostrow DG, VanRaden MJ, Fox R, et al: Recreational drug use and sexual behavior change in a cohort of homosexual men: the Multicenter AIDS Cohort Study (MACS). AIDS 4(8):759–765, 1990

Pillard RC: Sexual orientation and mental disorder. Psychiatric Annals 18(1):52–56, 1988

Pillard RC, Weinrich JD: Evidence of familial nature of male sexuality. Arch Gen Psychiatry 43:808–812, 1986

Pillard RC, Poumadere J, Carretta RA: A family study of sexual orientation. Arch Sex Behav 11:511–520, 1982

Saghir M, Robins E: Male and Female Homosexuality. Baltimore, MD, Williams & Wilkins, 1973

Silven D: Behavioral theories and relapse. FOCUS: Guide to AIDS Research and Counseling 8:1–4, 1993

Smith DE, Smith N, Buxton ME, et al: PCP and sexual dysfunction, in PCP: Problems and Prevention. Edited by Smith DE. Dubuque, IA, Kendal-Hunt, 1982

Stall R: The prevention of HIV infection associated with drug and alcohol use during sexual activity, in AIDS and Substance Abuse. Edited by Siegel L. New York, Harrington Park Press, 1988, pp 73–88

Stall R, McKusick L, Wiley J: Alcohol and drug use during sexual activity and compliance with safe sex guidelines for AIDS: The AIDS Behavior Research Project. Health Educ Q 13:359–371, 1986

Vaillant GE: The Natural History of Alcoholism: Causes, Patterns, and Paths to Recovery. Cambridge, MA, Harvard University Press, 1983

Weinberg M, Williams C: Male Homosexuals: Their Problems and Adaptations. New York, Oxford University Press, 1974

Ziebold TO, Mongeon JE (eds): Gay and Sober: Directions for Counseling and Therapy. New York, Harrington Park Press, 1985

Chapter 20

Seronegative Gay Men
and Considerations of
Safe and Unsafe Sex

Walt Odets, Ph.D.

For human immunodeficiency virus (HIV)–negative gay and bisexual men, safe sex is certainly central to their biological—if not psychological—survival of the acquired immunodeficiency syndrome (AIDS) epidemic. Yet among all the problems affecting gay men, unsafe sex has been the one whose discussion has been most prohibited; the morality of safe sex has made the topic of unsafe sex a taboo. This situation has developed partly out of concern with the reduction of HIV transmission, but it is also the product of a complex psychological, political, and economic situation that has badly obscured the human issues connected to safe and unsafe sex. Too much of the public conversation about safe and unsafe sex is directed at assuaging the anxiety and doubt of gay men, ensuring HIV funding, understanding the responsibility of the gay community, and bolstering the respectability of homosexuality itself.

In this chapter I use the term *safe sex* because it is still the mostly widely used term in education about AIDS and among gay men in general. The term *safer sex* is more accurate, but for many reasons, which I discuss in detail, it has been shunned. Still more accurate is the term *unprotected sex,* for it concretely describes the nature of the act without the prejudice introduced by the inference of danger. For example, unprotected sex between two men who are truly HIV negative is not unsafe sex; it is unprotected sex.

Political efforts by the gay community to promote safe sex are directed largely at the heterosexual community, and much of them seem to be a displacement from what were previously sexual or political issues. For gay men, so long on the outside of mainstream values, safe sex has provided a virtually pious position. In some it is a piety that has replaced gay political activism. In others, safe sex—and AIDS in general—have provided them with their first opportunity to experience a respectable position in the world that does not rest on concealment or denial of one's homosexuality. Unfortunately, this concern with piety and respectability, made credible by genuine concerns about HIV transmission, has often led to the widespread exploitation of shame and guilt. This is particularly noteworthy in a population that has been historically burdened with the shame and guilt about sexuality that have been promoted by a disapproving society; what now is occurring is that much of the shame about being homosexual is being displaced by shame about having unprotected sex. Within both the gay community and heterosexual society there is now widespread moral disapproval of those who newly contract HIV. The obvious ethical issue of protecting others from HIV exposure aside, unprotected sex that puts one's self at risk is now publicly characterized as a betrayal of one's social, ethical, and moral responsibilities as a gay or bisexual man.

The use of shame and guilt to ensure individuals practice safe sex ignores both social and psychological experience. The exploitation of these feelings has rarely been effective in keeping homosexual men from homosexual behavior and has never been effective in changing feelings. Similarly, this exploitation is equally unlikely to keep gay men from having unprotected sex, or thinking about it, or having complex feelings about it. Shame and guilt have worked to keep gay men closeted and quiet about their homosexuality; now, more than 2 years into the "third wave" of the AIDS epidemic, it is apparent that shame and guilt have been working on a large scale to keep men silent about their unprotected sexual activities. This silence is immensely destructive: unprotected sex is a common occurrence among gay men and unless it can be talked about rather than merely prohibited and ridiculed, gay men will not be able to make clear, conscious decisions about what they are doing.

Discussion of the politics of safe sex is not, obviously, aimed at discrediting safe sex. Rather, it is aimed at lifting the political burden from the reality and the psychology of the issue. The facts about unprotected sex are alarming, and they are not really new. In 1989, Moulton et al. published the results of their survey of 160 gay and bisexual men. They found that 11% were seronegative and 33% did not know their status. Nevertheless, "slightly more than 30% said they practiced safe sex seldom or half the time" (Moulton et al. 1989, p. 94). Additional studies of 1,898 gay and bisexual men in San Francisco, Chicago, and New York have shown consistently that "perhaps as many as one in three continues to engage in some high-risk practices" (see Dilley and Boccellari 1989, p. 139, for a review of these studies). In 1990, the Centers for Disease Control estimated that each year 40,000 gay men in the United States are being newly infected with HIV (personal communication, V. Zonana, *Los Angeles Times,* San Francisco Bureau, April 1990). In 1991, the executive director of the San Francisco AIDS Foundation reported that "the level of [HIV] infection is a staggering 40% in young gay men 20 to 24 years of age" (San Francisco AIDS Foundation 1991). Finally, a 1992 Australian study found that 33% of gay men reported unprotected anal intercourse within the previous year (Gold 1992).

Despite such figures, there continues to be widespread disbelief that gay men could be having unprotected sex, and, when the fact is acknowledged, a lack of education or complacency continue to be offered as the major explanations. Psychological and psychosocial issues have gone largely unmentioned and unexplored. As we are told by the 1992 safe sex campaign of New York's Gay Men's Health Crisis, "Safe Sex Is Just Common Sense." Such education programs are almost exclusively conceived by non–mental health personnel. When research is done, it is generally commonsense analyses of surveys that questioned gay men about their reasons for practicing unprotected sex.

Psychological Implications of Unsafe Sexual Practices

At a public policy level, the treatment of safe and unsafe sex as political and moral issues may well make some kind of pragmatic sense. At a psychological level, political taboos and social moralities serve only to obscure and deny complex feelings and behaviors. Psychological insights about unsafe sex must be considered as relevant background in public education programs and must be central in any psychotherapy with a man engaging in unsafe sexual activity. The psychotherapist has a responsibility, particularly when unsafe sexual activities are known to be taking place, to help the patient clarify the meaning of his behavior as he would any self-destructive behavior. Unsafe sex is one obvious way of not remaining a survivor of the AIDS epidemic. Clearly this potential consequence is failing as a deterrent for many men, and common sense will make no sense of their feelings and motivations.

A psychological description of unsafe sex will reveal that although its potential lethality sometimes is a deterrent, sometimes it is also a significant, though often unconscious, motivation to practice it. In other words, although public policy continues to assume that unsafe sex is practiced despite its dangers, it is clear that some men engage in it precisely because it is dangerous. Other self-destructive behaviors, such as abusing chemical substances, are also common among survivors of the AIDS epidemic, and they too should be considered in the following discussion of unsafe sex.

With the exception of very young men and older men newly coming out in gay society, ignorance about unprotected sex no longer appears to be a significant problem in the gay community. When educated men in 1993 engage in unprotected anal intercourse, the psychotherapist must assume the behavior to be of psychological significance. The practice of safe sex is the uninfected man's most convincing statement that he more or less accepts his identity as a survivor of the AIDS epidemic, and that he can live a life in survival that is reasonably healthy, intimate, and life affirming. Ambivalence about unsafe sex must be interpreted, in part, as ambivalence about one's identity and about life as a survivor; the practice of unsafe sex must be interpreted as, in part, the usually unconscious desire not to survive. The complexity of this issue was revealed in a personal communication a facilitator of HIV-negative gay men's groups in San Francisco, when he related the following about a recent group session:

Case 1

Mr. A had been talking—and it was the first time in the history of the group that anyone had been willing to bring it up—that he was often feeling like having unsafe sex. After he talked for a few moments, Mr. B blurted out, "I can't believe you're talking like this. I don't know about you, but I intend to stay alive, and you're going to commit suicide." Another member of the group then said to Mr. B, "You know, I don't think I heard Mr. A say he wanted to commit suicide, I don't think that's a good analogy. I don't think Mr. A is talking about committing suicide. He's talking about wanting to have sex, and I think that's what's making you so agitated."

I was sitting listening to this, and my mind went into a sort of free fall. The more I've been facilitating this group, the more I realize that I don't want to live without risk—that would not be living. And sometimes the group makes me think that we're hiding behind these prohibitions about talking about one thing or another as a way to hide out against life. I realized, with regard to this issue of sex, how complicated it is. What it comes right down to is life, and death, and sex, and these things mixed up together make quite a brew. At that moment with the group, I couldn't talk about it, because my feelings on this subject are just too complex. I couldn't keep my personal sensibilities out of my responsibility as a facilitator.

Although the potential lethality of unprotected sex may sometimes serve as a motivation to practice it, this is not always true. The intense focus on safe sex has obscured the fact that unsafe sex is just ordinary human sex and is often motivated by traditional, positive, human values (Prieur et al. 1988). That such instinctual and well-motivated behaviors now may also transmit a lethal virus is, of course, one of the important reasons for the psychological complexity of unsafe sex. It is my experience that, although unsafe sex certainly occurs in the context of impulsive or anonymous sexual encounters, it is most often reported by psychotherapy patients as a part of ongoing, intimate relationships. Within gay male relations the exchange of semen anally or orally is often experienced as an important expression of intimacy in precisely the way that the giving and accepting of semen vaginally or orally is an aspect of intimacy within heterosexual relations. In fact, this exchange may hold an especially important position in gay male relationships, for it has always stood for many men as a concrete gesture of the powerful intimacies that stand in defiance of mainstream prohibitions. Now that a decade of prohibition has made semen exchange relatively unusual and "special," it has become all the more powerful and meaningful. The promotion of safe sex has in fact caused its proponents to simply deny that semen exchange is as important as other positive aspects of ordinary, fluid-exchanging sex.

One of my patients, who grew to gay sexual maturity in the age of AIDS, voiced his feelings on safe and unsafe sex as follows:

> I have never had anyone come inside of me. By the time I got into sex—well, it was all over, it was all just safe sex. I've thought a lot about it with my partner, because some day I'd like to make love with him, and have him come in me, you know, like a prize, like something to take home with me. Sunday morning we went to breakfast and we were sitting talking, and I fantasized that he had come in me the night before. And I was just sitting there, like nothing was going on, but I knew there was still this part of him inside of me from the night before. I felt very close to him because of that, and the idea just made me feel very warm and special and close to him. I felt very privileged, I'd say. I felt like I could feel it inside of me.

The ease with which anal intercourse has been treated as a dispensable aspect of gay sex by the scientific and medical communities—as well as by many members of the gay community itself—and the widespread promotion of condoms as a minimal intrusion on sexual intimacy suggests that many do not appreciate the analogy between vaginal and anal intercourse. The proposal that the heterosexual population abstain from vaginal intercourse to curb HIV transmission would not even seem a possibility to most people. And more than a decade into the epidemic, no one would be surprised at the waning use of condoms in this population. If heterosexual couples had found the condom, as safe and effective as it is, to be only a minimal intrusion in vaginal sex, it seems unlikely that birth control methods to replace the condom would have received the research attention or public acceptance that they have. The heterosexual public, judging by statistics on sexually transmitted diseases and unwanted pregnancy, has resoundingly rejected the condom, and it is hard to see why public policy makers have assumed that the homosexual public would feel differently. As another one of my gay patients expressed it,

> When I was a kid, my uncle—who was elected by my parents to do the sex education—told me that using a condom was like taking a shower with your raincoat on. That's my feeling precisely. Of course my uncle was talking about straight sex, and his solution was that the woman should take care of the contraception. But I do find condoms a complete breach of intimacy, and if they remind me of anything, it's sticking a dildo up someone's ass. You're not there, your dick is there—with his raincoat on. In sex, touch is the most important thing to me, and that means skin. That's how I connect to another person. I find this whether I'm getting fucked or doing the fucking. It's almost the same thing to me: no skin, no connection. It just changes the whole experience.

The inability to see the analogies between vaginal and anal sex, although the two are obviously not identical in some respects, is based largely on homophobic aversion to anal sex, which is seen as primarily a homosexual behavior. The emotional and interpersonal import of the two is the same, and it should not surprise us that gay men are no more adaptive to abstention from an important, basic form of sexual intercourse or to the use of condoms to make that sex "safe" than would be the heterosexual population. (For a much more detailed discussion of the importance of anal intercourse in gay relations, the anus, and homophobia, see Odets, in press.) Psychotherapists working for insight cannot collude with the denial of these feelings.

One of my patients, a gay male in his 30s, addressed his feelings on the matter of safe sex and the conflict that it generated in him as follows:

> I was one of those people who said very early on that if oral sex transmitted AIDS then the guys from General [San Francisco General Hospital] could come and haul me away right now. Oral sex was all I had left, and so far as I'm concerned, it's not enough. Fucking meant a lot to me, and it's been almost impossible since the epidemic

started. I usually can't stay hard with a condom, and I know a lot of guys like that. The whole thing is incredibly frustrating and disappointing. I can't stand the things. They've been a disaster for me, and I know I'm not the only one. The only thing I can say for them is, they're a little bit better than being dead. And that's not much to say for something that used to be so important in my relationships. That's what I'd call the booby prize.

The fact is that many men are making choices between perceived sexual and emotional needs on the one hand and survival on the other. Denial of this cannot help clarify the issues surrounding safe and unsafe sex. There is no doubt about the danger of unprotected sex, but unsafe sex often also expresses the desire to be intimate and to love another human being in ways that feel meaningful and powerful to those involved. These issues and attendant choices must be made more conscious and clearer: Is it true, one must ask, that this expression of intimacy, of love, and of connection to another is as important or more important than survival itself? Although such considerations may be inappropriate as an explicit element of public policy, in psychological work there must be room for them.

That the public is so incredulous at the level of unprotected ("ordinary") sex now occurring in the gay community must be traced, in part, to homophobia. The AIDS epidemic has spawned unconscious confusions of too many powerful ideas. Often buried in the internalized homophobia of gay men themselves are feelings that gay men should not have been having sex with each other to begin with; that gay men have made their beds and now they must lie in them; that gay sex will be punished and AIDS is the punishment; and that abstention from sex will make reparations with whomever is so indiscriminately dispensing HIV. In other words, AIDS has provided new unconscious motivations—as if more were needed in this community—for gay men and their AIDS educators to introject the projected self-hatred of homophobic individuals, many of whom are in political and social power. Identification with such mainstream homophobic individuals and their values must, for many, offer the unconscious promise of a life of safety, respectability, and freedom from the torments of AIDS.

Motivations for Having Unsafe Sex

The Desire Not to Survive

Because unsafe sex is such an available and meaningful way of not surviving, it is surprising how difficult it has been for many in both AIDS education and the mental health field to acknowledge that some men engage in unsafe sex for precisely these qualities. There are many psychologically comprehensible reasons that men might not wish to survive the AIDS epidemic. These include depression, anxiety, and guilt (including guilt about surviving); lives emptied by loss, isolation, and loneliness; loss of social affiliation and psychological identity; and anticipation, more than a decade into the epidemic, of a future that holds more of the same. Despite the incredible impact of the AIDS epidemic on many parts of the gay community, many continue to doubt that its consequences could be sufficient for a man who is not otherwise depressed or suicidal to not want to survive. This doubt is at least partly rooted in denial of what AIDS has wrought for its survivors, a denial not unrelated to that experienced by a man after his first HIV-positive blood test or AIDS diagnosis: It seems simply impossible that AIDS could end his life. The doubt also arises from homophobic attitudes that the AIDS epidemic is justice meted out for transgressions; because the willing acceptance of punishment is part of how reparation is paid, gay men are expected to take the epidemic graciously. In addition, when the desire of some not to survive is expressed in suicidal or other self-destructive behavior, there is an implicit threat to the powerful, shared, social version of reality that allows one the optimism to entertain a personal, as well as communal, future. Tempting suicide by, for example, engaging in unsafe sex, is felt to be an act of betrayal that nettles one's own unconscious and "treasonous" feelings.

Human disasters—whether conflicts with other men or with microbes—have always produced a number of survivors who feel so troubled about the event and are so identified with nonsurvivors that they sacrifice themselves in various ways to the needs or cause of the nonsurvivors. In some cases, as with those who sacrifice their lives during a communicable plague by nursing the ill, we attach significance to the social contribution and ignore the self-destructiveness. To the extent that the self-destructive element is acknowledged, we understand the sacrifice as generous and altruistic rather than as reckless or suicidal. Such individuals are often heroes—not a threat to the social fabric, but its champions. The fact remains that the nurse is often making a conscious or unconscious decision to end his or her life, and society does not define that as pathological. To further the analogy it should be clarified that the nurse is also more personally and socially identified with the patient than with other survivors, and that identification is an important motivation for the sacrifice.

In other instances of self-sacrifice there is no material contribution to society, but rather, by the fact of one's death, a statement of social, political, and ideological allegiance. Every country and party has such heroes. The captain who goes down with his ship and the soldier who runs headlong into enemy fire are among them. The death need not contribute anything aside from its subjective and public meanings. That the gay man in San Francisco, New York, or Sydney is profoundly identified with his community and strongly feels such allegiance is undeniable. Such feelings are particularly common among men in larger gay communities that are poorly integrated into mainstream society and that have had large numbers of deaths from AIDS-related illnesses. To the extent that parts of the gay community are unable to develop a life and identity that includes more than AIDS, the gay identity will remain confused with AIDS. As long as that is the case, a death by AIDS will, for some, continue to serve as an important expression of their identification with and allegiance to the gay community, as illustrated in the following case example.

Case 2

In the following dialogue, Mr. C, a psychotherapy patient, and I discussed his having unprotected sex with his current HIV-positive lover and his former lover, who had died several years before from an AIDS-related illness.

Mr. C: I feel an obligation to stick around for other people, not for myself—except for my lover. My mother is hysterical with the idea that he has HIV, and of course I wouldn't think of telling her about what kind of sex we have. But I spent my first 2 years here [in therapy] figuring out how I'd spent my first 33 years living for other people—and especially for my mother and sister. I won't do that anymore.

Therapist: Do you think I suggested that?

Mr. C: No, I suggested that—felt that. People are saying to me all the time, "Oh, I hope you won't get sick because we don't know what we'd do without you." I love my friends, and they have been very good friends to me, especially when my former lover was sick, but they can't come over in the middle of the night and get in bed with me when I'm wondering what we're doing here—what I'm doing here. My commitment to my lover comes from my heart and most of the rest of this comes from my guilt. I won't live that out anymore.

Therapist: Won't live what out?

Mr. C: My guilt. I meant my guilt. And I meant I won't live that out, like, I won't survive because my mother needs that. I will live in my heart, not my guilt. It is other people who want me to survive, and it's only part of me. The other part wants to live in my heart.

This patient's allegiance to the gay community was expressed in several ways. His desire to "live in my heart, not my guilt" is developmentally about living as a gay man rather than the heterosexual his mother and others wanted him to be. In the context of the AIDS epidemic, this patient's commitment became one not only to being gay, but to contracting HIV and experiencing an early death rather than responding to the conventional fears of his mother and heterosexual friends. He felt that these "outsiders" had no perspective about what it meant to be gay, and this is reflected in their doubts about his choice of partners and his engaging in sex—much less unsafe sex—with an HIV-positive man. For the patient, being gay meant living in a heart that loves another man and that accepts infection with HIV if that is what it takes to express his gay love.

The Feeling That One Will Not Survive

There is a complex feeling commonly seen among survivors of the epidemic that is rarely discussed—the sense of inevitability that so many gay men feel about "catching" AIDS. Many men with consistent HIV-negative test histories do not believe they will survive. Psychotherapy patients often say they "know" they are uninfected but "feel" or "believe" they are HIV positive or will somehow inevitably become so. The belief may be inconsistent over time and rationally unconvincing, but is often persistent and compelling. This phenomenon has become more common as the epidemic has spread into its second decade and has remained unabated in the gay community. The following case example presents how some gay men have this sense that they will inevitably be infected.

Case 3

Mr. D, a 22-year-old, HIV-negative psychotherapy patient, had been experiencing an undiagnosed genital dermatitis (that seemed unlike an HIV-related problem) for several weeks. He talked about his feelings shortly after finding out that a man whom he had been dating and with whom he had had a single, "safely" conducted sexual experience was HIV positive. This was Mr. D's first personal encounter with HIV.

Mr. D said, "When I found out that he was positive, it freaked me out—not for myself, but just the whole thing. I don't know how to live with this, because I feel afraid to kiss him, even if I know that's okay, because it just plays into my whole fear about HIV. Over the weekend I wanted to call my mom and talk to her, but I thought, you can't talk to her about this because she's going to tell you that you're going to get AIDS because you're gay. When I moved out here [to California] she didn't want me to go, she said I didn't belong there, because I would get AIDS there, and what she meant was, I would be gay there—and for that matter, that I would be leaving her alone to have her lonely life with my father, who's so out-to-lunch. I feel like all this is stacked up against me. I mean, I had enough trouble with sex and being gay without this—and now I find myself feeling just like my mother. And in my rational mind I know this isn't true, but I keep feeling, you are going to get AIDS because you're gay. And his being HIV positive confirms that. I know how people get AIDS, but I also have this feeling that it's out there—that my life is already written and out there—and that I will get AIDS because I'm gay—that if you're gay, you get AIDS. When I went to

the dermatologist last week, he told me not to sit on anything because he didn't know what I had and he didn't want to get it all over
the place, and I just felt like he was saying to me, 'You're a homosexual, and God knows what you filthy people have, but I don't want
it.' When he did that, my first thought was, Well he's probably
right—I'm dirty, I'm a queer, and I have AIDS, and I don't want to
contaminate his other patients. Then I got mad." Mr. D left the
dermatologist's office, but his feelings that he had AIDS or was destined to have it left with him.

Experiences such as Mr. D's should be distinguished from hypo-
chondriacal anxiety. With the latter, attention to physical symptomatology is more fully conscious, the focus is on signs and symptoms
of disease, and both symptoms and the contracting of disease are more
ego dystonic. In contrast, the belief that one will not survive—though
resting logically, if not psychologically, on the idea that one is already
infected or will unavoidably become so—involves more complex, elu-
sive, and destructive beliefs than the interpretation of signs and symptoms and the fear that one has illness; and they seem associated less
with anxiety, than with processes of introjection and identification,
guilt, and depression.

Introjection and Identification

Mourning and the feelings of loss, grief, and emptiness that accompany it are often fended off by an introjection of the dead individual. *Introjection* is the process in which parts of the dead individual
are taken on by the survivor, who thus keeps the dead individual
"alive inside of himself." This process reduces the experience of
separation and the need to mourn. This is seen most clearly in survivors who take over the deceased individual's home, clothing, and
possessions, living in the house like its former tenant, and often
taking over that individual's mannerisms, habits, attitudes, and activities. Introjection is often thought of as a relatively primitive defense against mourning. The survivor does not take on the deceased
one's form of life, attitudes, or aspects of his identity through personal development, but simply takes them over, whole and unas-
similated. Primitive or not, introjection is often necessary to ward

off unmanageable grief. Introjective fantasies are also a normal part of healthy adult experience. For example, they are one aspect of the power and emotional significance of sexual intercourse, whether it be oral, vaginal, or anal.

Identification is considered a more mature and constructive process than introjection, but one that accomplishes some of the same purposes. In identification one grows through a more complex developmental process to be like the individual one is identifying with. One comes to understand another individual, to appreciate his tastes, attitudes, ideas, and character, and to incorporate them, where desirable, into his own development as a person. Such identifications are an assimilation of the dead individual without taking him in whole, an incorporation of another that is relatively integrated into who one is and is becoming.

In practice, introjection and identification are not always discrete processes, nor is one usually the sole approach to grief to the exclusion of the other. Both work in fending off the experience of separation and loss by making one feel as if he is the person he is trying to hold on to. When that person is dying or dead, both introjection and identification can make the survivor feel that he too is dying or dead, a particularly likely consequence of introjection because it is global and indiscriminate and because it is often an early, impulsive response to an overwhelming loss. A gay patient, immediately after a lover's death, may feel quite consciously that he is sick and dying. It may not even occur to him that he isn't, so violent may be the introjection. A person experiencing such feelings is very likely to expose himself to unsafe sex. What difference would it make for someone already infected and dying? Schochet, a San Francisco psychologist, told me of a study she had conducted among HIV-negative gay men:

> Highly significant relationships were found between post-traumatic stress symptoms and experiencing many deaths of acquaintances, *not really believing one is HIV-negative* [emphasis added], and having unsafe sex in the past year. . . . Experiencing many losses of lovers, friends, roommates, and acquaintances also correlated with not really believing one's serostatus. (R. Schochet, personal communication, June 1992)

Guilt

To this point, the discussion has implied that introjection and identification, in making the survivor feel like the deceased individual, only incidentally make him feel he is HIV-infected, ill, or dying. That is frequently true, but in coming to feel like the deceased individual, one also reduces the differences between one's self and the deceased, and these are not quite the same thing. It is the difference between the survivor and the deceased one that forms the basis of guilt, including guilt about survival itself: "The greater the discrepancy between one's own fate and the fate of the loved person one failed to help, the greater the empathic distress and the more poignant one's guilt [about surviving]" (Friedman 1985, p. 532). As one becomes more like the deceased individual, the discrepancy is reduced and so is the guilt. HIV-infected men, of course, rarely feel guilt about other HIV-infected men.

In addition, there are ways in which guilt about surviving—often including the feeling that one is not worthy of surviving—leads more directly to the feeling that one is somehow fated not to survive anyway. The sense of fate may simply fulfill the wish not to survive, but it also often includes the feeling that one will not be allowed to survive because of one's unworthiness. Thus the belief that one will not survive can be a passive form of not wanting to survive. Such beliefs rest on largely unconscious, primitive, magical thoughts, sometimes associated with conscious or unconscious beliefs in an omnipotent being—God or parent—who sees to it that people get what they deserve. Such magical thinking is an expression of the helplessness, passivity, and depression that those living in a plague understandably experience. No longer feeling in control of life, they are tempted to assign control, in fact or in fantasy, to someone else. In both cases, such passivity may well become a self-fulfilling prophecy of HIV infection.

This complicated mix of introjection, identification, and guilt can be seen in the following case example.

Case 4

In one psychotherapy session, one of my patients, Mr. E, talked about the weeks following his lover's positive HIV test. At that time

Mr. E had not yet been tested for HIV. He said, "It was about a month ago, right after my partner got his HIV test—you know, that's when we started having unsafe sex. When I think back on it, it was just that—I guess, if he was positive then I was positive. I just never thought otherwise about it. It didn't seem that we could be different in that way. Our sex then was very powerful—it was my way of holding on to him, saying that AIDS could not have him, it was how we stayed together. We were in it together."

I asked Mr. E at this point what he meant by their being in it together. "Were you trying to contract HIV from your partner to stay together? Because when you talk about holding on to him, not letting AIDS have him, it sounds as if you knew you didn't have it."

Mr. E responded, "It was that we had HIV together, we had everything together, that HIV couldn't separate us, that it couldn't break us apart. It wasn't that I was trying to get it, I just had it. Maybe I was trying to get it, but I didn't know it. I knew I was positive. But a couple of weeks later when things had cooled off a little bit, a friend asked me if I was worried about myself. I couldn't think for a minute what she meant, and then she said, 'Well, are you worried that you might have gotten HIV from him?' Well, I was completely amazed. It was the first time that I thought that I might not have it, that there might really be this big difference between us, and that we weren't in it together. Then I went to get tested, and when the nurse read me the results [which were negative] on Tuesday, this awful thing just went through me, and I thought, Oh my God, this can't be true, because my partner has it, and it can't be that I'm negative. I just started crying, and the nurse kept saying, 'Oh, that's good, negative is good,' and I just kept crying, and I said to her, 'No, you don't understand, because my lover is positive.' I just felt like this awful thing had happened, like someone had cut us in half."

Because they lacked any reasonable basis, Mr. E's early feelings that he had HIV were the result of an introjection and primitive identification with his partner. As we continued in therapy over the following months, a more complex identification with his partner developed and was expressed in Mr. E's increasing desire to have HIV as an expression of his devotion and his desire to support him. The feelings of guilt were also clarified as the psychotherapy continued. Mr. E said, "My partner has never said anything like this, but I know that I had the feeling after his test that if I were negative, he might be mad at me. I never thought that consciously, but I can see it now when I think back on it. And I didn't want to be negative either. So, if I thought he might be mad at me, I know that I had the idea that I might be negative. But there was something else about our [unsafe] sex then, and it was like, Oh, what the fuck. If he is positive, then everything's out of control, our lives are completely fucked up, and what difference does it make if I have it or not?"

"So your sex was a combination of thinking you had HIV and wanting it in order to stay with your partner?" I asked. "But it was also a way of making sure you had it so that your partner wouldn't resent you."

"It was all those things," he said. "But you forgot the other part—that everything seemed so fucked up, that I was thinking, there's nothing you can do about anything anymore, this is just all out of your hands—if you get it, you get it, and there's nothing you're going to do about that or anything else. It was, like, if the garbage is in [the kitchen] stinking, or the plants are dropping dead, well those are just the things you have to put up with in life."

Depression

Chronic depression may produce a sense of discouragement and hopelessness that can easily make life seem impossible. Unable to talk about the sheer unhappiness of their survival because they have had the good fortune to escape AIDS, many surviving men begin consciously or unconsciously to attribute their difficult life experience to their own "illness." This may serve two purposes. For the survivor himself, at an unconscious level, the belief that he is ill helps make sense of the fact that he is feeling so bad, and it allows him to feel a shared, publicly recognized source of misery. This is a process related in some senses to other somatizations, when psychological conflict is displaced onto physical conditions. Physical symptoms are often more acceptable than psychological ones, and this is particularly true in the midst of an epidemic.

The survivor may also feel that his unhappy condition will have more plausibility to other people—particularly HIV-infected men—if he has or is thought to have HIV illness. This can motivate a man to consciously misrepresent his condition or, less consciously, to slide into the feelings and behaviors—often the form of life—of an infected man. This is commonly seen in HIV-negative men who live as a dying man does, without a sense of the future or any responsibility to it, moving within the scope and scale of a life that may end any day. For those who are not dying, as well as for many who are, the experience can be quite liberating because it allows one to live with an immediacy and intensity generally denied those who are assumed to have a normal life span. Some of the depression experienced by survivors can be ameliorated by this liberation and, for some, the liberation may make the complex burden of an expected normal life span unacceptable.

The conscious misrepresentation of one's HIV condition is described in the following example.

Case 5

Mr. F, a depressed, HIV-negative patient, was having dinner with three HIV-positive friends. He related the following incident: "We were in a booth by the window in a deli, and all these guys were going by on Market Street, and every now and then someone would go by, and you'd say to yourself, Well, he has really bad AIDS. He looks terrible. I wonder what the poor guy's got."

"Who would say to himself?" I interrupted.

"Well, I would. I'm sure everyone was doing it. You know, Maybe he's got CMV [cytomegalovirus] or, I guess that's KS [Kaposi's sarcoma] on his neck. You know, you see those kinds of things. But what I wanted to tell you was, this guy goes by and my friend waves at him and he waves back, and then my friend says to us, 'That guy and I are in the same [medication] trial at General [San Francisco General Hospital].' And another friend says, 'Oh yeah, what are you on?' The next thing I know, we're sort of going around the table talking about who's taking what, and I'm thinking, What the fuck am I going to say when it comes to me? I was going to get up and go to the toilet, and just as I started to stand up, my friend says, 'What are you taking?' And I said, 'Oh me? Just AZT [zidovudine].'"

Mr. F started to laugh at this point. "Just AZT?" I queried, too surprised to laugh.

"Right. Just AZT."

"And then what did you do?"

"I went to the toilet," said Mr. F.

"That doesn't seem like a complete resolution to me."

"To say the least. In fact, they all think I'm positive now. I sat down in the toilet—it's so small in there you can hardly breathe—and I didn't know if I was going to start crying or laughing. I kept thinking, Just AZT? What the fuck did you say that for. Just AZT? Just AZT? I went over this again and again, and I knew I was going to have to go back out and sit down and look at them, and I didn't know if I could do it."

"What were the feelings that made that seem so difficult?"

"I was embarrassed. And ashamed."

"Why ashamed?" I asked.

"Because I've been so depressed about the epidemic and I don't have a good reason to be depressed. I don't have AIDS, and people I know who do aren't as depressed as I am."

"And did you feel some guilt at that moment?"

"Yeah, I was very guilty. It was like I was . . . I started to say bragging, but that doesn't seem right."

"What about the feeling though? The feeling that it was bragging?"

"I was claiming that I was part of things when I wasn't. I couldn't come out to them as negative. It wouldn't have made any sense. In some ways I realized that I've been pretending—I realized this while I was sitting in the bathroom—I've been pretending that I'm positive. Not by saying anything, but by little things. By being *affected* by the epidemic. I mean, my friend, who is positive, is taking the epidemic a lot better than I am. And I could just see myself saying, 'Oh well, I'm not taking anything. I'm negative.' I know my friend's mouth would just have fallen right on the floor, and he'd be thinking, Well, then what the hell is he so depressed about all the time? I'd have to say, 'Well, I know I'm not as affected as you guys, but I'm upset about it too.' I couldn't see myself saying that."

Denial and Counterphobia

Psychological denial is a defense that attempts to simply disavow the existence of unpleasant reality, and it has surely touched every corner of the AIDS epidemic, including the practice of unprotected sex. Simple denial about unprotected sex seems particularly operative in the men in their teenage years and early 20s who continue to ride the familiar postadolescent sense of omnipotence and immortality, mistakenly believing that HIV-related illnesses are spread not by contemporary behaviors but by membership in the gay society of the 1970s. Although they became sexually active after HIV was discovered, an astonishing number of young men are seroconverting. When they reflect in therapy about the behaviors that likely infected them, their most common remark is, "I don't know what I was thinking."

Older men also exercise simple denial about unprotected sex. Many surviving members of the gay society of the 1970s seem also to believe that HIV infection is a product only of those years. They often deny the possibility that younger men could be infected, an idea based on the obviously faulty logic that younger men became sexually active after the discovery of HIV and practice safe sex. Older patients often report unsafe sexual encounters with younger men who, because of their limited sexual history or merely because of their age, were assumed to be uninfected. Younger men involved with other younger men often share such assumptions too.

Last among simple forms of denial leading to unprotected sex is the denial of gay identity. In my experience, men who identify themselves as heterosexual or bisexual but engage in homosexual behaviors are at a particularly high risk for contracting HIV. These men do not consider themselves members of high-risk groups. Although the specific behaviors of such men may entail very high HIV risks, denial obscures the significance of the behavior. Thus the denial of homosexual identity colludes with denial about how HIV is transmitted. Many AIDS educators, the popular press, and the public continues to believe in the importance of risk groups. The idea that one contracts HIV because of a particular psychological and social identification is obviously incorrect. It is an idea powerfully driven by hatred and self-hatred and the projection or internalization of all that is hated. When a gay patient reports that he feels regret for being gay because "that's how I got AIDS," one sees how powerfully the confusion and self-hatred of others may be internalized and unleashed on the self.

In contrast to the straightforward uses of "simple" denial just discussed, denial appears to support unsafe sexual activity in an entirely different way. Among gay men in general, the psychological—as opposed to the intellectual—confidence in safe sex is extremely low. It is difficult to find any real consensus on what safe sex is. There are "safe" activities, but a lot of what people desire and now commonly do are much more accurately defined as "safer" or "possibly safe." Furthermore, epidemiological and biological models for HIV are bewilderingly complex and inconsistent. This all adds up to small reassurance when the transmission of a lethal virus is in question. Because of these reasonable, as well as other completely irrational and often unconscious, sources of fear, many men are quite afraid of safe sex, even in its stricter definitions. At an unconscious level, most gay men are afraid of safe sex even when they behave within their own safe sex guidelines. Although the risk involved in much safe sex is probably comparable with that of many well-accepted daily activities (e.g., automobile travel), the voicing of any fear about safe sex is nearly as politically unacceptable in the gay community as the confession of having had unsafe sex. If safe sex does not work, everyone will be infected and gay men will be banished to lives of celibacy. Without the possibilities allowed by safe sex, the epidemic would be unendurable.

Given such fears, conscious and unconscious, safe sexual activity requires the exercise of some denial about feelings, plausible and ridiculous alike. Once the denial necessary to allow safe sex has been accomplished, denial about the possibilities of unsafe sex is, for many, easier than is readily acknowledged. The defense is in place, a climate of denial around sexuality in general has been created, and if there are significant motivations to engage in unsafe activities denial serves admirably. Denial is one of the few psychological defenses with enough primitive, reality-distorting muscle to allow unsafe sex in a man who has not consciously initiated a plan of self-destruction. I believe there is a high correlation within gay men between conscious and unconscious fears of safe sex and the practice of unsafe sex. Men who express conscious anxiety about safe sex and a stated reticence to engage in it seem often the most likely to engage in sporadic, impulsive episodes of unprotected sex, as in the following case example.

Case 6

Mr. G, a psychotherapy patient in his late 30s, was an intelligent and well-educated man who worked as an engineer. His character suggested schizoid tendencies, and he had a long, pre-epidemic history of anxiety problems, including anxiety about his homosexuality, sex in general, and emotional intimacy. His fears about HIV infection had greatly aggravated these problems, and he often feared even casual kissing because he felt HIV transmission was possible from it. For several years, Mr. G had been unable to have an orgasm unless involved in solitary masturbation.

One day Mr. G came into a regular therapy session following a weekend in Los Angeles, where he had stayed in a gay hotel. "Saturday night I got fucked," he announced as he sat down for the hour.

"Really?" I said.

"Not only that, but without a rubber."

"Do you know what this is about?" I asked.

"Well, of course, I've replayed it a thousand times. I can tell you the facts, and they are pretty straightforward. I met this very attractive guy by the pool. He asked me if I wanted to come back to his room and, without hesitating for a minute, I said yes. We went to his room and though I was a little anxious at first, at some point he asked me if I would like him to fuck me—and at that moment, I clearly just switched into some altered state of consciousness. I was there for almost 2 hours, and it felt like 10 minutes. It was as if I'd become someone else, as if I were watching us in the room, rather than being in the middle of it. Unfortunately I got fucked without a condom, and I've been obsessing over it ever since. I just roll it over and over again in my mind, and I have the idea that if I can just go through it one more time, I'll realize that it never happened, that my memory has played a trick on me, and that none of it happened."

"But it happened, apparently," I said. "And it seems that it was you."

"No doubt about it."

"And do you understand what this 'altered state of consciousness' was, what it is that was going on with you?" I asked.

"I can tell you that being in L.A. had something to do with it, that I felt far away from home and from myself, and that it all had the quality of a dream—very timeless and a world in itself in some way. It was that feeling that I was not in my real life that let me do it. And probably not in my real body. Shit, I hardly. . . . "

"Hardly what?"

"I started to say that I've hardly let anyone kiss me in 6 years. And here I am getting fucked on a hotel bed without a condom—it's really unbelievable."

In its most extreme form, denial and other dissociative defenses may support counterphobic behavior, as appeared was the case with Mr. G. It is not uncommon for those who are depressed, anxious, and immobilized by fear to impulsively engage in precisely the activity that they fear. Such counterphobic behavior is not only conducted impulsively, but also often recklessly and compulsively, which raises the risks of the behavior well beyond what they might have been had the activity been conducted with more conscious consideration of its meaning. Counterphobic behavior is often, at least in part, an attempt to counter feelings of anxiety and helplessness by "mastering" the feared activity, and to express tension and anger about one's helplessness and the situation that produced it. It is certainly an element in some unsafe sexual activities and there is often a correlation between those men most fearful of sex and the counterphobic and impulsive engagement in unsafe sex.

Poor Self-Esteem

Self-esteem issues are often developmental in origin, and in the lives of many gay and bisexual men they certainly predate the AIDS epidemic. In addition to an accumulation of developmental deficits, some gay men experience the epidemic as more of a narcissistic injury. For many gay men, but particularly for those whose self-esteem has been derived heavily from their identity as members of the gay community, that identity may suddenly be experienced as a narcissistic liability. With all the acceptance that gay men have gained because of the epidemic in some segments of society, it is also true that this is a community now plagued by disease and death and one subjected to the wrath of much of society for the very existence of AIDS. Illness, disfigurement, death, and abusive or indifferent treatment by government agencies, health providers, insurance carriers, and the popular media may deal a serious narcissistic injury.

Whether narcissistic deficits result from developmental problems alone or from an interaction of developmental issues and the epidemic, including reactive chronic depression, poor self-esteem supports unsafe sexual activity. Simply put, a sense of self-worth is part of what allows a man to make choices about sex and life, to feel a sense of control, and to feel that he contributes to the course of his future. People take better care of things and selves that they feel a part of, feel responsible for, and value.

Unsafe sexual behavior is no more likely to be completely eliminated from the gay community than any of the other self-destructive behaviors in which humans have perpetually engaged. As psychotherapists, however, we must be as free as possible of political agendas and the distortions and denial that they encourage. Only by so doing will we will provide ourselves and our patients an opportunity to make unprotected sex and feelings about it as conscious and intelligible as possible. We may thus help replot the future of a community that has too long shouldered the social and psychological consequences of being sexually different, and that, in the United States, has now borne too much of another dark and awful event. One of my patients, who was in his mid-60s, felt this way about it:

> I'm afraid this epidemic has really thrown ice water on my sex life. I never thought a little piece of rubber could do that, but condoms have created in me a real sense of grief, a sense of loss about what used to be. I can't mess around with those things, and all the other problems involved with sex now, and I'm pretty sure now that I'm too old to ever outlive the need for all these precautions—my God, you go to the bedroom with an arsenal of pharmaceuticals in the hope that you won't kill each other making love. The good part for me is that I'm old enough to take an early retirement on sex. But young people, I don't know what they're going to do about it. I'm glad I'm not in their position. Even at my age, I've begun to wonder who I am. I say I'm gay, but, you know, I don't have sex with men anymore. That leaves me wondering just what it is that constitutes my being gay these days. When people ask me now, I'm tempted to say, Oh I used to be gay, but I'm retired now.

Summary

As with every aspect of the epidemic, each man must find and negotiate his own suitable path through his conflict about sexuality. That task requires the gay community's acknowledgment that unprotected sex is not the only danger now facing gay men: Too many live in fear, sexual dysfunction, and isolation, and too many now destroy themselves from within through the internalization of the sexual and HIV-driven self-hatred of others and the displacement—internal and external—of homophobia onto AIDS.

The loss of our capacity for sexual, human intimacy is surely one of the three great dangers of the epidemic, third only to the physical suffering and the loss of life. Many of us will find paths that conserve or restore our capacity for intimacy while allowing biological survival. But we must ask a question on behalf of those who harm no others, and for whom sexual intimacy in its ordinary, and now dangerous, form is the path of choice: Why is it that we mourn those who are ill or who have died because they fulfilled their passions and needs for intimacy in an age when it appeared to cost nothing, but now censure and ostracize those who only do the same in a new age when it must cost them their very longevity on earth?

References

Dilley J, Boccellari A: Neuropsychiatric complications of HIV infection, in Face to Face: A Guide to AIDS Counseling. Edited by Dilley, Pies, Helquist. San Francisco, CA, AIDS Health Project, University of California at San Francisco, 1989

Friedman M: Toward a reconceptualization of guilt. Contemporary Psychoanalysis 21:501–547, 1985

Gay Men's Health Crisis: The Basics. New York, Gay Men's Health Crisis, 1991

Gold R: Unprotected intercourse in HIV-infected and non-HIV-infected gay men. Unpublished paper, June 1992. Available from Ron Gold, Ph.D. Faculty of Education, Deakin University (Geelong Campus), Victoria, 3217, Australia

Moulton J, Sweet D, Gurbuz G, et al: Do groups work? evaluation of a group model, in Face to Face: A Guide to AIDS Counseling. Edited by Dilley, Pies, Helquist. San Francisco, CA, AIDS Health Project, University of California at San Francisco, 1989

Odets W: Life in the Shadow: Being HIV-Negative in the Age of AIDS. New York, Irvington Publishers (in press)

Prieur A, Andersen A, Frantzen AH, et al: Gay men: reasons for continued practice of unsafe sex. Paper presented at the First International Symposium on Information and Education on AIDS, Ixtapa, Mexico, June 1988

San Francisco AIDS Foundation: The Epidemic's "Third Wave." Impetus, San Francisco, CA, San Francisco AIDS Foundation, 1991

Chapter 21

Survivor Guilt in Seronegative Gay Men

Walt Odets, Ph.D.

During this second decade of the acquired immunodeficiency syndrome (AIDS) epidemic, one hears a great deal in mental health circles and in the popular press about gay men and survivor guilt. Nevertheless, the term *survivor guilt* has remained too imprecisely defined to be truly useful to the clinician in diagnosing or treating this condition. Although the mental health clinician may recognize the reality of the phenomenon, for the nonpsychotherapist the idea of survivor guilt is most often denied entirely on the premise that it does not make sense: "What would I have to be guilty about?" is the most common retort heard from gay men surviving the epidemic.

Despite such obfuscations and denials, I am convinced that survivor guilt is one of the clinical cornerstones of a psychological epidemic that is sweeping the surviving, seronegative gay male community. Survivor guilt is especially destructive for many reasons, but particularly because it erects barriers to the survivor's recognizing, acknowledging, and communicating his psychological distress.

In the San Francisco mental health community serving gay men, and particularly in the larger agencies, there has been tremendous resistance over the past decade to addressing seronegative psychological issues. This is just now beginning to change in San Francisco, and it is my impression that, with the exception of some individual psychotherapists, the resistance exists in all urban areas with large gay populations. The reasons for this situation are numerous, and because psychotherapists and patients seem often to collude in the resistance, it is important to clarify some of them.

Resistance to Recognizing Psychological Impact of Seronegativity

There is no doubt that earlier in the epidemic we needed money and resources for treating human immunodeficiency virus (HIV)–positive patients and those with AIDS, and that we kept these populations as our priority. In addition, in the earlier years of the AIDS epidemic it seemed possible that the epidemic would be brought under control medically, which would have both limited the psychological damage to survivors and allowed us to tend to the survivors after the event was over. Things have not gone as planned. The epidemic is likely to continue for decades, and survivors and nonsurvivors must coexist. Survivors will not live through decades of unaddressed psychological distress and then be successfully treated when the epidemic is over. Too much damage will have been done.

A second source of resistance to recognition of seronegative psychological issues has been more purely political. Many individuals in the larger HIV service agencies in San Francisco privately recognized what was initially called *recidivism*—a term borrowed from criminology to describe a return to unsafe sexual practices—several years before they made any public acknowledgment of the fact. It was feared that such revelations would damage funding. It was felt that existing AIDS funding had to be spent on people who had AIDS or who were at first-time risk for contracting HIV. This consideration did not include people who were merely devastated by the social and personal impact of AIDS, nor those who knew how to protect themselves from HIV infection but were not doing it. In the May 1990 edition of *Impetus,* the newsletter of the San Francisco AIDS Foundation, the correspondence section contained only the following two anonymous letters. It was apparent that this political situation was coming to a head:

I am writing in response to your recent newsletter [which discussed sexual recidivism]. I am a gay woman who lost my only brother to AIDS and have since watched two very good friends die.

I've been active in fundraising and have donated personal money to various AIDS organizations and will continue to do so for the ever-increasing needs of those who are ill. But I will not give money to your organization because of your stance to reeducate gay men in safe sex practices. I can't even believe you put this in your newsletter.

If men who are now aware of the practices that spread AIDS choose to engage in unsafe sex, their risk is their own responsibility, and I resent being asked to give time or money to support this issue.

The second letter represented the opposition:

I read with grave interest your latest edition of *Impetus* where you discussed "relapse." I say "grave" because I am one of the people you are talking about. I've . . . practiced only safe sex activities since 1987.

Unfortunately, several months ago, I slipped once and practiced high-risk sex. I have never done it since, and slipped just once, but I just found out that I am now infected with the AIDS [virus].

I can't tell anyone about this since everyone I know seems to think that people who do this deserve what they get.

I really believe that if I had been able to talk about the problem of relapse, I might not have had unsafe sex. . . . I hope you can get to others so it's not too late for them.

It is clear that unexplored feelings and politics are obscuring the issues underlying this interchange, and as psychotherapists we have a responsibility to clarify such feelings and to abstain from politically motivated psychotherapeutic interventions.

Finally, the mental health community's own survivor guilt and denial must be cited among the reasons it has resisted acknowledging seronegative problems. If a man feels guilt for having had the good fortune to survive when another has not, it seems clear that he will be resistant to recognizing his own distress and doubly resistant to talking about it. Denial separate from survivor guilt may include denial of the personal and social impact of the AIDS epidemic on the gay com-

munity in general, denial about the complexity of feelings surrounding safer and unsafe sex, and denial of the likelihood that the epidemic
may take an irreparable psychological toll from many survivors, especially those with multiple losses. Many in the mental health field continue to refer to HIV-negative men with psychological issues as "the
worried well." But the facts of this epidemic make a mockery of the
very term. In cities with concentrated gay populations, some men
truly find themselves in the position of lone survivors of families lost
in the Holocaust. Would we refer to a Holocaust survivor as someone
fortunate and "unaffected" by the Holocaust? Would we wonder what
needs he or she had for psychological services? Yet HIV-negative gay
men with comparable losses are routinely treated with such dismissive
questions.

By 1988, more San Franciscans—mostly gay men—had already
died from AIDS-related illnesses than if one took the number of all the
San Franciscans who died in the four wars of the 20th century and
doubled it (Baker et al. 1988). In the spring of 1990, San Francisco
Mayor Agnos opened the International AIDS Conference by announc-
ing that the updated figure could be arrived at by *tripling* that war toll.
It is inconceivable that the survivors of this event might be accurately
characterized as merely worried or well. In his study of 745 New York
gay men, Martin (1988) found there was "a direct dose-response relation between bereavement episodes and the experience of traumatic
stress response symptoms, demoralization symptoms, and sleep disturbance symptoms" (p. 858). In addition, Martin found that recreational drug use and sedative use also increased proportionately to
bereavement episodes, and that men with one or more bereavements
were four to five times more likely to seek mental health assistance in
connection with concerns and anxiety about their own health than
were men who experienced no bereavements.

In another study of gay men in New York, Dilley and Boccellari
(1989) initiated structured interviews of 236 AIDS and AIDS-related
complex (ARC) patients, using 139 asymptomatic gay men as control
subjects. They discovered that 39% of this "healthy" control group
qualified for a DSM-III-R (American Psychiatric Association 1987)
Axis I diagnosis of adjustment disorder with depressed or anxious
features.

Dilley, Director of the AIDS Health Project at the University of California at San Francisco's, summed up the situation up as follows:

> A critical concern is the impact of bereavement and anticipatory grief on a variety of populations: PWAs [people with AIDS], PWARCs [people with AIDS-related complex], seropositives and *those in their social networks* [emphasis added]. . . . Indications are that people undergoing stress of this magnitude show high levels of psychological distress, as well as physical illness. Among those harmful health outcomes are demoralization, a sense of helplessness, sleep disorders, irritability, increased use of tranquilizers and sleeping pills, and reliance on mental health and medical care. (Quoted in Baker et al. 1988, p. 38)

Identifying Symptoms of Survivor Guilt

Depression, anxiety, isolation, substance use and abuse, dissociative experience, and sexual, interpersonal, and occupational dysfunctions are all familiar to any mental health provider working with gay men. Such signs and symptoms, however, are seen in men both with and without survivor guilt, and the clinician must be able to distinguish survivor guilt within such complex presentations.

Depression, anxiety, and dysfunction of all types may be an essentially direct response to the AIDS epidemic. Loss, anger about that loss, and helplessness to do anything about it, resulting in a depression, are commonly seen. Fear for one's own health and that of loved ones may produce anxiety. However, survivor guilt may be an important *mediating* element in the development of depression and anxiety. Such guilt is largely unconscious, is generally denied or rationalized, and it is virtually never an explicit part of the presenting complaint. If psychotherapists—a group, as will be discussed shortly, perhaps particularly prone to the experience of survivor guilt—collude with patients in the exclusion of guilt issues from therapeutic attention, the outcome of that therapy will be unsatisfactory.

For the psychotherapist it is important to distinguish between directly produced depression and anxiety on the one hand and guilt-mediated depression and anxiety on the other. Seen in the context of grief and mourning, both appear to involve a struggle to separate from the lost object, but there are important differences in this regard. "Direct" depression and anxiety are often part of normal grieving, whereas guilt-mediated depression and anxiety are complicated and entrenched by survivor guilt. I believe that normal grieving does not, by definition, include survivor guilt, and that survivor guilt is most clearly understood as a complication of the normal grieving process. In normal grief, depression and anxiety are seen to be largely about the loss; in grief complicated by survivor guilt the feelings will also be about the loss, but the patient has additional feelings not seen in normal grief alone. These may include feelings that one would like to take the deceased individual's place, bewilderment at having survived the deceased individual, irrational feelings that one may die or is responsible for the death of the deceased individual, feelings that one is not worthy of survival, and an apparently inordinate extension of the grieving process in which the mourner is apparently not able to let go of the lost object. This last distinction is important, because much of the remorse is not about the loss of the object—an event that is in reality finished—but about the survivor's survival, an event that is ongoing and therefore cannot be "grieved."

Likewise, normal grief may be distinguished from grief complicated by survivor guilt by the type of anger present. Anger at the deceased for leaving the survivor behind is a common experience in normal grieving, but it is rarely found in the individual experiencing survivor guilt. Rather, the latter experiences remorse and sadness at being left behind and feels that it is his own fault, rather than the deceased individual's, that this has occurred. Finally, those experiencing normal grief usually wish the deceased individual to be back in life, whereas those who are feeling survivor guilt generally wish to join the dead.

It should be clear from this brief discussion that the relationship of survivor guilt to grief and mourning is a complicated one, but space limitations prohibit much expansion on this theme here. (For a further discussion of this issue, see Odets, in press).

Interpretations of Survivor Guilt

Interventions for the grieving psychotherapy patient differ depending on whether the individual's experience includes survivor guilt. Survivor guilt is a complication that can substantially inhibit or arrest the mourning process, and it often increases the risk of self-destructive behaviors.

There are certainly many gay men for whom the symptoms related to normal grieving and direct depression, such as anxiety and dysfunction, will become chronic and permanent to some extent, regardless of the degree to which therapy is able to clarify the meaning of the feelings and the events from which they arise. Such profound psychological transformations are created by severe, repeated losses and by other trauma characteristic of wars, plagues, and other significant, destructive social events. Although such transformations are of a magnitude generally associated with early developmental experience, they are also familiar as a consequence of very severe stressors in later life. The Holocaust and the Vietnam War are perhaps the most recent events that have produced such severe stressors on such a large scale, although to some extent the impact of these events was more evenly spread throughout society. Experienced by many, rather than largely by a minority, these events were given social form and meaning from which many individuals benefited psychologically. Such social sharing helps make sense of a tragedy. For the gay man in America, the AIDS epidemic has often seemed like a huge, ghettoized hell invisible to most of society. The lack of broad social support and acknowledgment, and the widespread ignorance of the meaning of the event has exacerbated gay men's personal costs. Although the AIDS epidemic can be shared within the gay community, elsewhere, such as with family and heterosexual friends, it can seem virtually a nonevent.

Direct depression and anxiety, depending on the severity of the stressor and psychological resilience of the patient, may or may not persist in the face of therapeutic intervention. In contrast, although guilt-mediated grief may be especially dangerous if unaddressed, it is my clinical experience that it is often responsive to psychotherapeutic intervention. Guilt, and the depression, anxiety, and dysfunction that it generates, may be ameliorated by clarification and interpretation, often producing substantial improvements in the experience and functioning of the patient. The following case example powerfully illustrates the guilt-mediated toll that this epidemic can take:

Case Example

Mr. A, a long-term therapy patient and a professional writer, spoke to me about a visit with Mr. B, a former lover and close friend who had been diagnosed with AIDS a few months earlier. At the time, Mr. A thought himself HIV negative. He said, "[Mr. B] was tired and was lying on the bed napping. I was watching him, from across the room, staring at him, and suddenly I imagined I could actually see the virus, like tiny dust particles, pumping through his veins and lodging in muscles and other parts of his body, contaminating him. I suddenly felt so completely repulsed, as if he had actually become physically repulsive. Can you imagine—my friend, who was once so beautiful to me? I felt afraid to touch him because he was diseased and I was afraid I would catch it just by touching his arm, or that he would wake up and want to touch me. He was still sleeping, but this panic just swept over me, and I felt, literally, like running out of his apartment. I started feeling so awful about these thoughts, of fearing him, of finding him repulsive, and of thinking about abandoning him while he was sick, that the idea came to me that I could be sick myself, or that I should be, that I could talk him into infecting me or do something else to get infected so that I would not have to feel torn between these feelings. I had the idea that if I lay down on the bed beside him, to take a nap with him, that would do it, and it seemed irresistible. I would just lie down and nap with him and not wake up." Mr. A eventually died from an AIDS-related illness.

Clearly there are many ways to understand the feelings expressed in this example. Many clinicians reading this transcript may note an attempt at introjection to ward off mourning, a desire to "merge" with the dying friend and thus prevent his loss. This interpretation might well be useful. But guilt is a very important unconscious feeling here and should also be opened to interpretation. The introjection serves not only to prevent Mr. B's loss, but to make the patient "like" Mr. B, to allow the patient to share Mr. B's HIV condition and thus have nothing to be guilty about. Characteristically, the patient has no explicit sense of guilt: he just "feels bad" about Mr. B. Also noteworthy is the unacceptability of the ambivalence about Mr. B, and the fatal solution to that ambivalence. The patient will share Mr. B's fatal illness and he will not be a survivor.

Indications of survivor guilt are seen in many similar forms outside of psychotherapy. For example, a positive HIV-antibody test or AIDS diagnosis results in a decrease of anxiety symptoms in some patients (Dilley and Boccellari 1989). Conversely, at HIV test sites one often sees significant distress in response to negative blood test results. The former executive director of Wellness Networks, Michigan's largest AIDS service agency, and current executive director of Pacific Center for Human Growth of Berkeley, California (which, among other services to sexual minorities, provides HIV testing), cited four common, "paradoxical" responses to negative HIV-antibody test results (S. Walton, personal communication, February 1989):

◆ My lover is positive, now what am I going to do?
◆ If anyone deserved it, it is me.
◆ All my friends are positive, how can I relate to them?
◆ Now I'm going to have to deal with my life.

He estimated these made up approximately 1 in 20 immediate responses at the test site, but that the number of such responses rose significantly once patients had left the test site. According to Walton, *crisis responses*—those requiring special psychological intervention by a supervisor—were generated by negative HIV tests by approximately a 3 to 1 margin over positive tests.

Other expressions of guilt among seronegative men include many seemingly irrational behaviors. A binge of unprotected sex, especially after the death of a friend or lover, is a phenomenon not uncommonly reported to me in therapy sessions. Such behavior often seems motivated by guilt and the self-destructive impulse arising from it. Although the fact that gay men are returning to unsafe sex is now widely acknowledged by AIDS service providers, it is still largely treated as a problem of complacency or a need for renewed safer sex education outside of this domain. With very few exceptions our AIDS education programs in the United States continue to ignore psychological issues as one source of unsafe sexual behaviors. (See further discussion of safe and unsafe sex in Chapter 20 and Odets, in press.) It may be stated here that as mental health practitioners we would be naive to accept the popular view that the possible dangerous consequences of unprotected sex serve only as a deterrent. For some—those who are depressed, anxious, and living a life that often seems not worth living—the potentially self-destructive nature of unsafe sex clearly serves as an incentive to practice it.

Characteristics of Survivor Guilt

Guilt is a diverse and complex phenomenon. Although survivor guilt, as one form of guilt, is discussed above in its relationship to grief, it is important to try to separate out and refine the idea of survivor guilt in its own terms. The following description of survivors by a Berkeley psychiatrist will be familiar to those living in the AIDS epidemic— although the description is actually about survivors of the Holocaust. In this passage, Friedman (1985) discussed the work of another researcher, Niederland:

> Typically, after struggling to begin a new life and often succeeding, these people succumbed to a variety of symptoms like depression, anxiety, and psychosomatic conditions. . . . Niederland believed these symptoms to be identifications with loved ones who had not survived. His patients often appeared and felt as if they were living dead. Niederland believed that these identifications were motivated by guilt, which he called survivor guilt. The survivors experienced an "ever present feeling of guilt . . . for having survived the very calamity to which their loved ones succumbed." (p. 520)

Friedman expanded this understanding by describing survivor guilt as including not only guilt about the fact of having survived, but also feelings that one

> could have helped but failed. . . . It is a guilt of omission. It is the guilt of people who believe they have better lives than those of their

parents or siblings. The greater the discrepancy between one's own fate and the fate of the loved person one failed to help, the greater the empathic distress and the more poignant one's guilt. (p. 532)

In suggesting that some survivor guilt is not simply about public events but is connected to developmentally earlier guilt about parents or siblings, Friedman touched on some of the etiological underpinnings of survivor guilt. Obviously one brings to public events one's personal history and development. This is a central insight in Erikson's "psychosocial" description, and it is a fact, I think, about every psychological development. It is not only our past and present that are connected, it is our private and our sociocultural worlds too. Particular problems with guilt in an individual's developmental background may fuel the guilt attached to public events in later life.

Mr. A, the patient from the case example, grew up with a mother who had been mildly crippled by polio as a child and walked with a cane throughout Mr. A's childhood. His feelings about her were the subject of much conversation, and clearly he had identified his Mr. B with her. The following dialogue is taken from another session with him:

Case Example *(continued)*

Mr. A said, "My mother called last night and I noticed this feeling that I often have with her—you know, I had friends over for dinner and we were having a good time, but when I heard it was her on the phone, I noticed that I toned down—as if I didn't want her to think I was having a good time."

"Do you know why you would do that?" I asked.

"Well my guilt about her, which we've talked a lot about," Mr. A responded.

"But how do you get to wanting to sound as if you're not having a good time?" I wondered.

"Well if she's not, then I shouldn't be, I guess. It would be like pushing it in her face, you know, 'You may be depressed, but I'm out here in California having dinner with my boyfriend and having a ball.'"

"So you would be sort of showing her up by having a good time?"

"Yes, definitely," said Mr. A.

"And abandoning her to her bad times?"

"Well I have abandoned her . . . just by going to California, so far as she's concerned. I can tell you that she calls me up because she's depressed and she wants me, as you call it, to 'fix' her. This has been a lot of our relationship. My dad certainly isn't going to do it. He's out bowling or yukking it up with his friends, anything to stay out of the house."

"And did you 'fix' her last night?" I asked.

"Well, of course not."

"And because you couldn't fix her, you thought it better to seem depressed yourself?"

"When you put it that way it sounds silly of course," said Mr. A. "But if I can't do anything about her depression, the next best thing seems like being depressed myself—to keep her company so to speak."

"This is like your self-consciousness about running around in front of her or walking too fast when you were a child. We have speculated about your foot pain and limping." (Mr. A often had foot pain as a child, and this sometimes kept him from normal play activities.)

"Yes—if she couldn't run I did often feel that I shouldn't run in front of her. Showing her up again."

"And perhaps literally running away from her, leaving her behind," I suggested.

"Yes, exactly. Running away and leaving her behind, because that is what I often wanted to do. I often pretended I wasn't with her because of my embarrassment about her [being crippled] in front of other kids—I'm embarrassed by these feelings even now, as much as we've talked about them, it's disgusting really that I did this to her—but I would run ahead so people wouldn't think I was with her."

"You feel a lot of remorse about this, that this was something you did to her," I stated. "Almost as if your feelings of embarrassment caused the disability."

"It is only because I was a child that I can excuse myself."

"And it occurs to me that you still bring these feelings—I'm referring here to your disgust for yourself—to your relationship with [Mr. B]."

"I don't see that," Mr. A responded cautiously.

"I'm thinking of the day you watched him sleep, of being disgusted by him, afraid of him, of wanting to run out on him, and how much that sounds like your feelings about your mother. And about feeling so much guilt about those feelings, and about coming up with the idea that you could have HIV too, that you could be crippled like your mother."

"Well, I'll take your word for it, but I don't really see this."

"I wonder if it isn't harder for you to look at your feelings about [Mr. B] than about your mother," I suggested. "That you are having difficulty with this because it's still hard for you to look at those feelings."

Mr. A did not respond to this suggestion, and it was only over the following period of several months that this line of interpretation began to provide him clarification of his feelings.

Other Developmental Sources of Guilt in Gay Men

Developmental descriptions of gay men and speculation about the origins of homosexuality have been very politicized, even within mental health circles. Developmental description is often shunned as a reductionistic effort aimed at pathologizing homosexuality, and any etiologic explanations that imply choice are shunned as a political compromise and an untruth. In fact, developmental description is often of interest in connection with heterosexual development and need not imply pathology in the case of gay men at all. Furthermore, it still seems correct to me that childhood experience has a role in homosexual development and that any element of choice this might imply introduces no political compromises that could damage the purposes of gay rights. In many instances, including religious and political observation, legal and human rights are defined as including chosen, voluntary behaviors. The idea that homosexuality is "legitimate" and deserving of social acceptance and legal protection only if it is the result of uncontrollable causes—and is thus immutable in the individual—is a profoundly homophobic position. Is it possible that homosexuality is, in and of itself, so reprehensible that it must be "involuntary" to qualify as acceptable and deserving of civil protection in a humane society? The psychotherapist who adheres to such political views forecloses on too much meaning in the pursuit of legitimacy—both for himself and his patients.

The following developmental sketch is intended as a brief summary of clinical observations about a kind of family the author has observed in numerous psychotherapies with gay men. I believe that, as a group, gay men in psychotherapy experience an inordinate problem with guilt early in life as compared with the general population. Such guilt often seems to be the result of an absent or otherwise available father who leaves the son, his wife, and perhaps other siblings emotionally abandoned, lonely, and depressed. The son, often the youngest or oldest of the siblings, may take on the task of trying to repair not only his mother's loneliness and depression about her unavailable husband, but also the depression of younger siblings who are in turn neglected by their mother. He becomes an emotional caretaker for the family, often describing himself as the family's mediator or psychologically most responsible member. If the homosexual son is the youngest of the siblings, the task seems most often centered on the mother's depression alone as older siblings having separated themselves from the family system.

Guilt enters this developmental picture because the son, now working to be husband and sometimes parent, understandably fails at the task. In such families the son is "given" to the mother in exchange for the father's freedom from emotional ties and responsibilities. Through identification with the father, the son may thus bear the father's guilt towards his wife, and he will certainly feel guilt about failing his mother in his task as substitute spouse and father. Elements of such a family organization are seen in the history of Mr. A, above. Also seen in that patient's history are a number of other developmental events typical among gay men that exacerbate problems with guilt. Although they can only be mentioned here because of space limitations, I have discussed them more fully elsewhere (Odets, in press). These include the guilt about abandoning the family in order to live a homosexual life-style and guilt about others who are affected when the gay man comes out, thus abandoning his largely false heterosexual self and those to which it was cathected.

Men with such developmental backgrounds grow up with a sense of unworthiness, failure, and guilt about relationships in general, guilt about their sexuality, and often guilt about making livers for themselves that are less lonely and depressed than those of their mothers or siblings—in other words, guilt about having successful relationships. These are all aspects of survivor guilt, and this guilt provides a predisposition that, given the synergistic support of real-world adult circumstances like the Holocaust or the AIDS epidemic, can become a devastating, often fatal experience.

Other Developmental Problems

Other developmental problems also interact with and exacerbate the psychological resilience of seronegative men living in the AIDS epidemic. Histories of mood disorders, particularly difficult conflicts about sexuality, and long-standing personal isolation (including schizoid character trends) will all interact destructively with the public event. At the more troubling end of this interactive spectrum, we see men with extensive, serious conflict about their sexuality and consequent isolation. These men, in the midst of the AIDS epidemic, find new reasons for remaining isolated (and perhaps sexually dysfunctional); AIDS may be enlisted unconsciously to displace the conflicts from the private to the public sphere. In the middle of the spectrum we see men with similar developmental issues that were either less severe or were better worked through in adulthood, and for them the AIDS epidemic may be a test of psychological "progress" or may entail some regression. Still other men, nearer the benign end of the developmental spectrum, may find themselves with developmentally unprecedented issues of loss, guilt, depression, isolation, or sexual dysfunction that are largely reactive to the epidemic. The problems of these men are more easily addressed than those of men in the first two groups. Finally, at the extreme end of the spectrum are many men who possess a fortuitous combination of relatively benign development and a good psychological "constitution," which combine to allow for a weathering of the AIDS epidemic with a minimum of serious disturbance.

Psychotherapeutic Treatment

The psychotherapeutic approach to patients experiencing survivor guilt is relatively straightforward; in fact, much "ordinary" psychotherapy is about survivor guilt in the broadest sense of the concept. All psychotherapists work with problems about separation from the family, ambivalence about success, and a sense of inadequacy in relationships. These issues always involve survivor guilt, even when seen in an individual not living in an epidemic.

In general, the defenses against experiencing guilt about the current events must be clarified and the patient's pain, expressed in resistance to that clarification, interpreted. Few patients have any conscious experience of guilt per se, and the more serious the unconscious guilt, the more powerful will be the resistance to having it described clearly. Typically, those experiencing the most serious guilt about survival will deny guilt, presenting with some combination of anxiety, hypochondriasis, depression, and social or sexual dysfunction. They may acknowledge some question about why they are among the survivors—the "Why me? question in reverse," as one patient called it—and they will often be found to be engaging in unsafe sex, substance abuse, or other self-destructive behaviors.

Such men strongly identify with particular HIV-infected men, perhaps partners or best friends, or with HIV-positive men in general, and they may feel that their seronegative status has created a breach in their particular "mixed-antibody status" relationship, represents a violation of their allegiance to the gay community, or threatens their identity as gay men. These feelings are summed up strikingly by many of my psychotherapy patients who are in the process of coming out saying that they will truly and finally be gay and part of the gay community when they have contracted HIV. Though often said jokingly, these feelings are profound, especially in older men coming out later in life. Finally, men with significant guilt about survival are often found working in AIDS services, often at "burnout" levels. The sublimation of depression and anxiety arising from guilt into such useful "acting out" is a common—and not entirely pathological—expression of life in the epidemic.

When these signs and symptoms have been clarified as aspects of survivor guilt, the therapist may then begin to interpret such feelings, and this will involve beginning to connect the current guilt to developmental issues and conflicts. As in all therapies, this connection making, when supported by real insight, is powerful and is the basis for reducing the grip and the power of self-destructive feelings. When it is understood that guilt about surviving those who are lost to AIDS is irrational and unrealistic, and that it is compelling because it connects so powerfully to earlier conflicts characterized by guilt, the patient may then begin to feel that he has a right to have the best life he can—at any rate a decent one—and that trying to do so is not violence against, betrayal of, or abandonment of those less fortunate. "To a degree not generally recognized, psychopathologies are pathologies of loyalty" (Friedman 1985, p. 530).

Summary

In closing, a word about survivor guilt and countertransference is warranted. Those in the helping professions, including psychotherapists, and perhaps gay male psychotherapists in particular, have chosen a profession that provides an opportunity to help repair patients (and the self!) in a way that they were unable to do as sons or siblings. Such motivation is surely near the heart of the "curative" impulse. But the psychotherapist may also use his or her work to remain attached to failed parents and siblings—and thus to his or her own failure—by remaining inordinately attached to the troubled lives of patients. She or he thus avoids the abandonment of mother, father, or siblings for a better life and the exacerbation of guilt that such an abandonment would induce. Such acting out of survivor guilt in the countertransference is evidenced in psychotherapy practices overwhelmed by HIV problems and by the psychotherapist who seems unable to maintain any reasonable separation from the despair and hopelessness of his or her patients. Just as life itself becomes a betrayal of the dead, a life happier than that of one's dying patients feels intolerable. This is sometimes the psychological foundation of "burnout," but it is in all cases an approach with a limited future for both therapist and patient. If a gay psychotherapist in the second decade of our epidemic is going to help others clarify their feelings about survival, he must clarify his own feelings about guilt, abandonment, and the lives of seronegative gay men. The latter may be especially difficult for the seropositive therapist.

There are many reasons it is now crucial that we address survivor guilt in the gay community. At the most pragmatic level, healthier survivors make better caretakers of those who have AIDS, and today this is important work in the gay community. In addition, there are the issues concerning the survivors themselves. Many possible survivors will not ultimately survive because of the self-destructive behaviors that guilt, depression, and anxiety can fuel. For those who will survive in a biological sense, there is already an immense amount of psychological damage wrought by the AIDS epidemic, and this damage is only compounded and exacerbated by guilt. The psychological futures of countless survivors, as well as the future of the gay community as a whole, depend partly on the ability of mental health providers to deal with the intense issues arising in both seropositive and seronegative gay men.

Although services for HIV-negative gay men have been controversial in many parts of the gay community, it must now be clear to any astute observer that we have to address the pain of potential survivors and nonsurvivors concurrently if we are to intercept what has already been allowed to grow into a psychological epidemic among HIV-negative gay men. If we are asked why AIDS resources should be directed to those who are "unaffected" by the AIDS epidemic, as psychotherapists we must answer that lone survivors of families destroyed in the Holocaust—albeit alive—cannot properly be described as "unaffected" by the Holocaust. The Holocaust lasted 6 years; the AIDS epidemic has already lasted twice that long. We cannot wait until the epidemic is over before we begin our work with HIV-negative men, and if attention to this population arouses our own guilt or anger or that of others in the gay community, those feelings must be clarified in order to allow this necessary work to begin.

If we are not able to adequately address the issues of seronegative men the costs may be unendurable. As a 23-year-old patient, 2 weeks after an HIV-positive blood test, said, "I'm sometimes glad to think I won't be around in 10 years because by then the only gay people left will be those whose lives were ruined by watching the rest of us die." Surely there is much potential truth in these words, and mental health providers are among those in a position to help see that this does not happen.

Reference

American Psychiatric Association: Diagnostic and Statistical Manual of Mental Disorders, 3rd Edition, Revised. Washington, DC, American Psychiatric Association, 1987

Baker R, Moulton J, Gorman M: An Epidemic of Loss: AIDS in San Francisco's Gay Male Community, 1988–1993. San Francisco, CA, San Francisco AIDS Foundation, 1988

Dilley J, Boccellari A: Neuropsychiatric complications of HIV infection, in Face to Face: A Guide to AIDS Counseling. Edited by Dilley J, Pies C, Helquist M. San Francisco, CA, AIDS Health Project, University of California at San Francisco, 1989, pp 138–152

Friedman M: Toward a reconceptualization of guilt. Contemporary Psychoanalysis 21:501–547, 1985

Martin JL: Psychological consequences of AIDS-related bereavement among gay men. J Consult Clin Psychol 56:856–862, 1988

Odets,W: Life in the Shadow: Being HIV Negative in the Age of AIDS. New York, Irvington Publishers (in press)

Section IV

Impact on the Therapist

Chapter 22

Empathic Challenges for Gay Male Therapists Working With HIV-Infected Gay Men

Steven A. Cadwell, Ph.D.

The acquired immunodeficiency syndrome (AIDS) epidemic has thrown therapists and patients into relationships that trigger intense mutual issues of morality, sexuality, disease, and mortality. These issues are especially poignant for those of us who are gay male therapists working with gay male patients with AIDS. In this chapter, I present the results of a study done on the specific challenges facing gay therapists working with HIV-positive gay patients. A closer look at our experiences offers an opportunity to understand better the specific identification issues and the ways in which we are currently managing. This exploration also has more general implications for understanding the impact of identification on the therapeutic relationship and how it may be managed.

AIDS has had a profound impact on psychotherapy. Those psychotherapists who both work with a growing number of people with AIDS (PWAs) and have friends, lovers, and relatives with AIDS have been in a difficult position. Stress theory identifies variables affecting stress levels applicable to work with AIDS: stressor pervasiveness and persistence, the timing of the experience within one's life course, the limits of resources or opportunities to assert control, the personal meaning one attributes to the stress (Benner et al. 1980), and the level of uncertainty or importance of outcomes (Beehr and Bhagat 1985).

Research on burnout in hospice work has isolated features also inherent in AIDS work: the nontraditional nature of the work, the idealism of those attracted to the work, the repeated formation and termination of relationships with patients, the high level of ambiguity in the work, and the possibility of matched characteristics of the worker and patient (Cherniss 1980; Thomas 1983; Vachon 1979). In this chapter I focus beyond the sociopsychological level to the relevance of identification as a concept for understanding the internal dynamics of the therapist. I emphasize understanding both the dynamic nature of the identification between the gay male therapist and his patient and the coping strategies the therapist uses to deal with his identification.

Identification Issues in Psychotherapy With HIV-Infected Gay Men

Ideally, psychotherapy allows the patient an opportunity to engage in a process of merging and separating, identifying and distancing with the therapist to strengthen his boundaries of identity (Little 1950). In this paradigm, the principal work of the therapist is empathic in nature. Little (1950) described empathy as follows:

> The basis of empathy, as of sympathy, is identification, and it is detachment that makes it distinct from sympathy. The detachment comes about partly by the use of the ego function of reality testing with the introduction of the factors of time and distance. The analyst necessarily identifies with the patient, but there is for him an interval of time between himself and the experience which for the patient has the quality of immediacy—he knows it for past experience, while to the patient it is a present one. (p. 35)

Gay therapists are particularly vulnerable to their own immediate exposure to AIDS as a painfully present phenomenon. Clearly, as gay male therapists, we can easily identify with the experience of HIV or AIDS patients. But how are we able to detach and introduce the factors of time and distance to sustain empathy? A great risk for the gay therapist is what Racker (1968) defined as *concordant identification:*

> Based on introjection and projection, on the resonance of the exterior in the interior, or recognition of what belongs to another as one's own (this part of you is I), and on the equation of what is one's own with what belongs to another (this part of me is you). (p. 134)

The gay male therapist may repeatedly experience concordant identification with a PWA because of the therapist's vulnerability, which may be manifested on at least four levels. First, the therapist may be medically vulnerable to infection by HIV: he may become infected or he may already be infected. Furthermore, he may or may not know his HIV status. Second, he may be vulnerable to homophobia— the irrational dread of homosexuality (Weinberg 1971). As gay men search for reasons for the disease, they may think moralistically. The response of American society to the AIDS epidemic further reinforces this homophobia. Third, the gay therapist is vulnerable to grief in response to death and illness caused by AIDS. The magnitude of his loss extends to his collegial support network, to a large portion of his practice, and to his personal and social network. Finally, he is socially and politically vulnerable because of the loss of a powerful portion of his community. In the gay community of San Francisco, 50% of the gay men are infected with the virus. In the population at large, 20% to 25% are infected with the AIDS virus (Boffey 1988). The actual and potential social and political loss to the gay community is enormous.

In the Boston gay community, gay PWAs and other gay men often request gay therapists because there is both an ample supply of gay therapists and sophisticated patient demand. Consequently, PWAs generally make up a higher proportion of gay therapists' caseloads than of straight therapists' caseloads. Although lesbian therapists have borne and continue to bear a tremendous piece of the HIV work with gay men, and some dynamics in their work are similar to that of gay male therapists, in this chapter I explore the dimensions and impact of the shared vulnerability of only the gay male therapist and gay PWAs he treats. A second focus of this chapter is to describe the means these gay therapists have found to maintain their empathic stance.

Identification:
Empathy and Countertransference

Although no one has focused exclusively on the topic of identification in gay therapists working with patients with HIV spectrum illnesses, the literature on identification and countertransference offers a theoretical framework for describing the dynamics of the therapeutic relationship. I discuss identification in therapy in terms of empathy and countertransference.

Identification in Empathy

Despite controversy over the nature of empathy and the role of identification in empathy (Basch 1983; Buie 1981; Deutsch and Madle 1975), psychoanalytic ego psychologists integrated affective and cognitive viewpoints. Schafer (1959) defined *generative empathy* as "the inner experience of sharing in and comprehending the momentary psychological state of another person" (p. 345). The affective component involves the ability to temporarily flex one's ego boundaries enough to regress in order to reexperience affective experiences in one's own past. After experiencing one's own affective states, these feelings are projected onto the other individual and then tested by observation for validity.

The ability to regain a sense of self-other differentiation and observe the other within the context of what is known of the other person involves the use of cognitive capacities, such as attention to cues, memory, the differentiation between past and present, the differentiation between projection and reality, and analytic and synthetic functions. "Affect operating with too little cognition would not achieve comprehension of another's experience; it would lead to confusing and intolerable reactivity involving an illusion of identity, fusion of the ego with the object" (Schafer 1959, p. 349). By definition, empathy entails healthy ego development and secure self-other differentiation, not an experience of merging (Buie 1981). The ego is the executor of empathy (Buie 1981). In this chapter, I use identification in its nonmetapsychological, descriptive sense. Empathy is seen as having a component of identification but as also having crucial components that are cognitive and ensure self-object differentiation.

Identification in Countertransference

Although identification is crucial to the therapeutic process, it is also potentially hazardous. The failure of the trial identification (Fliess 1942) is countertransference. Here most theorists agree. But they differ as to the clinical utility of the countertransference that results. One theorist's failed trial identification is another's useful countertransference tool. Kernberg (1963) joined Little in suggesting that this emotional experience of the analyst may be useful in that it "duplicates" the experience of the patient. Kernberg held that these emotions can be used by the analyst because the therapist has important compensatory mechanisms operating: aspects of his ego remain intact whereas others are involved in the empathic regression. However, Kernberg went on to acknowledge that the therapist may not always be able to "snap out of" the countertransference position created by a certain patient. Severely regressed patients may precipitate a permanent emotional distortion and a "fixed" countertransference position in the analyst, resulting in "reappearance of abandoned neurotic character traits of the analyst in his interactions with a particular patient; 'emotional discontinuation' of the analysis; unrealistic 'total dedication'; or 'micro-paranoid' attitudes toward the patient" (Kernberg 1963, p. 54).

Other authors have delineated the different, difficult countertransference reactions to psychosis (Kernberg 1963; Little 1950; Reich 1960; Winnicott 1956), to suicidality (Buie and Maltsberger 1974), to terminal illness (Adler 1984), to cancer patients (Slaby 1988; Weisman 1981), and to dying patients (Le Shan and Le Shan 1961; Sanders 1984; Weisman 1973). Therapy with PWAs is difficult because the inevitability of death is brutally apparent, as is the specter of deterioration, waste, and excruciating pain. Furthermore, therapy with patients with AIDS may include all of the following difficult clinical challenges at once: primitive issues (if the patient has characterological problems or regresses under stress), the issues of psychosis (stemming from organic complications), issues of suicidality, and the issues of terminal illness.

Dunkel and Hatfield (1986) and McKusick (1988) outlined countertransference issues they found common among both straight and

gay clinicians working with gay men with AIDS: 1) fear of the unknown, 2) fear of contagion, 3) fear of dying and of death, 4) denial
of helplessness, 5) fear of homosexuality, 6) overidentification,
7) anger, and 8) need for professional omnipotence. Of these issues,
Dunkel and Hatfield noted that the gay clinician may be particularly
vulnerable to anger and overidentification, but they did not mention
the risk of homophobia for gay clinicians. The gay therapist is no more
immune to homophobia than the straight therapist. In fact, the gay
therapist may have had less chance to work through his homophobic
response because it is not "politically correct" in the gay community
to acknowledge such feelings.

With all these complex countertransferential feelings fomenting,
the work for the gay psychotherapist with a PWA is tremendously
challenging. How does he manage his anger or the pull to overidentify,
as so many of his characteristics match his patients'? Because no studies exist in this specific area, I looked to situations where other therapists share traits with their patients.

The extensive empirical literature on shared characteristics in the
therapist and the patient is motivated primarily by concern that dis-
similarity between the two leads to bias and lack of efficacy in the
treatment. I am focusing less on perceived external similarity and
more on the experience of internal match (i.e., the shared feelings of
vulnerability to the AIDS epidemic and subsequent high probability
of identification). The identification of countertransference vulnerabilities when therapist and patient are matched is just beginning to be
researched. The dearth of literature addressing this specific countertransference problem is in itself curious and may be explained by the
ambivalence therapists have had for countertransference as a treatment tool.

Most existing research has been conducted by women about female therapists' countertransference to female patients in treatment
(Ruderman 1986; Shainess 1983). Ruderman suggested that feelings
that derive from society's negative attitude toward women become ac-
tivated in a female psychotherapist's countertransference, leading to
powerful and complex identification with the patient. She also makes
a strong case for the mutually reparative experience and achievement
of new and significant levels of personal integration for both female

patient and female therapist when countertransference themes are explored as fully as possible.

In conclusion, empirical and theoretical studies contribute to a sense of the convergence of issues that must be managed by the gay male psychotherapist working with gay male patients with AIDS.

Study Method

I conducted this study in Boston, Massachusetts, from January to May of 1989. Questionnaires were mailed to therapists listed in the Massachusetts Department of Public Health AIDS Resource Guide; respondents were included in the study if they were gay, licensed clinicians who had worked with HIV or AIDS patients for at least 6 months. Semistructured interviews lasting 90 minutes were taped, and content analysis was employed to discern common themes and differences in the manifest content from line-by-line analysis of interview transcripts. I made two assumptions from these interviews: 1) for the most part, respondents commented only on conscious countertransference, and 2) on balance, the therapists had the capacity to view their patients as differentiated others.

Sample Description

In the final sample ($N = 15$), the average age was 42 with a range from 32 to 55. All were white, gay males. The therapists were from similar sociocultural backgrounds and they were either HIV negative or did not know their HIV status. (One clinician who had AIDS-related complex withdrew from the study because of health concerns.) Seven were psychologists, 4 were licensed independent clinical social workers, and 4 were psychiatrists. Their clinical experience ranged from 7 to 28 years with an average of 15 years, and their experience working with HIV patients ranged from 3 to 7 years, with an average of 6 years. Twelve of the subjects were in full-time private practice; 3 had combined private and hospital practices. In their practices, they currently had between one and eight HIV-related cases, with an average of five cases. The percentage of gay patients in their practice ranged from 30% to 95%, with the average being 63%.

Results

Data analysis revealed the gay psychotherapists' felt vulnerability to identification in three areas: 1) vulnerability to contagion, 2) vulnerability to death and grief, and 3) vulnerability to homophobia.

Vulnerability to Contagion

Each of the therapists described anxiety about his health, although the intensity of their anxiety and defenses vaiied. One therapist described his terror after having worked with gay men with AIDS for a year. He became sick with fevers and swollen lymph nodes that lasted for 4 months and was convinced that he had AIDS. His illness turned out to be "cat scratch fever." Although the onset of his anxiety was triggered by real symptoms, he reported that it was exacerbated by his work with gay men who have AIDS.

The therapists universally described as most difficult those patients who expressed their destructive impulses sexually. Distressed patients with AIDS who acted out in unsafe sex or suicidal patients who sought HIV infection stimulated the therapist's own fears of contagion. One therapist described a self-abusive patient who was compulsively trying to get AIDS:

> I wanted to shake him or slap him. I know what the guy's issues are, and I know this doesn't have to do with him. This has to do with me. He doesn't need to be shaken or slapped. He has his own way of torturing himself. What stirred me up was the way in which he really wanted to get AIDS to give a certain kind of meaning to his life where there was nothing but emptiness. And the opposite of that is what is true for me. AIDS threatens the meaning of my life. The conflict of our two issues is always present. And sometimes it feels unbearable.

Vulnerability to Death and Grief

The therapists described experiencing deaths in numbers that did not fit the norm for men between the ages of 30 and 45. Many described knowing between 30 and 50 people who had died of AIDS—friends, lovers, ex-lovers, patients, and colleagues. Often several crises converged on the therapist all at once: the death of a patient, the death of a friend, and the diagnosis of AIDS for another person in his life. Death affected the therapists in different ways. One practitioner said,

> Every time a new patient walks in, I have this sort of Ray Bradbury hallucinatory type experience for a minute, and I see the skull behind the skin on the face. And I imagine what he might look like dead.

Other therapists described intense grief reactions: "It feels like it's so endless. You don't get a chance to recover from one before the next death hits." Because their professional role inhibited many therapists from attending their patients' funerals, several described the difficulty of finding alternative opportunities to grieve. As one therapist put it:

> This October, I went to the quilt in Washington. And the reason I really went was because one of the panels is of my first patient who died. You would have thought he died yesterday. I cried and cried and cried and cried. He'd died 5 years before!

Most (12 of the 15) of the men interviewed were between ages 38 and 45, a predictable time for mid-life concerns. Mid-life issues combined with the numbers of deaths intensifying their grief reaction:

> I realized in a sort of "Oh, wow!" moment that I was losing friends at approximately the same rate my grandmother was. And that was premature. It reminded me of a quote from a world history teacher that times of war change the order of things and force parents to bury their children. This is a similar distortion of the natural order.

Because of the numbers of deaths, gay therapists experience loss of personal and community supports. Many of the study therapists talked openly about being in the midst of their own "unremitting grief reaction," a trauma that one man compared with the reaction to the atom bomb drop at Hiroshima. The social significance of the loss was experienced in various ways; the "transformation of gay sexuality" was mourned. One therapist grieved that his celebratory community of liberation had become a community of mourning. Their "unfinishable" grief was for people lost and for the potential of more people dying.

Vulnerability to Homophobia

Being gay themselves, the therapists' own experiences of oppression and stigmatization made them all the more sensitized to their patients' dilemmas, thus triggering the therapists' shame, rage, and dedication to care for HIV-infected people. One therapist put it as follows:

> What it means to live an affirmative gay life in America, probably in most of the world, is that you are an outlaw. . . . If this epidemic had first appeared in white straight men who were congressional leaders, the entire mind set of the epidemic would be different.

After a decade of affirming gay pride, the experience of the AIDS epidemic has stirred unresolved feelings of shame and rage for both patients and therapists. As one therapist put it,

> Being diagnosed HIV positive is a devastating experience. It's also a shameful experience. In listening to therapists who are homophobic about their HIV-related cases, I am reminded how much moralistic stigmata is attached to HIV status. It's no surprise that patients bear enormous shame. I know their shame, but because of my own issues, I find it very difficult to talk with PWAs about how shamed they feel.

Consequences of Vulnerability

Many of the psychotherapists noted that their identification was also the source of their motivation to do their work. Most drew on their personal experiences to understand their patients' experiences better. As one therapist noted,

> I know my patient knows that I have a visceral understanding of who he is and what he's dealing with. I know he knows that I un-

derstand from the inside out what he's dealing with and that he feels very understood.

The obvious risk they felt was that this "passion" may go unmanaged with serious adverse consequences. Some therapists described losing perspective because of too much intimacy or too much distance—boundaries lost or never approached. They talked of being overprotective at times. A therapist whose lover died of AIDS told about being confronted by his patient after the therapist had been unusually overbearing in cautioning him against becoming involved with a man who was HIV positive, even though they were practicing safer sex and the relationship showed promise.

The therapists also talked about joining the patient's tendency to avoid exploring feelings out of fear of their own. One therapist described the pull to be "the patient's friend, or the patient's patient, or the patient's parent" and to act out his countertransference in some unobserved way. In this enactment, the patient's transference wish and the therapist's countertransference both remained unexplored.

Some therapists may try to manage intense identification by distancing themselves from the patient. A hospital-based social worker described his struggle with the "everydayness" of the work. He feared that he was avoiding his feelings and worries about his numbed approach. One therapist had supervised other gay therapists who "take on AIDS cases willy-nilly, to the point that they become machinelike. They're talking as though they're doing a heroic duty but they're not there for any of them, and they're losing themselves day by day and it really worries me."

Management of Vulnerability to Identification

The study subjects displayed six different methods of managing their vulnerability to identification: 1) behavioral, 2) ego supportive, 3) political, 4) personal growth, 5) spiritual, and 6) cognitive. Each respondent used a combination of management techniques relying on one more heavily than another at different times.

Behavioral Management

Limit numbers of patients.   Early in the epidemic, many were not able to limit the number of HIV-positive patients because of limited resources and an unrealistic sense of the amount of the work they could manage. Although they could not predict the number of their ongoing patients who might seroconvert to being HIV positive, many reported that had their cases seroconverted in large numbers, they would have had to terminate and transfer patients. One therapist described his quota of HIV cases this way:

> I've settled on 25% of my patient load being HIV positive as a working model, after having at one point probably 50% or 60% HIV-related cases and finding that was too much. It required me for about 9 months to stop seeing people with AIDS completely. The personal impact and the amount of extra work associated with patients with HIV-related illness is enormous.

Absolute numbers of HIV-related cases or percentages of cases may be less important than taking the time out to assess one's own limits in terms of one's quality of life.

Break the isolation.   Some private practitioners organized to meet with other therapists in AIDS-related organizations, conferences, and in peer support groups. Therapists who were the solitary providers of HIV services in large hospital settings were working to achieve a more equitable distribution of cases and were creating support groups with their peers.

Choose other means of involvement.   The responding therapists listed a variety of activities as alternatives to direct clinical work, including teaching, administration, research, supervision, organization of conferences, development of videos, being an expert witness for public policy hearings, and writing. These activities gave the therapists distance from the intensity of their clinical relationships.

Personal life.   This included personal relationships with friends and lovers; an active social life; hobbies such as singing, reading, music, cooking, travel, or home improvements; physical exercise; having children; and leisure time doing nothing.

Ego-Supportive Resources

Supervision and collegial support.   The supportive and containing dimension of supervision and collegial support was crucial to the subjects:

> I had two patients who had just died of AIDS, had just gotten a new patient with AIDS, had a close friend who'd died of AIDS, and another close friend who just got diagnosed, and I'd this long-term patient who seroconverted all within a month. The supervision group gave me some feedback and advice. I wasn't hearing it because I was just so burned out. One person put it to me, "Your whole life sounds like it's nothing but shattered edges. You need to do something." I heard.

Supportive friendships.   Although friendships were sometimes precarious because the friends too were vulnerable, friends lent a vital sense of fraternity and community. As one therapist put it,

> I feel that I'm active in a community now in which there are substantial numbers of people that I love and feel loved by. I've got a fraternal group of men friends who I feel very safe and very happy with and that's new for me in the last 5 years. These are all people I can count on.

Political and Community Involvement

Political and community involvement provided the subjects with a means of managing resurging homophobic feelings that might have been experienced internally or externally. One psychologist described the sudden importance of declaring his gay identity at a national professional meeting. He had never felt the need to come out before. His experience of coming out seemed to be part of his politicization through his experience in the epidemic—of finding power in collective commitment, of asserting the rights of the disenfranchised by publicly identifying with them.

Although none of the gay therapists described becoming full-time political activists, they did describe heightened political awareness as they witnessed how politics affected the resources available to their HIV patients. Many participated through community action groups, such as the Boston AIDS Action Committee, or served on public policy boards related to HIV issues. This involvement gave them a sense of impacting larger systems that affected their patients and also enabled them to have some distance from the intensity of their clinical work. A psychiatrist put it this way:

> On the upside, work with HIV has involved me much more in the gay community than I was before. I'm not a big politico, but my involvement has helped my feelings of professional isolation and helplessness.

Management Through Personal Growth

Therapy dealing with issues of death, loss, and homophobia triggered the therapists' use of a range of intrapsychic defenses that they described as a means to negotiate distance. Some expressed concern that their own style of defensive management interfered with their clinical relationships. Some were returning to psychotherapy for themselves. Others were seeking alternative ways to "heal the healer." As one social worker described it, "I go to bioenergetics a lot and scream. I find a need to do very visceral work."

Spiritual Life

Some men talked about using traditional (e.g., Buddhist, Christian, and Jewish) spiritual practices to find more grounding to continue in their work. Others described difficulty achieving a sense of spirituality that gave them the support they needed. The loss and death in the pandemic were disrupting their earlier simple religious beliefs. As one therapist reflected,

To really understand the loss to the community was to challenge any notion of this being a benevolent universe. I then had to consider a spiritual view that incorporated not malevolence but pain. What I need to feel is that however I understand the world, which may change from day to day, I can buy into it.

Any therapist needs a center pin of a belief system, even if a shifting one, in order to face the uncertainty, pain, and death that he or she will encounter from his or her career, particularly if the work is with AIDS patients. Some of my respondents described meditation as a means to maintain their sense of balance.

Cognitive Management of Vulnerability to Identification

Role clarification.   In defining their professional role, other therapists seem to be negotiating the boundaries of the work. As one therapist stated,

At first we have an expectable role. When patients get sick, it tends to fuzz over. . . . Maybe you're more like a friend. Or maybe you're part of his medical care. Your role is not clear. So you carve out a niche for yourself.

The therapists working with HIV or AIDS patients have expanded their repertoire of treatment models. One psychiatrist talked of a "social casework" model, which he described as being more active and offering more concrete, confrontational advice instead of his usual objective, analytic role.

Time frame change.   Initially, the study therapists said they were as caught up in the immediate crisis as were their patients. Over time, many described a growing sense that their interventions were not temporary crisis management. As therapists, they were in the epidemic for the long haul, and they needed to reconceptualize their involvement to allow for sustained contact over time.

Specializing in the work.   Different therapists focused on different tasks that they felt they could manage. As one stated, "I really like seeing people who are difficult to diagnose and figuring out what's going on. I also like using medications and seeing people get better. That's enormously rewarding." Having a sense of mastery enabled many of the therapists to stay strongly grounded in their sense of providing care. They then were less apt to join the patient in hopelessness or panic.

Meaning found in the work.   The capacity to conceptualize their work as profoundly significant and as having an impact enabled several of the therapists to sustain their commitment. One therapist described the meaning he had found as follows:

> Maybe we shouldn't want to get away from AIDS. There's enough to be learned of life's real essence there: of helping people, seeing human's response to illness, which is such a basic thing. People confiding for the first time in their parents that they're gay, that they're sick. Lovers talking to each other. I think our gay community's response has been just awesome. . . . There's that strange dialectic between the sense of loss and the sense of gain. Feeling in the end helpless, but in the end very powerful that you can mobilize resources in yourself and among your friends.

Rather than expecting to cure their patients, the more successful therapists witnessed and cared for their patients through their pain. The therapists reported that the process of growth and gain was mutual. These therapists spoke of their increased capacity to sit with loss and to deal with a range of their own feelings: sadness, fear, and anger. One therapist affirmed the growth, stating,

> Having been in the middle of it now for 8 years, a lot of what I feel and learn I am indebted to my patients for. That's the other part that keeps me going. Patients have taught me things to pass on to other patients. I've been given a gift of insight into the ways of life that most people don't get a chance to have.

Variability in Adjustment

The most successful of the therapists had taken time off, limited their number of patients, developed very active personal lives with a range of involvements, attained collegial support, become clear about their work, and used a highly developed ego support system including colleagues, consultation, family, and friends. Others were less resolved and more caught in the negative consequences of identification such as overinvolvement or distancing. As examples, recall the quasi-hallucinatory skulls one therapist described, or another's description of avoiding his patient's affect out of fear of his own grief, or the therapist whose life was "all shattered edges." These less effectively adaptive positions were either acute reactions to difficult patients or to difficult periods in the therapist's own life or reflections of more chronic isolation and limited resources.

Discussion of Study Results

AIDS has unleashed devastation on therapists and their patients that challenges the therapist's capacity to manage identification issues. The study results describe a situation that has not changed in the intervening years; if anything the cumulative impact on surviving gay men has mushroomed. The conditions my respondents described match current experience. Unfortunately, as the rate of HIV infection grows in our midst, so will these experiences. Because of the array of shared vulnerabilities, gay male therapists seem much more apt to experience "concordant identification." This concordance can be experienced as sameness and sometimes as a bridge to deepened empathy. At other times, the concordance overwhelms the therapist, creating confusion about boundaries. In these moments, therapists are liable to slip into a deeper countertransference in which the therapist's experience intrudes, resulting in overidentification or defensive detachment.

In order to offer resources to the traumatized patient, the gay therapist must adhere to boundaries that define his separateness from that trauma. Intrinsic and vital to all therapy (Fliess 1942; Freud 1910; Little 1950), this exercise is not unique to therapy with HIV patients. What is unique to therapy with HIV patients is the continuing, unremitting exposure to death and grief. The therapy delivers the pain of loss in a way that is qualitatively different from that experienced in most other therapies. In the epidemic the magnitude of loss is more on the order of war or some natural disaster. Here the gay therapist positions himself on the front line of a battle that threatens his gay peers and himself.

For the gay psychotherapist, the immediacy of death is as close as the thought, There but for the grace of God go I. To put this at the core of one's work puts the work on a level that challenges one's sense of self in the world. The impact of the trauma, the "crunch" (P. Russell, "The Theory of the Crunch," unpublished manuscript, February 1975), the mutuality of the vulnerability, coerces intimacy. At the same time, the therapy requires vigilance to sustain a separate sense of self. Achieving this sense of stable separation in the face of trauma is in itself a life task for every healthy individual (Horner 1984; Mahler et al. 1975). But here the task is formalized as one's daily professional life. Essentially, the therapist must choose boundaries in the service of better meeting the patient's needs rather than in the service of the therapist's need to disengage from the threat of engulfing pain and death. Put another way, the therapist must use identification in the service of understanding the patient rather than allowing himself to become lost in identification and thereby lose himself in panic (Beres and Arlow 1974; Little 1950; Reich 1960).

This experience reaches to the essence of how we understand others through empathy. To be too rigid about boundaries can also be to avoid through distancing, which can be experienced by the patient as lack of caring or even as hate. To be too identified can also be to join and lose vital differentiation. It is right at the boundary that the therapy is done. Tracking the therapy to this extraordinary permeable membrane of relatedness takes us to that place where self and other mix. To return to this inchoate place and come away clear and strong is the essence of identity. In this place, the therapist navigates, using multiple ways of knowing: joining and distancing, and identification and detachment.

These gay male psychotherapists speak about their real relationship with their patients as they talk about the passion and intimacy in their work with HIV or AIDS patients. Concepts of countertransference and transference fall short of describing these dimensions of their therapeutic relationships. Closer to their experience is Greenson's (1972) exploration of the genuine, nonfantasy relationship between analyst and the patient—the real relationship—which is heightened in instances of therapeutic need such as illness and death. As many of the gay psychotherapists described, their HIV patients have had a profound need for a more real relationship with the therapist within the alliance.

The real relationship between therapist and patient can be healing to both. The experience of being in the relationship that some theorists call "containment" (rather than the feature of insight revealed through transference) is most crucial to the treatment relationship (Modell 1976; P. Russell, "The Theory of the Crunch," unpublished manuscript, February 1975; Winnicott 1956). That mutual growth is an inherent and healthy part of the work resonates through many of their descriptions. This also illustrates Searles's (1975) notion of the "mutually growth-enhancing" therapeutic process.

However, the sanctuary the gay therapist and HIV-positive gay patient find together also has its limits. To be too isolated in the therapeutic relationship is a risk for both therapist and patient. For the therapist, the containing, holding environment is by necessity larger than the dyadic treatment relationship, and extends to other levels of support: supervision, therapy, and involvement in organizations. Therefore, I propose a complete description of the treatment relationship that includes all these dimensions.

Vital aspects of generativity are also inherent in the work.

One therapist says he is passing along what previous patients taught him to his next patients. This sense of "passing along" speaks to a sense of legacy that is critical to the success of many survivors of trauma (Lifton 1979). This "telling of the story" is the same witnessing function in which Holocaust survivors found affirmation. This dimension captures some of the Eriksonian stage of generativity versus stagnation.

But there is a way in which these therapists also speak from a depth that reaches the challenges Erikson (1950) described at an even later stage of life—ego integrity versus despair:

> Although aware of the relativity of all the various life styles which have given meaning to human striving, the possessor of integrity is ready to defend the dignity of his own life style against all physical

and economic threats. For he knows that an individual life is the accidental coincidence of but one life cycle with but one segment of history; and that for him all human integrity stands or falls with the one style of integrity which he partakes. The style of integrity developed by his culture or civilization thus becomes the "patrimony of his soul," the seal of his moral paternity of himself. In such final consolidation, death loses its sting. (p. 268)

Those gay therapists who describe themselves as most capable of joining and accepting the work also report that they have reached a depth of compassion that comes from a clarity of acceptance and a steady, balanced dedication to defend the therapist's life-style against all the physical and economic threats that the HIV epidemic has thrust upon his life.

Summary

This study points to ways to strengthen the gay clinicians' ability to do this work: 1) assess the therapist's vulnerabilities to identification over the course of AIDS work and 2) develop resources to sustain the work at all levels of the therapeutic relationship and holding environment—from the patient's level to the therapist's level to the sociopolitical level.

Although this chapter focuses on the gay male therapist and gay male patient with HIV-related illness, attention to the crucial issue of identification is applicable to other pairings of therapists and patients. Understanding the helpers' vulnerabilities may be a more generally useful prophylaxis against the infectious hazards endemic to this "impossible profession": burnout, suicide among therapists, and sexual abuse perpetrated by therapists, to name a few.

For all the difficult challenges of psychotherapy with HIV and AIDS patients, therapists are tremendously rewarded for their involvement. This is the good fight, and many are strengthened by it. With the numbers of HIV-infected people growing daily, increasing numbers of mental health professionals are needed. The best application of this study will be to equip these people better by alerting them to several specific pitfalls and satisfactions in the work.

References

Adler G: Special problems for the therapist. Int J Psychiatry Med 16:91–98, 1984

Basch MF: Empathic understanding: a review of the concept and some theoretical considerations. J Am Psychoanal Assoc 31:101–126, 1983

Beehr TA, Bhagat RS: Introduction to human stress and cognition in organizations, in Human Stress Cognition in Organizations: An Integrated Perspective. Edited by Beehr TA, Bhagat RS. New York, Wiley, 1985, pp 3–19

Benner P, Roskies E, Lazarus RS: Stress and coping under extreme conditions, in Survivors, Victims, and Perpetrators: Essays on the Nazi Holocaust. Edited by Dimsdale JE. Washington, DC, Hemisphere, 1980, pp 219–258

Beres D, Arlow J: Fantasy and identification in empathy. Psychoanal Q 43:155–181, 1974

Boffey P: Spread of AIDS abating, but deaths will soar. New York Times, February 14, 1988, p 1

Buie D: Empathy: its nature and limitations. J Am Psychoanal Assoc 29:281–308, 1981

Buie D, Maltsberger J: Countertransference hate in the treatment of suicidal patients. Arch Gen Psychiatry 30:625–632, 1974

Cherniss C: Professional Burnout in Human Service Organizations. New York, Praeger, 1980

Deutsch F, Madle R: Empathy: historic and current conceptualizations, measurements, and a cognitive theoretical perspective. Human Development 18:267–287, 1975

Dunkel J, Hatfield S: Countertransference issues in working with persons with AIDS. Soc Work 31:114–117, 1986

Erikson E: Childhood and Society. New York, WW Norton, 1950

Fliess R: The metapsychology of the analyst. Psychoanal Q 11:211–227, 1942

Freud S: The future prospects of psychoanalytic therapy (1910), in Collected Papers of Sigmund Freud, Vol 2. Edited by Jones E. New York, Basic Books, 1959, pp 285–296

Greenson R: Beyond transference and interpretation. Int J Psychoanal 53:213–217, 1972

Kernberg O: Notes on countertransference. J Am Psychoanal Assoc 13:38–56, 1963

Horner AJ: Object Relations and the Developing Ego in Therapy. New York, Jason Aronson, 1984

LeShan L, LeShan E: Psychotherapy and the patient with a limited life span. Psychiatry 24:318–323, 1961

Lifton R: The Broken Connection. New York, Basic Books, 1979

Little M: Countertransference and the patient's response to it. Int J Psychoanal 31:32–40, 1950

Mahler MS, Pine F, Bergman A: The Psychological Birth of the Human Infant. New York, Basic Books, 1975

McKusick L: The impact of AIDS on practitioner and client. Am Psychol 43:935–940, 1988

Modell A: The "holding environment" and the therapeutic action of psychoanalysis. J Am Psychoanal Assoc 24:285–308, 1976.

Racker H: Transference and Countertransference. New York, International Universities Press, 1968

Reich A: Further remarks on countertransference. Int J Psychoanal 41:389–395, 1960

Ruderman E: Gender-related themes of women therapists in treatment of women patients: their creative and reparative use of countertransference as a mutual growth experience. Clinical Social Work Journal 14:103–126, 1986

Sanders C: Therapists, too, need to grieve. Death Education 8:27–35, 1984

Schafer R: Generative empathy in the treatment situation. Psychoanal Q 28:342–373, 1959

Searles H: Countertransference and Related Subjects—Selected Papers. New York, International Universities Press, 1979

Shainess N: Significance of match in sex of analyst and patient. Am J Psychoanal 43:205–217, 1983

Slaby A: Cancer's impact on caregivers. Adv Psychosom Med 18:135–153, 1988

Thomas VM: Hospice nursing—reaping the rewards, dealing with the stress. Geriatric Nursing 4:22–27, 1983

Vachon MLS: Staff stress in care of the terminally ill. QRB Qual Rev Bull 5:13–17, 1979

Weinberg G: Society and the Healthy Homosexual. New York, St. Martin's, 1971

Weisman A: Coping with untimely death. Psychiatry 36:366–378, 1973

Weisman A: Understanding the cancer patient: the syndrome of caregiver's plight. Psychiatry 44:161–168, 1981

Winnicott D: On transference. Int J Psychoanal 37:386–388, 1956

Chapter 23

Countertransference, the Therapeutic Frame, and AIDS: One Psychotherapist's Response

James M. Fishman, L.I.C.S.W.

In 1981 I took a job as clinical social worker at the Fenway Community Health Center in Boston, Massachusetts, which at the time specialized in treating sexually transmitted diseases in gay men. The overlapping medical and psychosocial stresses patients experienced from chronic hepatitis B or venereal warts warranted a referral to our fledgling mental health department of two. By the end of 1981, however, reports began to trickle in from health clinics in New York, San Francisco, and Los Angeles about a new, virulent disorder initially known as *GRID* (gay-related immune disorder) that was killing previously healthy young gay men. Being the only gay-oriented outpatient treatment facility in Boston, we bolstered ourselves for the coming onslaught as we watched some cities responding with too little, too late. We were caught between the media fanning the flames of hysteria on the one hand, and the gay male community, which was still in denial about the need for safer sex practices or uninformed about what was in store, on the other. In response, we held public forums, which evolved into a grass-roots organization later known as the AIDS Action Committee of Massachusetts. It is in this context of many unknowns that I was assigned my first case of a patient with acquired immunodeficiency

For Don B. and Jeff C.

syndrome (AIDS) (see below). At the time, fewer than 10 cases of AIDS had become officially diagnosed in Massachusetts.

In 1985, after several years of involvement with the Education and Mental Health Subcommittees of the AIDS Action Committee, as well as much clinical experience with Fenway patients who either had AIDS or experienced an acute anxiety that they were about to contract it, I decided to move to San Francisco to assume the directorship of a mental health program for gay men. When I took the administrative and supervisory job as head of the men's clinical program of Operation Concern in 1985, I entered a community that was not in denial. With more than a 50% human immunodeficiency virus (HIV)–infection rate among gay men in a city long viewed as a mecca for sexual minorities, San Francisco was a city numbed by continual, repeated loss. Along with a casual acceptance of something terrible, I saw in the gay community a renewed commitment to making positive changes in physical, medical, and spiritual well-being.

The difference in the two cities' responses to the epidemic was most evident in their vastly differing attitudes towards taking the HIV-antibody test. In 1985, only a small minority of gay men in Boston had elected to take the enzyme-linked immunosorbent assay (ELISA) test. The psychiatric and medical communities stressed extreme caution, addressing the community's anxiety over confidentiality, uncertainty of prognosis, and potential stigmatization. The same professionals in San Francisco, on the other hand, emphasized empowerment, advocated new drug trials, and criticized the untested as being in denial. Each city had something special to offer; yet both seemed, in a way, off balance. If Boston's view seemed overly cautious, then San Francisco's seemed a bit cavalier.

Amid this climate of deepening crisis, my role at Operation Concern required me to nurture the staff therapists, clinical volunteers, and interns. Staff frequently expressed concerns that they were not doing enough to meet the demands of the epidemic. We started monthly meetings to address our internal HIV concerns, countertransference issues, and educational needs. In the process, we discovered we were already doing quite a lot. Each clinician, in fact, had been carrying a caseload of predominantly HIV-positive men, some of whom had advanced AIDS. We wrestled with the changing boundaries of the therapeutic frame—whether or not our roles extended to hospitals, home visits, or funerals. One of our conclusions was that we need not become an AIDS agency (San Francisco already had several). We had existed as a clinic before AIDS, and just by continuing to serve the mental health needs of the community we were preserving critically needed services. However, two structures that we eventually set up helped: a clinicwide memorial service to honor all Operation Concern staff who had died of AIDS, which has become a yearly tradition, and a bimonthly support group for gay male therapists, known as the HIV Networking Committee. These helped because unconsciously we had become numb, almost blasé about the enormity of the tragedy affecting us all. We needed to reclaim our sense of integrity, of purpose and vision, of having something to offer. Thus we were able to acknowledge the pain and the losses we were enduring, yet to continue with the work.

In this chapter I present several case examples of countertransference in working with gay male patients with AIDS. The first case example is that of my very first AIDS patient in 1982, to whom I was introduced in the hospital by his Fenway physician. Here, against a backdrop of media and community hysteria in Boston, I was forced to confront my irrational fears and defensive coping style. The second case example concerns a long-term gay men's psychotherapy group in San Francisco where, in the course of the group, a member in seemingly good health was diagnosed with AIDS; in this example I examine the choices and snap decisions made about roles and boundaries in response to a quickly unfolding group crisis. Third, I discuss the case of a man with AIDS-related complex (ARC) whose progressive illness evoked in me responses of distancing and blaming until I regained the empathic vantage point and could acknowledge my own fears of abandonment. In each example I attempt to connect the countertransference to the unfolding therapeutic goals, and to demonstrate that a healthy interplay must exist between maintaining the therapeutic frame and being willing to place one's self in awkward, uncharted terrain.

It is important for me to make two acknowledgments. First, I write this as an openly gay man; it is this identification process that no doubt has shaped some of my own responses and reactions. The nongay clinician will, of course, have to wrestle with many of the same responses, but will also have his or her own other set of issues, biases, perspectives, and contributions. Second, I am fortunate to have had a supportive group of professional peers, as well as two agency consultants who volunteered at Operation Concern. I felt safe enough to expose my vulnerabilities, fears, and needs to these men. The two volunteer consultants—gay male psychiatrists who were experts in their respective specialties—were both diagnosed with AIDS and eventually died. Their premature deaths have created a profound vacuum in our community.

Treating an Early Case of AIDS

This first case example illustrates how I was forced to confront my own anxieties and irrational responses to AIDS in the early days of the epidemic.

Case 1

Mr. A was frail, scared, and looking older than his 37 years when I met him in his hospital room. He did not look well. I had been briefed by his primary care physician at Fenway that he was in denial about the eventual fatality of AIDS-related illnesses. His lover of 7 years was quite distressed from the caretaking aspects of AIDS. Mr. A expressed repeated wishes to stay at home, but the Pneumocystis carinii pneumonia (PCP) required his hospitalization. Mr. A focused mostly on his hopes and plans following his discharge from the hospital. A self-described "suburban gay" whose dream was to stay at home, garden, and cook, he recounted to me his occasional "wild" forays down to New York City without his lover. Theirs was an open relationship that had evolved into a loving, nonsexual partnership. The trips to New York invariably included a night out at the baths. Mr. A claimed to be able to pinpoint the actual trip in which he contracted the virus. He seemed resigned rather than regretful about having been exposed to the virus. I wondered to myself if his resignation—which disturbed and puzzled me—was merely a disguised belief that he "got what he deserved" (i.e., a form of internalized homophobia). I wanted to explore this line of thought, but he did not give me an opening. I probed a bit about his strict religious upbringing, but it soon became clear that his having acquired AIDS was not the problem; to him, it was a mere inconvenience, an interference with his plans. Although I saw my initial goal as helping Mr. A come to terms with his AIDS diagnosis, he continued to use denial to defend against impending loss. Our focus eventually became one of exploring his past and looking at his hopes for the future. "We're a feisty lot, my family," he said. "We're fighters."

During our second session in his room, the magazine lying on his bed fell to the floor. Reluctantly I forced myself to pick it up, irrationally fearing contagion. By my third visit, his face began to resemble the photographs taken of concentration camp survivors: his wrists were thin and his cheekbones hollow; his facial complexion was red and flaking. Inwardly, I was shocked and horrified. I was also informed by his physician that he had developed toxoplasmosis—a parasitic infection that can grow in the brain and cause mental status changes. His lover was the first to notice him in a state of utter confusion; he and I had an informal family visit outside the room as I was leaving. I ended up connecting him with a surviving lover of a person with AIDS who had been through what he was confronting.

When I arrived for his next session, Mr. A did not recognize me. He kept staring in my direction, obviously confused yet alert enough to be frightened by his own mental state. I repeated my name and purpose, and by the time he seemed to comprehend, he had drifted off to sleep. By his fifth session, he was asleep for the whole visit.

These being the early days of the epidemic, the visits for me resembled wading through a mined harbor. The unpredictability of the course of the disease, the fact that from one week to the next I could not anticipate his mental status or even his appearance, coupled with the fact that here was another gay man, a member of my own community about my age, appearing helpless to this onslaught, sent my anxiety surging. A couple of times I left with a cold, internal chill and I could not warm up. Typically after each session I headed for the nearest rest room and compulsively washed my hands.

The world outside of the hospital seemed unsafe as well. Few of my gay colleagues seemed to be grasping the enormity of the epidemic. To them, AIDS was a distant cloud on the horizon. The media attention, meanwhile, sent waves of paranoia through the heterosexual community. One anxious mother called the clinic asking whether to allow her gay son into her home during his upcoming visit. "He's coming in from San Francisco," she explained. And I lost my temper with a television news anchor who demanded, "Can you get me an AIDS victim by seven o'clock tonight?" Yet

many gay men continued to have unsafe sex. Some activists pro-
claimed that all this hysteria was just a ploy of the medical establishment, which was "antisex and shouldn't be heeded anyway." I found
myself in the single gay man's dilemma: any potential source of
physical comfort was also a potential source of infection. And, when
on occasion I did venture out to a bar, inevitably some patron recognized me from one of my speaking engagements and grilled me
on the details of safer sex. The only oasis was the AIDS Action Committee meetings, especially the potluck meals. These informal sessions provided a safety zone where I could get support from peers.

After my fifth session with Mr. A I had the following dream: I
was walking on a country road alongside a wooded area when I
noticed a small brushfire rapidly beginning to spread. Nobody was
paying any mind. The townsfolk were going about their business. I
could not get anyone to respond to my plea for help, so finally I
called the fire department, who took their time as well. The
brushfire turned into a blazing forest fire. When the firefighters arrived, they rigged up a garden hose that barely reached the fire. I
woke up in a state of terror.

The epidemic, like the fire, was raging out of control. The number of cases had doubled every 6 months. I found myself dreading
going back for one more session with Mr. A. I told his physician that
I did not think I could handle it. He encouraged me to talk it over
with my supervisor; he also informed me that Mr. A's health was
rapidly declining and that it looked like he had no more than a week
to live. After sharing my fears and leaning on two colleagues for
support, I went back for my final visit before Mr. A's death.

At first glance Mr. A looked better than he had in weeks; his face
was shiny and smooth, almost youthful. But as I took a seat he gave
no signs of recognition. His eyes appeared frightened; he moved
them rapidly first toward me, then away. I forced myself to sit and
talk to him despite my doubts that he could comprehend. Most difficult of all for me was that I could not help noticing his hands
making involuntary, staccato movements under the bedsheets. Was
he masturbating? Had he lost all voluntary control? I stayed a bit
longer, then said good-bye. This was my final visit, on a Thursday.

After Mr. A's death, I flew down to New York City as planned to
spend the weekend with two close friends. The headlines of a gay
magazine gave us pause: "1,000 Cases and Counting." We pondered

what it all meant, where it might all lead. And the next night, I, who gave lectures to gay men about safer sex, risk reduction, and AIDS anxiety, proceeded to have unsafe sex with an anonymous partner who I had just met in a Village bar. In fact, I had among the least safe kinds of sex in the riskiest city of them all. "He's young and from the suburbs," I rationalized.

I know about survivor guilt and counterphobic behavior (i.e., rushing headlong into danger as a way of attempting to master anxiety). What I did not know, however, was that these maneuvers could apply to me and could be so unconscious and swift. I soon realized that I was dealing with my lack of control by trying, unconsciously, to get AIDS and get it over with. If I made sure of whom, where, and how I contracted the virus, there would be no more worrying. Luckily, I grasped the meaning of my acting out. I was fortunate enough to eventually test negative for the HIV antibody.

And yet that very role of luck haunted me—why this person? Why that? Why did his lover, who had had many more partners than he had, test negative? And why the volunteer who had hoped to make a documentary for us about AIDS? The virus was indiscriminate. Where did one direct one's anger? At the virus? The medical establishment? The government? My gay brethren? The apathetic public? Toward God?

My work in Boston gave me much in return: a sense of accomplishment, purpose, professional expertise, visibility, and community. But in the end, I decided to take a job in San Francisco that was not in a health setting, in part to escape the accumulated heaviness of AIDS and its increasing prominence in my life. There were bigger fish in the San Francisco AIDS pond; I hoped to become, once again, anonymous. I sought to reclaim my former role as clinician and let others carry the torch. I arrived in a new city knowing very few people—my buffer against loss—and surveyed a compassionate, progressive medical community. I had traveled, I soon learned, into the eye of a hurricane.

AIDS Enters a Psychotherapy Group

When AIDS enters a group as the topic of discussion, it can transcend immediate concerns of health and be a metaphor about other immediate dangers within the group. For example, in the beginning phase of a group when members are making a contract to become a working group, someone may bring up AIDS as a way of testing out group safety in terms of confidentiality, level of disclosure and vulnerability, boundaries, and group norms. AIDS can serve as an early metaphor for issues of abandonment or even engulfment. In a later stage, when competition and leadership issues emerge, AIDS may represent the dangers of aggression. Just as AIDS can be viewed as a destructive, uncontrollable menace outside the group, so too can competition for power present as an uncontrollable, uncontained force within the group. Thus all levels of AIDS as metaphor must be explored depending on the developmental stage of the group.

Revealing a new member's HIV or AIDS status to a group from the start can be less disruptive than sitting with the anxiety of wondering, Who among us will be next? The dynamics are different for the member who seroconverts after he is an established part of the group and attachments have been formed. Those who enter with HIV can serve as role models of people who are coping and trying to integrate it with their lives. Or they can be painful reminders that even in the safety of the group, no one is immune from loss.

Disclosure of one's antibody status to a group has many parallels to the coming out process, when the risks of being discredited by others must be weighed against the potential benefits of healing a split-off part of the self. The experience of being scapegoated for one's difference is a seminal experience for the gay man. To come out as HIV positive or as having AIDS can reawaken old fears of stigmatization or ostracism, especially from one's peers. Tales abound of people with AIDS being abandoned by friends, loved ones, employers, and roommates after such a disclosure. The highly charged nature of AIDS—the fact that it associates sex with death—often results in the surfacing of deeply embedded underlying conflicts. As illustrated in Case 2, a group faces and integrates AIDS when the illness intrudes into an ongoing group process.

Case 2

In 1986 I began to lead an ongoing psychotherapy group for gay men in my private practice in San Francisco. Of the seven members

I initially accepted into the group, only one of the potential members, a formerly married man in his early 40s, had tested positive for the virus (several had never taken the test but were contemplating doing so). Virtually everyone had AIDS on his mind. It was woven into the fabric of each man's life. The health crisis impacted members' sexual behavior quite radically. All professed to be practicing safer sex or doing without sex altogether. Without the easy outlet of anonymous sex, many were now facing their deep-seated difficulties in forming lasting, intimate bonds with others. Isolation, low self-esteem, the fear of commitment or rejection, a sense of not fitting into the gay scene—these were the catalysts that brought them to group to learn new, healthier ways of relating. Many had lost close friends, coworkers, or former lovers to AIDS. Two members reported having lost former psychotherapists. In agreeing to join a group that focused on the fear of loss, or on unresolved accumulated loss, members knew they were risking the intrusion of AIDS through a number of possible doors.

With the exception of being an openly gay therapist, as facilitator I disclosed very little about myself to this group and then only after exploring members' thoughts, fantasies, and feelings. The transference had been a central dynamic in my groups. My orientation was psychodynamic within an interpersonal, group-as-a-whole, and intrapsychic context. My frame did diverge from the analytic stance, which views socializing between members as a form of acting out. I neither encouraged nor discouraged outside contact, but simply made two provisos: first, that any significant interactions must be brought back into the group and explored; and, second, that members ought to discuss and explore intragroup sexual attractions rather than act on these desires.

Seven members began the new group together, and in session 3 I added an eighth to complete the group. The newest member, Mr. B, was 25 and easily the youngest. He lived rent-free in his uncle's house and was not "out" to any family members. A former substance abuser, he had been in recovery for over a year and was in individual therapy as well. Living in a conservative suburb, he had few gay friends. Sexually he had been celibate for almost 2 years, partly out of a fear of AIDS but mostly because of his newly acquired sobriety and fears of intimacy. His cherubic, Italian good looks suggested he might have become the "baby" of the group, been envied, or become the object of someone's crush. Instead, he emerged as an articulate, forceful, and demanding member of the group—in fact, he served as catalyst for the surfacing of issues of inclusion and exclusion. Other members vied for his attention; one member in particular— Mr. C—felt threatened by and rivalrous toward Mr. B.

Eight months into the group Mr. B began to complain of bronchial symptoms, including shortness of breath. He had not been for a medical checkup in over a year and casually mentioned his aversion to hospitals and doctors. He was somewhat estranged from his parents, whom he described as "dysfunctional and erratic, like untreated alcoholics"; he was loath to confide in his parents about his symptoms, and he had particular contempt for his father, whom he described as a "wimp" who was "all bark and no bite."

On hearing about his symptoms, the group reacted with concern bordering on alarm. Members insisted that he get a checkup at once. When Mr. B finally went to a health clinic later that week, the physician on duty immediately admitted him to a nearby hospital as having PCP, one of the opportunistic infections that is diagnostic of AIDS.

When my answering service gave me the hospital room extension for Mr. B, I took in the worst at once. I called him without thinking, and he shared the news over the phone. With his encouragement, I arranged to stop by later on in the day to visit him in the hospital. Because distinct clinical boundaries had existed up to that point, I knew that this visit would be a break in the therapeutic frame. Whether in part as a result of my own anxiety or partly in response to his need for support, I headed over to the hospital with a mixture of dread, grief, and forced calm. Suddenly, AIDS had intruded into the group with indiscriminate force, striking down its youngest member. Would he recover? Probably. Would AIDS return? Yes.

The hospital seemed too close to my office; I somehow wanted more time to compose myself. I did not want to cry. I thought, Why Mr. B? and then, selfishly, Will the group turn into an AIDS group? The fact that Mr. B had entered the group as a presumably healthy young man and had gotten sick so quickly eroded the illusion of control even further.

The visit itself was not thought out—it was somewhere between a visit and a session. Mr. B sat up slightly and shook my hand. He was quite weak and was talking softly in an even tone of sadness and relief. I stood by his bedside, scanning the room for a seat, but the only chair had a bedpan on it. I sat on the bed, wondering if this was too intimate—but decided it was less awkward than standing and safer than dealing with the bedpan. Without my role as therapist to protect me, I was left knowing a great deal about Mr. B, except how to act; he helped me by filling me in on the details; he apparently had had a close brush with death. He chose to go to a gay-oriented health clinic in San Francisco rather than risk exposure with his family doctor, who did not know Mr. B was gay. The lung biopsy at the hospital confirmed what the clinic doctor already had suspected. In addition to telephoning me, he had called his mom and one member of the group. He had had the double task of coming out to his mom as gay and as a person diagnosed with AIDS. She had been coming to visit daily, but his father could not handle it and stayed away. "He's wounded," explained Mr. B.

I asked Mr. B how he wanted me to handle this with the group, and he stated that he would welcome any visitors. He actually seemed relieved to be under the care of a hospital. At this point there was a knock on the door, and a woman in a trench coat entered whom he introduced as his mother. Suddenly, I was in no-man's-land, without any rules, and I had to wing it. I wondered what his mother must have been thinking about this man sitting on her son's bed. "He's my group counselor," he told her. She smiled. I was safe. I stood up and shook her hand.

"How's he doing?" she asked me. "He's talking a lot," I answered. "Well, I was just about to leave. I'll be in touch." As I exited, I saw her face—there were no words to describe her pain and her love.

The following week I steeled myself to tell the group. "I have some difficult news, . . . " I began but started to cry. "Mr. B is hospitalized with Pneumocystis. He has AIDS." The group was in shock. After prolonged silence, members started offering comments, slowly building their remarks into some cohesive whole. Two members visibly withdrew—one tucked his feet under him on the couch, as a child would. "He welcomes any visitors from the group," I added. Someone suggested buying a card. Numbingly, we stitched something together. Some plan. Everyone had been through this before, but this time it was different. This was group. Finally, I regained my composure and remembered that I was the therapist; something automatic took over. I was not just a friend or another gay man or a peer. Later I realized that I had not been neutral, that I had tacitly encouraged people to visit. I asked, "Maybe some of you aren't ready, or may choose not to visit. What would it be like to dissent, to choose not to go?"

One member who had never taken the HIV-antibody test but who had had frequent bouts with herpes over the past 10 years, spoke up first. "I'm sick of talking about this. Are we going to turn this into an AIDS group? I had to watch my lover die in the hospital, and I don't want to go through this again." This was his first time expressing anger directly in the group. He was unapologetic. Mr. B's hospitalization had allowed him to unleash pent-up feelings about the unfairness of the virus, unresolved grief over his lover's death, and resentment at how AIDS had eclipsed other, equally valid forms of suffering in the gay community. Another member expressed it this way: "It took me 20 years to learn to separate sex from death—I went to Catholic schools. Now AIDS ties them back together again. When straight people think of us, all they think of now is disease, death, and promiscuity."

The subject of the AIDS virus had been usurped, for a moment, by the immediate reactions to Mr. B the individual. Mr. C, the emotional leader of the group who had had an uneasy truce with Mr. B from the beginning, brought the discussion back. He wondered if he would have to walk on eggshells around Mr. B when he returned. "Or will I be allowed to confront him on anything? Will we all be superpolite? Besides, it might be Mr. B who rejects us. He may not want to come back. Maybe he'd rather be in a group just for people with AIDS. He may find us irrelevant."

The group expression of grief found many forms. Each member dealt with the news in his own, characteristic way: anger, denial, loss. In a way, each member's voice carried an aspect of grief for the entire group. "We're at a pivotal time in the group," I told them. "How we handle our feelings will make a big impact on how we cope with this crisis." The most dangerous reaction would have been to isolate one's self. I was thinking of all the unresolved losses in the room—both AIDS and non-AIDS related. With the exception of the AIDS quilt, gay men are not encouraged to grieve openly.

Many in the group decided to visit Mr. B in the hospital. One member who had become a close friend of Mr. B's and who had become the unofficial ambassador between the group and Mr. B was the first to weep openly in the group. He announced that Mr. B would be returning to group in a couple of weeks. My own contact with Mr. B during this interim period was limited to phone calls every few weeks. After a 12-week absence, Mr. B finally returned to the group. He had recovered from PCP and looked well. "I feel like I know you all so much better—even you, [Mr. C]," he said. Although his feistiness was there, a new tone of vulnerability and dependency was also evident. He shared how his parents were coping, and then he dropped a bomb: "My uncle has evicted me. He's afraid of catching AIDS."

A sense of outrage swept through the group, then vulnerability to abandonment by one's own family. The formerly married member, who was seropositive, expressed the fear that his ex-wife could keep the kids from visiting him should she find out about his antibody status. His anxiety escalated: "She thinks she's a good Christian. I'm sure I'd lose the court case in the Midwest. Will I lose my visitation rights? I could see her using this against me—she hates the fact that I'm gay."

Another member recounted how his own sister, who had generally been pro-gay and had met his past lovers, refused to invite him home over the holidays because her fiancé was afraid of catching AIDS. "We're re-diseased," he said. Thus the fear of being ostracized for one's real or perceived HIV status reawakened earlier risks of being rejected for being gay. The group wrestled with some of its deepest fears, fears that had been perhaps only semiconscious up to that point. Who among us will be left? Who will take care of me if I get sick? Would the group visit me in the hospital? Will there be anyone around left to visit me? The fear of abandonment stretched from one's own community to one's biological family.

Mr. B crystallized the increased sense of dependency and vulnerability within the group when he stated, "You guys have been more of a family to me than my family. Who knows if I'd be alive today if you hadn't pushed me to go to the clinic? I was too scared. Deep down, I thought it could be AIDS." In this instance the group became both his literal and his symbolic family. It began to dawn on people that they did care for one another, exposing the lie in the internalized stereotype that all gay men really care about is sex.

Mr. B's reintegration into the group did not take long. Contrary to the group's and my fears, the group did not become an "AIDS group." AIDS, of course, had become visible in our midst, but the fear of it eclipsing other, less life-and-death issues proved unfounded. Eventually, however, Mr. B decided to leave San Francisco in order to pursue his dream of traveling abroad. He knew that I could not hold a space open for him for 6 months, but he was always welcome to reapply. The group members, worried for his health, probed him on the efficacies of such an arduous trip. But his feistiness won out. He had to travel while he was strong.

Although all terminations evoke issues of death and loss, Mr. B's leaving the group marked the first stage of mourning his eventual death. As Mr. C put it, "[Mr. B]'s leaving is a death for me, as I know he and I won't become friends." In his presence, any anger the group felt about his leaving remained unacknowledged. "It seems as if the group feels safer with its angry feelings towards me than towards Mr. B," I offered. They could admit their fears of abandonment by me more easily than they could acknowledge their dependency on each other. After Mr. B left, however, considerable resentment and envy surfaced. One member pierced the posttermination glow around Mr. B when he said, "Everyone keeps saying [Mr. B] did such a great job of working on his feelings; but he didn't do that much of it in here. And he was better calling other people on their stuff than he was at copping to his own shit." Sibling rivalry surfaced. The group perceived that I gave Mr. B carte blanche to come and go as he pleased. And once I finally let him go, it became evident that I was not powerful enough to protect the group's integrity from this loss. These feelings required much working through.

Eight months after having left for Europe, Mr. B returned to the Bay area and died shortly thereafter. Because I had lost touch with Mr. B, and perhaps to protect myself, I chose not to attend the memorial service held in his parents' home. The group held its own memorial of sorts, reviewing Mr. B's life and final months. Several years later, Mr. B's death was still mentioned in the group by those members who were around to remember; it had not gone away.

In retrospect, as I look back at my own role and choices, I reflect that some mistakes were made. However, I am glad I veered on the side of loosening the therapeutic frame with Mr. B and the group. Perhaps I served as a role model as someone who did not have all the answers, but who muddled through as best he could; as someone who could eventually help steer the ship into calmer waters. Shifting from "in role" to "out of role" proved to be a challenge. At times, it threatened my own sense of control and identity; there were times when I needed the role to hide behind, for I could not be, and could not let myself become, a peer. For that kind of support, I had to go elsewhere. My own exhaustion, despair, and grief were emotions I lived with, discussed with peers, or repressed.

I lost five more patients over the next 2 years. Another patient's lover died, and two patients started on zidovudine (AZT). Several colleagues at the clinic were diagnosed as well. And late one afternoon, after a long day of seeing eight private patients, it hit me that all eight were coping with HIV. I understood how this community had become numbed. There was more grieving in store, but also more lessons.

Abandonment: A Therapist's Fear

The last case example illustrates the unconscious temptation to distance patients because of the therapist's own fears of abandonment.

Case 3

Mr. D presented for individual psychotherapy with depression and a lack of direction in mid-life. He was 48, on medical leave from his clerical job, and diagnosed with ARC. His medical leave centered on a work injury that he said had been exacerbated by his employer's neglect. A worker's compensation claim had been filed against the company and was pending. His ARC symptoms had abated and his health was more or less stable. He swam several times a week, and he bolstered his fragile self-state through a series of anonymous sexual encounters. Underneath, he felt empty and fraudulent, admitting his worker's compensation claim was somewhat of a scam.

Mr. D had moved to San Francisco at age 25 to study nursing, but he found the studies to be too grueling, so he dropped out. In its place, he discovered and embraced the counterculture life-style of the hip dropout. After many years of living communally, he moved into a small apartment by himself. Coming from a lower-middle-class Italian background, he never did fulfill his parents' dream that he would become a lawyer. Mr. D traced his ambivalence toward success to his father's undermining any real attempts of his to separate and become a full, functioning human being. In fact, his older sister still received weekly handouts from Dad. His mother, who had died of a heart attack 10 years prior to our beginning therapy, was pictured as the benign figure of the household who watched father and son spar, but who was helpless to intervene.

Mr. D had a legendary network of friends, some of whom complained that he was overly dramatic and demanding. Initially, I became caught in the transference-countertransference, treating him as an intractable child who always needed more. Opposed to my psychodynamic style—which he found withholding—Mr. D wanted hugs, instant catharsis, and longer therapy sessions. Some of his requests seemed legitimate, such as his wish to change rooms to one spacious enough for him to lie down on the floor (his back necessitated that), but many requests merely seemed like a testing of boundaries and seemed to originate in a sense of entitlement. Our initial sessions were stalled in a series of skirmishes.

When I made a conscious switch from a Kernbergian stance of viewing him as a borderline patient with an angry wish to flounder to a Kohutian perspective of him as a person who lacked mirroring selfobjects, our relationship improved. As I adopted a more empathic vantage point, I saw his requests less as demands and more as attempts to assert some control without being undermined by an authority figure. He had never been mirrored as the potential hero; his grandiosity had been stifled and shamed. I tried to hear his requests from this perspective rather than weighing his every need with a skeptic's eye. As a result, our work deepened. When he faced his first major crisis and felt suicidal we switched to twice-weekly therapy to get him through. His worker's compensation claim had been turned down, and his own physician had betrayed him. He felt useless and in a panic. Part of each session included a 15-minute update on his plans to get rehabilitation counseling.

But Mr. D never followed through with rehabilitation because he developed PCP and became an official AIDS patient. The official switch from ARC to AIDS diagnosis meant that he had instant access to numerous support services: financial, emotional, and social. Most important, AIDS provided him with a new identity, and he became a warrior fending off the ineptitudes of the medical system. AIDS was his way out, and he confessed to feeling guilty at how relieving it was to finally have AIDS. This was more than the typical relief of a person with ARC converting to AIDS and finally being legitimized by the system. Mr. D had been taken off the hook of his mid-life crisis.

Mr. D's friends rallied around him in a fiercely loyal and committed fashion. They formed a nucleus of helpers who would meet monthly first among themselves and then with Mr. D. The group included men and women, gay and nongay men, elders and teenagers. As his health declined, these friends took shifts being "on call." The meetings included the processing of feelings, and sometimes Mr. D was criticized for his tendency to demand.

In our individual sessions Mr. D frequently obsessed over his tendency to push people away through his heavy demands. "How can I be angry with such a loving group of people?" he would ask. His anger created a furious superego backlash. While on the subject of his fears of abandonment, I raised the issue of our relationship and wondered if he had any concerns on this score. He said he trusted me now, that I had been with him for over a year. I started to address the issue of his failing health, noticing how sometimes he had difficulty climbing the stairs to my office. I offered him the option of eventually switching our sessions to his home, should his health worsen. He thanked me and said he would keep this in mind.

A month after this conversation I prepared to leave for a 3-week vacation. I asked if he had any feelings about my leaving at such a pivotal time. "No. You're entitled to a vacation. You always ask me that question. Besides, I have my support group." Although Mr. D still wrestled with issues of feeling too selfish and demanding, he rarely if ever raised concerns about being dependent on me. Yet, on my return, I received a note in my box saying he had canceled that day's appointment. The message said to please call. On the phone Mr. D informed me that he had not been feeling well all morning; he had had diarrhea. I resisted getting pulled in. He's trying to get me to give him a session over the phone, I thought to myself. Yet he won't come in. I became chilly on the phone. He's probably angry with me about my vacation and exaggerating his symptoms; he's acting out, I thought. I stopped listening to him.

At our session the following week, I interpreted his cancellation as his anger over feeling abandoned. He became furious. "I almost didn't come back," he said. "After our phone conversation. You were so cold on the phone—you didn't even take the time to ask what was happening with my health. I had been having terrible cramps and diarrhea—it took me a half an hour to cross the room to reach the bathroom. You and your interpretations!" At this point I realized that he was not exaggerating.

I said, "Perhaps I'm scared you're getting sick on me; maybe I'm scared of your dying."

These words come out unbeknownst to me, and they rang true. I realized, in retrospect, that my defenses went up during the phone call, and my skepticism was my protection, my armor. He was not the one with the abandonment issues—I was. I had grown attached to him and did not want to face the prospect of loss. I had seen too many go quite suddenly. This marked another turning point in our therapy and a barrier on both our sides fell away. I had been using

my professionalism to hide my feelings. Mr. D appreciated my owning my defense mechanisms. My being human allowed him to continue the work. Both of us were on the verge of tears.

Eventually Mr. D did request to move our sessions to his studio.
Inwardly, I resisted slightly, resenting the extra traveling time. But
by now I also knew the complex sources of such resentment. The
sessions in the home remained 50 minutes long; he sat on his bed
and I sat on a pillow on the floor. Sticking to the 50-minute hour
helped us both to remember that these were indeed sessions rather
than visits. By virtue of our meeting in his home, our sessions grew
more intimate. The boundaries were there, but they were altered by
my entering into his space. I could see by the rotating photos on his
wall his latest decorating attempts; a photo of his support group; his
favorite flower. He honored these sessions by making sure that his
friends and I did not collide; we were not interrupted. He made
excellent use of the time. He proved to be a fierce advocate for himself in battling the health care system. A good deal of our work then
focused on his rapprochement with his father. Father and son grew
closer with the advancement of AIDS. His father even attended one
of Mr. D's support group meetings.

Occasionally the old suspicions arose in me. Was he really sick
enough to justify these home sessions? If he were hooked up to an
IV, then I could see it. In these instances, I reminded myself that the
mistrust arose in direct proportion to my fears of impending loss. Of
course Mr. D could be demanding and entitled—these were real
sides to his character. But they were part of the bargain.

Mr. D hesitantly took one last trip to visit his father, but the trip
was cut short because of rapid deterioration in Mr. D's health. He
knew he was going to die soon; I knew it. Even to the end, he had
some criticisms of a few members of his support group—and the
self-recrimination. I blurted out, "Yes, you're demanding! But you're
still lovable." He had managed not to alienate any of his support
group; he kept his demands in check. He feared isolation more than
he feared death.

Scared as I was, I needed to raise the subject of our impending
termination. "We need to be able to say good-bye," I told him. "Let's
talk about us."

"Our relationship?" he asked inquisitively. "I never thought of
it as all that important. I mostly think of my group." I questioned
his denial, but left it at that. I did tell him how much I have valued
knowing him and working with him. And at that point, the doorbell

rang and in walked his Shanti practical support volunteer, to my dismay. Mr. D chose to let her stay, thus cutting our session short for the first and only time.

One can tell on one's answering machine when a friend or colleague is letting you know of a death. They have a disguised, overly polite tone. In my case, 3 days after our last session, Mr. D's best friend left a message for me to call him. I knew that Mr. D had died. It was over. Although I was prepared, you are never really prepared. It doesn't get any easier. I was invited by his friend to a potluck supper memorial in her home. I declined. Confidentiality does not end in death and, besides, Mr. D's extended family was not mine.

But where could I go with my grief? In this case, I had a patient sitting in the waiting room for our 9:00 A.M. appointment. I informed him that I would be 15 minutes late. I then sought out a trusted colleague down the hallway who, luckily, was free. I went into his office and broke down. Once I regained my composure, I continued with my professional routine for the day. But I was left with a jumble of grief, resentment, guilt, and, finally, numbness. I needed someone to help me heal this wound that had injured my personal and professional self-esteem. It was only through having a whole hour with peers and a consultant the following week that I was able to finally comprehend the depth of my anger over my last session with Mr. D—his refusal to give me some final acknowledgment of the importance of our relationship. It was only through my peers' validating my sense of woundedness that I could release my anger and acknowledge that there were times when I had wished that Mr. D would just hurry up and die and my guilt at having gotten my wish. Only then could I let Mr. D go. I could even let in that he might have needed to distance me in order to separate or to keep his sense of control intact.

And with all of this, I was able to give back to myself the credit for caring for a dying man as long as he had lived.

Conclusions

The gay male therapist faces many challenges in terms of countertransference and therapeutic frame when working with people with

AIDS. Identification, accumulated loss, and numbing make introspection, reflection, and collegial support crucial to maintaining a sense of perspective and wholeness while doing the work. In my own case, I was lucky enough to get—and determined enough to ask for—such support. Some of the hazards of unconscious countertransference can be seen in my own defenses of counterphobic acting out (hazardous to myself) and pathologizing my patient. Helplessness seemed to be the common trigger.

The therapeutic frame must remain fluid enough to accommodate the shifting paradigms involved in crisis work and in AIDS work in particular. Yet, for the work to retain its focus, the therapeutic frame must be able to contain unexpected disruptions and not go too far afield. In the group that I ran, I needed to know that, after breaking down and crying, I could pull back and thus make it safe for others.

Finally, there has never been an epidemic quite like AIDS; therefore, a degree of comfort with the discomfort must be maintained—a cutting edge, if you will. My own belief is that the therapist who has all the preordained answers and interventions is robbing his patients of a special gift, and cheating himself or herself of a powerful nexus with truths. These truths only become evident when the therapist is open and ready.

In my own case, I will miss these patients dearly. By reminding myself of their deaths, I reclaim my memories of their lives.

Chapter 24

Peer Supervision and HIV: One Group's Process

Abraham Feingold, Psy.D.

F or mental health providers and private practitioners in particular, peer or collegial supervision[1] is both an economical and effective approach to receiving assistance on clinical matters that arise within the course of conducting psychotherapy. Providers engaged in such an endeavor meet on a regular basis for the purpose of listening to, examining, discussing, and sharing their mutual problems of psychotherapy in the hope of helping one another cope more adequately with patients who have difficult cases. Meetings are interactive and mutually supportive, permitting the sharing, ventilation, and exploration of feelings induced through contact with a patient. Repressions, denials, and fantasies may be addressed and the painful anxieties and burdensome responsibilities of the therapist lessened, contributing to an improvement in the quality of care. Meetings may also assist therapists in stabilizing during times of emotional upheaval engendered by their own personal crises (Todd and Pine 1968).

---

[1] Use of the term *supervision* in this context, although common in the psychological literature, is technically incorrect. Supervision implies that a participant is a supervisor of other participants and so assumes the liabilities inherent in a supervisory relationship. The process may be more accurately described as peer or professional sharing, with the presenting party alone responsible for the direction of the therapy (Berkowitz 1993). This important distinction will be reflected in the terminology used throughout this chapter.

Peer sharing helps participants overcome professional isolation (Brandes and Todd 1972; Danto and Mazzella 1988; Evans and Cohen 1985; Kline 1972; Nobler 1980), offers a vehicle for transmitting information on advances in clinical theory and practice (Schreiber and Frank 1983), and more generally promotes professional development (Brandes and Todd 1972; Nobler 1980; Remley et al. 1987; Schreiber and Frank 1983; Winstead et al. 1974). At times, peer sharing may be the approach of choice, if not necessity, when the clinical matters arise that are outside the realm of what is usual or expectable in the community of providers available to the practitioner.

In the early years of the acquired immunodeficiency syndrome (AIDS) epidemic, peer sharing was vital to the small number of providers who were offering clinical services to people infected with and affected by the human immunodeficiency virus (HIV). Expertise with these issues is, of course, growing in the major urban centers and can now be purchased on either a supervisory or consultative basis (Bor et al. 1992). Nevertheless, peer sharing remains a vital enterprise in groups that were formed years earlier and continue to meet as well as new groups that are forming in communities that only now are beginning to face the intricacies of HIV-related psychotherapy.

As in other major cities, Boston's earliest reported AIDS cases were almost exclusively among gay and bisexual men. The first local volunteer AIDS service organization, founded in November 1982, quickly assumed the status of a standing committee within a community health center serving a largely gay and lesbian patient population. All this occurred at a time when there was only a handful of AIDS cases in the entire state of Massachusetts. Nevertheless, there was tremendous urgency in those early years to prepare for an anticipated, and now realized, inundation of HIV-infected or -affected individuals and families requiring medical and mental health services.

Among the pioneers in Boston AIDS care were two mental health professionals affiliated with the gay- and lesbian-oriented health center. Through these individuals and their successors, the mental health perspective has always been represented within the larger community's response to HIV. A volunteer mental health subcommittee was formed within our local AIDS service organization and had its first meeting in September 1983. Mental health professionals, many themselves gay identified, were active early on in the clinical, consultative, and policy-making work of the subcommittee, which shifted gradually from crisis intervention to a more measured and reflective response to the mounting devastation.

By June 1986, Boston was in a position to host one of the nation's first conferences to address the mental health challenge of AIDS and related disorders. The planning and delivery of this conference provided a rallying point for the subcommittee and offered a showcase for the achievements of Boston area providers who were attempting to respond to the psychosocial and neuropsychiatric impact of HIV. As the subcommittee prepared for the conference, a clinician and leader in our community's mental health response to HIV identified the need for a peer sharing group to assist those who were or would soon be providing HIV-related psychotherapeutic services. An open invitation was extended to members of the mental health subcommittee and, in March 1986, the first meeting of the group took place in the community leader's living room.

Nine clinicians (seven men, two women) attended that first meeting. The group included psychiatrists, psychologists, social workers, and counselors, the majority of whom trained and practiced within a psychodynamic theoretical frame. All had significant interest and experience in issues facing gay men and were entering into the treatment of HIV-related concerns from that perspective, but had varying degrees of experience in working with HIV. One member had no experience of this type prior to joining the group; others were already treating one or more patients in hospitals, clinics, or private practice. Most group members had been touched personally by the disease (all the men were gay identified and one of the women lesbian identified), although none was known to be infected at the time the group began.

What follows is a description of our first 7 years together. The unfolding process of this group has been heavily influenced by the perceived vulnerability of members and their loved ones to the disease that drew their professional interest. A chronicle of this peer group's continuing journey through the uncharted territory of psychotherapy with those affected by HIV offers insight into the profound impact this disease has had on the professional sharing practices of one group of trained and experienced mental health providers.

As a group member, my perspective on this experience is undoubtedly influenced by my participation in the process. The selection of facts and their interpretation are, therefore, my own; I cannot speak for the group as a whole nor for any other group member.

Action or Reflection?

In parallel to the formation of the mental health subcommittee, our peer sharing group came together out of a sense of crisis. Numbers of HIV-positive patients were increasing and knowledge of psychotherapeutic technique with this population was growing but remained relatively limited. By drawing on one another's skills and experiences through our meetings, we hoped to reduce our own uncertainty regarding how best to proceed with our clinical work and perhaps even have some fun in the process. There did not appear to be time to engage in a more elaborate exercise of defining the group's purpose and direction. In ways, the group has paid a price for this lack of clarity and has had to devote significant time and energy in subsequent years to this purpose.

And so, although the members of the group included trained and experienced mental health providers familiar with group theory and the importance of framing the work of a group, there was surprisingly little discussion of parameters in early group meetings; nor, for that matter, was there much of a focus on group process. Instead, members proceeded without hesitation into the safe and familiar routine of case presentation and discussion.

Clinical Feedback or Support?

As the meetings continued on a more-or-less monthly basis, and initial anxieties were quelled within the emerging cohesiveness of the group, members began struggling to clarify the primary function of the meetings.

Although the group was ostensibly organized as a forum to discuss the clinical work being conducted by its members, the fact that group members had been, and were continuing to be, personally touched by the illness and death of loved ones could not be ignored. Nor could the added burden of the gay group members, who harbored private fears of possible infection with the virus. The question of what was appropriate subject matter for group discussion emerged as a central issue during the first 3 years of the group's functioning, and its initial discussion and resolution resulted in a founding member's leaving the group.

Within the context of the group, a greater push for personal support was understandable as, from its inception, the group took on a decidedly supportive tone. Meetings took place on Sunday evenings, rather than during the workweek, were scheduled for a "leisurely" 2 hours, and were hosted by group members in their homes. Coffee and cookies gave way to pizza and, finally, to elaborate, home-cooked meals that members would both gleefully anticipate and fondly recall. When a member's father died suddenly within our first year, an entire meeting was devoted to reminiscences of the member's relationship with him without a second thought as to the relevance of this material to the group's purpose. Another member, whose patient died of AIDS, vividly described the shock of discovering this patient dead at home and the discomfort of attending a memorial service as the unidentified therapist of the deceased. That member was not only supported in the often lonely grief work of the therapist, but was discouraged from attending future memorial services unaccompanied and invited to call a fellow group member for this purpose should the need arise.

At certain points, the supportive nature of our gatherings caused some members to push for a greater frequency of meetings to allow for more timely and extensive feedback from the group. This movement was rejected by the group as a whole on the premise that to devote additional off-work time to this enterprise would unreasonably burden members who already possessed minimal leisure time in the face of multiple professional obligations. Similarly, a movement to broaden the scope of case presentation to include non–HIV-related material that achieved only peripheral relevance (e.g., cases involving gay men neither infected with or affected by HIV) or presented some parallels (e.g., a non–HIV-infected or -affected patient presenting with a character disorder) was discouraged for fear of taking the group off the mark.

Of particular note, however, during the group's early years, was its tendency to stifle the expression of feeling around HIV-related illnesses and deaths of people in the members' lives who were not patients. Although acknowledgment of these events was permitted, the expression of feeling was judged not to be group business but rather material to be taken up with the personal supports built into members' lives (e.g., partners, friends, professional colleagues on an individual basis). Members were limited to discussing grief only from the perspective of its impact on a member's work as a clinician; the group goal was to support the member in continuing that work, rather than explore the larger impact of the clinician's grief.

Norms minimizing the disclosure of details within members' personal lives are not unusual in peer sharing groups (e.g., Brandes and Todd 1972; Hunt and Issacharoff 1975). Closed systems of this type, however, self-equilibrate and can exact a high price to maintain feelings of belonging and acceptance among group members. Members are not permitted to deviate from group norms; expressions of doubt and disappointment are censured (Issacharoff and Hunt 1977). As noted, one member found the distinctions drawn around affective expression highly artificial, verbalized his opposition to the norm, and paid a price for his dissension through subtle pressuring to terminate his involvement with the group, which he did. His departure has preoccupied the group at varying levels since its occurrence. According to Billow and Mendelsohn (1987), "like a death, which hopefully makes one reevaluate living, the loss of a member can encourage overt or covert reevaluation of group purpose, and hence may foster change. The person who left may be expressing the wish or fear of many."

In retrospect, it is clear that the group had a great deal of difficulty with affect generated by the growing epidemic in general and by most members' perceived personal vulnerability to HIV in particular. Members were seeking some way of containing this affect so as to permit the group to conduct its overt business. Although the focus was, and continued to be, on HIV-related issues, the relative infrequency of the meetings and the relative abundance of food served to dilute affect and encourage the use of alternative supports for managing nonclinical manifestations of grief. Together, these measures helped to protect members from being inundated and immobilized through fear engendered by the capricious virus. They allowed the group to manage, albeit with some measure of denial, the reality that loved ones and, in some cases, the clinician himself or herself were as vulnerable to HIV as the patients being treated. Only in more recent times has the group shown increased tolerance for the discussion of nonclinical HIV-related grief. Of note, too, has been a general trend toward greater simplicity of meals served during meetings.

Are You In or Are You Out?

From the start, inconsistencies could be noted in the group's management of its own boundaries. Because the support of the group was considered adjunctive rather than primary, the group instituted and has maintained a "flexible" boundary within itself, with attendance at scheduled meetings encouraged but not required. On occasion, this arrangement resulted in members simply missing meetings without notice to the host or other members. To remedy the consternation of the host around planning meals, a rule was eventually established that the host should be notified in advance of an expected absence.

During the meetings themselves, participation was neither solicited nor deterred. Fleeting acknowledgment was made of the reality that almost every member had a professional and possibly personal relationship with almost every other member and that patients were frequently shared across treatment modalities (e.g., my individual patient was in another's group; two members saw individuals who were treated by a third as a couple). Such realities did not appear to cause undue complications, however, as personal relationships were, for the most part, excluded from group discussion. In addition, members were advised to obtain releases from patients shared among group members so that, even when not identified by name, the clinicians sharing the case would have free reign in discussing their respective treatments.

The boundary between the group itself and the external world proved, however, to be quite a different matter. Through its first months of coalescing, the group jealously, yet understandably, guarded its outer boundary. Clinicians who sought entrance to the group but were not known to the majority of founding members were turned away. Even the inclusion of a well-known and well-liked tenth member shortly before the end of the first year sparked controversy and confusion in the months preceding the new member's arrival; the group had not settled on a mechanism for deciding about additions in membership. And yet, by the time of an original member's departure described earlier, which occurred in the group's third year of existence, the subsequent introduction of a new member occurred with minimal disruption to the group's ongoing process.

Several months following the introduction of this new member, the group stumbled onto unsettled ground in a seemingly disjointed discussion of the advisability of gay patients working with nongay therapists. The discussion seemed to have a momentum of its own and continued without benefit of processing by the participating members. In our next meeting, it was observed by the group's lone nongay member that the discussion seemed to augur a renewed focus on the group's capacity for inclusiveness, a topic that remained incompletely explored and certainly unresolved since the group experienced its first loss in membership. Unknowingly (or perhaps knowingly at an unconscious level), the group was preparing itself for its next major transition.

To Test or Not to Test?

In the group's early years, controversy over HIV-antibody testing raged loudly, unrelentingly, and inconclusively. In 1986, when the group first convened, antibody testing was considered ill-advised among the majority of Boston's mental health practitioners. The meaning of a positive test result was unclear at that time, and there appeared to be little one could do with this information anyway. Medical intervention was unavailable and the psychological stress engendered by this knowledge was thought to be both unreasonable and unnecessary.

During this period, our group of heretofore "neutral" psychodynamic clinicians by and large actively discouraged HIV testing among their patients under circumstances that did not reach the standard of "medical necessity" (e.g., to confirm a presumptive HIV diagnosis; for decision making in advance of or during pregnancy). Urgency to test was attributed to "AIDS anxiety" and interpreted as a reflection of unconscious shame or guilt over past behavior, if not an outright manifestation of internalized homophobia.

As time passed, however, and early intervention seemed promising, a shift in clinical practice occurred as providers assumed a stance of promoting informed consent and personal decision making. Concurrently, members began to share their own struggles with the decision to test and the impact of this struggle on their work with patients dealing with the same issue. Over time, several members submitted to testing and those who were seronegative reported these findings in subsequent group meetings.

During this period, one member was curiously absent for extended periods of time and, upon returning to the group, spoke cryptically about being unable to make the group meetings a high enough priority to ensure attendance. This member was empowered by the group to make his own decision but was encouraged to continue coming; privately, members had already begun to speculate among themselves that this member might be seropositive and ill, presumptions which, for the most part, remained unverbalized within the larger group.

At about this time, another member who had been conducting an open-ended psychotherapy group for gay men sought assistance related to an announcement within his group that a member was seropositive and diagnosed with Kaposi's sarcoma. The issue within his group was whether a gay psychotherapy group could contain a member with HIV or AIDS.

As Kline (1972) observed, "all process must eventually be focused upon process within the [peer] group." Billow and Mendelsohn (1987) noted that peer groups go through phases and that derivatives of the process may appear in the clinical material presented, in the interpretations made to it, or in the way such interpretations are received. Groups that overtly attend to these phenomena are referred to as *dual-focus groups* in that they relate the here-and-now experience to specific cases under consideration or, often, the reverse. And so, although the potential, if not already latent, parallel process remained unaddressed, our sharing group soon had the opportunity to address directly an announcement of seropositivity and illness for itself.

In the same meeting in which our nongay member identified our group's struggle with inclusiveness, the episodically absent member disclosed his positive-antibody status as well as his concurrent medical and psychological difficulties. In addition to describing his shifting priorities in the preceding months, this member voiced his concern over how the group would feel about his continuing participation (i.e., whether he would be perceived as a burden to the group or whether members would feel uncomfortable discussing their HIV-positive patients knowing that a fellow group member shared this serostatus). This member received unqualified support for continuing with the group at his own discretion; any ambivalence remained unverbalized, though it was hoped that the group would have the strength and tenacity to process whatever ambivalence did exist as it arose.

In March 1991, the group celebrated its first 5 years of existence with an extravagant Polynesian banquet. Although a second founding member departed the group just prior to this event because of non–HIV-related changes in his own personal life, the group continued reasonably intact and unquestionably vital. The group first toasted its next 5 years together and, following that, the time when a group such as this would no longer need to be meeting. It soon became all too clear that such a time did not appear to be close at hand.

In our subsequent meeting, a second member disclosed his newly discovered seropositive status and his ailing partner's AIDS diagnosis. After our initial shock, the group entered into a process of negotiating its boundaries with its now two HIV-positive members. Members advanced personal support within the group meetings and professional support outside the meetings (e.g., offering to phone patients to cancel appointments with these providers during health emergencies; offering to see these providers' patients in crisis sessions should the need arise). Now that we could no longer deny our personal vulnerability to infection, the tolerance for sharing personal HIV-related grief grew considerably and continued to do so as the group rallied around its stricken members.

Integrity or Despair?

During its next 2 years, the group shifted from a format of case presentation and discussion, which occurred less frequently, to the processing of feelings with and about our seropositive members. On occasions when both these members were absent from a meeting, the remaining members acknowledged one another's discomfort with presenting HIV-related case material that highlighted severe illness in their patients or negative countertransference feelings related to these cases. Members feared engendering hurt feelings in our own seropositive peers or suggesting that illness might be experienced as a burden to individual members or the group as a whole. The group, lacking the capacity to express ambivalence openly to these members, remained supportive in spite of countervailing feelings that had the potential to prevent us from attending to our own needs within the group.

And yet these needs may have assumed a lower priority in the face of the unique learning opportunity afforded the group by the illness of two of its members. Group sharing is a phenomenon often associated with the self-renewing tasks of mid-life and mid-career (i.e., care for the caretaker) (McCarley 1975). Our group, however, bore witness to the working through of developmental issues usually taken up in later adulthood and described by Erikson (1950) as the stage of ego integrity versus despair. Our two seropositive members manifested widely divergent approaches to management of a therapist's illness and retirement from clinical practice as they each arrived at their own balance around these issues.

The first member to disclose his HIV status maintained a fair measure of denial around his declining health, unable to hear gentle suggestions from the group to consider planning for the time when he would no longer be able to work. As cognitive, emotional, and physical limitations became more evident, the group attempted to confront this denial, with little success. This therapist never revealed his increasingly obvious health problems to his patients and grew more depressed and bitter as his illness advanced. In the end he had to suddenly close his practice, notifying patients after doing so of his AIDS diagnosis and offering referral for those desiring to continue their treatment with another therapist.

Throughout this ordeal, group members offered help in a variety of ways (e.g., telephone support and clinical consultation for this member with individual group members; partial or full group meetings with this member in his hospital room). Group efforts were, however, largely rejected as this member sunk into despair over his illness; when able to join the group, he verbalized unrelenting guilt over how he had managed the closing of his practice. Members felt helpless to intervene around his depression and, at the same time, felt angry that this member's behavior was pulling the group to extend itself in ways that might have been avoided had this member prepared for his retirement from clinical practice. Further, although this therapist no longer conducted psychotherapy, his guilty preoccupation prevented him from "retiring" in the formal sense of the word. As a result, he was unable to accept acknowledgment from the group for the genuine value of his many years of clinical service to the gay and HIV-affected communities. He withdrew from all but the two group members with whom he had a close, preexisting relationship; retreated socially out of fear of encountering former patients, whom he believed would express anger over his departure from practice; and was a focus of group discussion when present as well as when absent from meetings until his death in July 1992.

Concurrently, our other seropositive member demonstrated a more integrated approach to this final phase of work and life. He elected to close his practice at the end of May 1992, and gave his patients 4 months' advanced notice of this event. In revealing his HIV status to his large caseload, which included a number of men who were also HIV infected, he bore both the anger and sadness of his patients well, using the sharing group for purposes of ventilation and emotional support. As his practice drew to a close, this gifted therapist was able to transcend the therapeutic process by sharing with his less ill seropositive patients the wisdom he himself was accruing through the experience of his own illness and reconciliation with the prospect of death. Group members sat with rapt attention as this therapist presented case material reflecting these caring exchanges and were moved to tears by the stories' poignancy. He was encouraged to share this material through writing, but was ultimately unable to do so because of the rapid progression of his illness following his retirement.

The group honored his service as a clinician with a luncheon on his last day of practice.

Between the retirement of this peer and the final illness and death of our other colleague, the group fragmented to some extent over a nearly 5-month period. We gathered together twice during that period: for the wake and for a memorial service for our first stricken member. The latter was organized and the space paid for by group members, as we had a need to bring together the colleagues, patients, and family members of this individual who had succumbed to despair and was so unable to integrate his life experience and the people within it.

The healing that occurred through this coming together allowed the group to resume regular meetings in the subsequent months. Our retired colleague joined us as we continued processing our loss and, as a group, began to anticipate his loss. He died in March 1993.

These experiences have taken the group to places never imagined when we first came together more than 7 years ago. Our work has been enriched by the processes we have shared and, no doubt, will continue to share. Like all those whose lives have been touched by HIV, we have received a glimpse of our own futures, of the developmental work that lies ahead for us as clinicians and as people. We can only hope this knowledge will have a positive impact on how we live our lives toward that future.

Summary

Peer-group sharing benefits the experienced clinician by reducing professional isolation and promoting professional development through interchange with supportive colleagues. Psychotherapists engaged in providing HIV-related services can, in particular, profit from discussing complex cases with interested and informed fellow practitioners.

The nature of HIV is such that providers may be prone, at the least, to be moved by the misfortune of young, infected individuals with whom they strongly identify. At most, clinicians may perceive themselves as being, if not actually being, as vulnerable as their patients to the conditions they are attempting to treat. Not surprisingly, the intense affect generated in clinicians by HIV can find countertransferential expression not only within their therapeutic interventions, but also within the process of the sharing group itself.

As I see our own experience, a sense of urgency to begin helping one another address knotty case material supplanted the more mundane yet critical task of defining the group's parameters. Without a detached observer available to comment on process, our unobserved and unverbalized anxieties propelled us forward, blurring our focus (e.g., Have we come together to provide clinical feedback or personal support?) and resulting in a member leaving the group. Questions around the group's capacity for inclusiveness eventually centered on its response to the announcement of seropositivity in two members. Their illnesses and deaths inexorably altered the course of our group experience, causing us to rethink previously established norms and tackle dilemmas not even imagined at the group's inception.

When the illness and death of colleagues from AIDS-related illness are not, as in our case, overtly anticipated at the start of the group experience, members are left to follow the group's own process to new levels of relatedness to the AIDS-related clinical material presented and, perhaps more importantly, relatedness to one another. Obviously, no amount of planning can truly prepare the group for the eventuality of such loss, and the emotional richness of the experience would be attenuated by any structured attempt to do so.

Nevertheless, the work of any peer group must be grounded in a clear framework built by consensus. As we discovered, learning can be enhanced through group process observation by the membership and cohesion heightened through the extension of personal support by participants to one another. At times, support and process observation will likely need to supersede the greater emotional safety of strict case presentation and discussion for members to feel the full benefit of the group experience.

References

Berkowitz S: Supervision or consultation? Newsletter of the Massachusetts Psychological Association 36:9, 20, 1993

Billow RM, Mendelsohn R: The peer supervisory group for psychoanalytic therapists. Group 11:35–46, 1987

Bor R, Scher I, Salt H: Supervising professionals involved in the psychological care of people infected with HIV/AIDS. Counselling Psychologist 5:95–109, 1992

Brandes NS, Todd WE: Dissolution of a peer supervision group of individual psychotherapists. Int J Group Psychother 22:54–59, 1972

Danto EA, Mazzella AJ: Peer supervision in occupational social work. Employee Assistance Quarterly 4:29–44, 1988

Erikson EH: Childhood and Society. New York, WW Norton, 1950

Evans M, Cohen PF: Borrowing a vision: a creative use of countertransference feelings in peer supervision to release barriers in the intuitive analytic process. Current Issues in Psychoanalytic Practice 2:111–121, 1985

Hunt W, Issacharoff A: History and analysis of a leaderless group of professional therapists. Am J Psychiatry 132:1164–1167, 1975

Issacharoff A, Hunt W: Observations on group process in a leaderless group of professional therapists. Group 1:162–171, 1977

Kline FM: Dynamics of a leaderless group. Int J Group Psychother 22:234–242, 1972

McCarley T: The psychotherapist's search for self-renewal. Am J Psychiatry 132:221–224, 1975

Nobler H: A peer group for therapists: successful experience in sharing. Int J Group Psychother 30:51–61, 1980

Remley TP, Benshoff JM, Mowbray CA: A proposed model for peer supervision. Counselor Education and Supervision 27:53–60, 1987

Schreiber P, Frank E: The use of a peer supervision group by social work clinicians. The Clinical Supervisor 1:29–36, 1983

Todd WE, Pine I: Peer supervision of individual psychotherapy. Am J Psychiatry 125:780–784, 1968

Winstead DK, Bonovitz JS, Gale MS, et al: Resident peer supervision of psychotherapy. Am J Psychiatry 131:318–321, 1974

Section V

When the Therapist Is HIV Infected

Chapter 25

Necessary and Unnecessary Disclosure: A Therapist's Life-Threatening Illness

Claire E. Philip, L.I.S.W.

I s there something about the human immunodeficiency virus (HIV) phenomenon that causes us to think twice before we regard it as generically as other life-threatening conditions in examining the impact of a therapist's illness on clinical practice? I think the answer is both yes and no. The portions of a health crisis that are generic among therapists are those that pertain to 1) the traditional stance of anonymity, 2) the fundamental assumption of both the health and the honesty of the therapist (Friedman 1991), 3) the recognition that it is the patient's fantasy and the meanings attached to the content that we pursue in treatment, and 4) the vulnerabilities that are engendered by serious and life-threatening illness. The part that may be viewed as more specific to the therapist who becomes HIV positive has to do with the scope and depth of emotional distress that accompany the diagnosis and that may anticipate it. The milieu in which the gay therapist belongs is today steeped in grief in both a social and a philosophical sense; this grief cannot be sidestepped.

Conceptualizing the Dilemmas

Coming to terms with my own ultimately fatal illness, a low-grade B cell cancer affecting the blood known as *Waldenström's macroglobulin-*

emia, I struggled to conceptualize the nature of the dilemmas facing me as a therapist who had been in private practice for 16 years. The view that made the most sense in retrospect was that illness ranges along a continuum of being acute and survivable at one end and chronic-acute and not survivable on the other (Philip 1993). The middle of the continuum describes a variety of prognostic differences and circumstances. At the time of diagnosis, one's condition may fall at any point along the line. Within this framework, I was able to locate myself over time at two points. The initial diagnosis of my illness was made in 1985 under nonacute circumstances, and I learned immediately that the illness would be fatal, but that a temporary remission was possible with the palliative treatments available. Three and a half years later I arrived at a point farther along the continuum. Treatment failure and acute complications landed me in the hospital for the first time, demanding an immediate plan to provide for the continuity of my patients' treatment.

Obligation to Disclose

One very significant aspect of my own experience was the delay in disclosure of the illness to patients and colleagues. The actual disclosure was compelled by an acute and life-threatening illness, secondary to the original diagnosis, that resulted in a 6-week absence from practice, and not by the fact that I knew in the beginning that the underlying cancer was fatal. Two major changes brought the issue of disclosure to the forefront: first, the possibility of a long disruption in work with patients demanded some explanation, and second, I resumed work visibly altered to those who noted the wig I wore. This brings us to the matter of necessary and unnecessary disclosure, a matter that is intrinsically linked to the issue of planning for the continuity of patients' treatment.

Patients are likely to recognize in retrospect the differences between an acute and survivable illness (e.g., its sudden and unforeseen nature, the time-limited healing process, illness with possible long remission) and the early stages of a chronic, fatal condition such as Lou Gehrig's disease, certain cancers, or acquired immunodeficiency syndrome (AIDS). These differences expose important dilemmas (Philip 1993). In other words, if we know we are going to die sooner rather than later, do we withhold that information until compelled to reveal it by circumstances? If so, by which circumstances? An episode of acute illness can happen to anyone, and generally speaking we follow our professional principles in attempting to minimize its impact on our patients; it is the disruption caused by that illness that precipitates action or explanation. However, when we become ill without disruption or visible evidence, we may be inclined not to disclose the fact of our illness, either to colleagues or to patients.

I now extend these criteria to a consideration of therapists who are already stressed by the illness of human immunodeficiency virus (HIV)–positive friends, companions, and patients and who then become HIV positive themselves. A problem of potentially much greater magnitude may exist for this population: emotional overload.

For most illnesses, we can say that the sense of a continuum begins with diagnosis of a particular condition or perhaps with the search for diagnosis in the face of symptoms. In the case of the HIV phenomenon, perhaps it is more accurate to speak of a "phantom section of the continuum," a segment that precedes notification of the presence of the HIV antibody. In my mind's eye, this segment is located as the foreground for the other continuum as though it were a pane of glass. For example, a gay therapist might identify himself as at high risk for HIV infection but may not have undergone any testing and is simply frightened though asymptomatic.

Both therapist and patient may silently share positions, therefore, that detach themselves from one another emotionally behind the "pane of glass." One might suggest that the real continuum begins with positive test results or, as with any other serious illness, the presence of diagnosable symptoms. But that phantom segment of the continuum is bound to impact one's personal and professional life; it amounts to a period of dread, perhaps not unlike the expectation of recurrence in cancer patients. Farther along the continuum, a person might have been tested, found to be HIV positive, but have a T cell count of 800; in other words, not be particularly debilitated. Any negative change in the markers for chronic illness likely brings a degree of fear and obsession related to it. A slipping of numbers becomes a major event. An example might be the downward shift of a T cell count from 800 to 600, not close enough by any means to diagnose the presence of AIDS, but more than enough to elicit an emotional reaction. Likewise, one might have a T cell count of 800 but contract an opportunistic infection that is treatable but distracting, painful, and frightening. In addition, it is not only one's own physical state but the vicissitudes in the well-being of lovers and friends that stress one's capacity to manage anxiety.

It is difficult even in hindsight for me to say with any certainty that the best time for disclosure of my own illness to patients would have been after some reasonable lapse of time following diagnosis—enough time to process the shock, assess the damage, think through the needs of self and patients, and so forth. I was distracted from that step partly by the death of a parent. In any event, what happened reflected a return to a state of "normal" denial claimed by reasonably healthy people that was encouraged by the invisible and nondisruptive nature of the illness and its treatment during the first 4 years. I had obliterated the possibility of an uneven, though temporary survival from a continuum I knew fully well would end in death. Thus I had rationalized away the need to plan for the continuity of my patients' therapy in the face of serious complications, or to include colleagues in or inform them about such planning (Philip 1993).

Role of the Professional Family

Silver (1990) wrote of the role of the "professional family" in relation to her own serious illness (also cancer), and the farther I travel along the continuum of my illness, the more convinced I am of its importance in mitigating the overwhelming burden of personal and professional agony that faces a clinician in a serious (and especially long-term) health crisis. Those who need the help have some responsibility for disclosure to colleagues, and those colleagues who would be helpers have some responsibility to reach out when something appears amiss or when asked. I imagine that the professional family is needed on an exponentially greater order by the therapist who has become HIV positive. The nature of the disease and the attitudes that accompany the announcement of its presence suggest that the therapist as well as his or her patients need protection from abandonment and help with grief and mourning.

It is surprisingly easy for therapists to rationalize "business as usual," in part because we are trained to withhold personal information, in part because health issues are often regarded as especially personal, and no doubt in part because we, as do our patients, attach particular meanings representing all ego developmental stages and powerful feelings to symptoms. In the case of HIV, meanings are loaded with shame, guilt, stigmatization, castration, a sense of loss of control, abandonment, material losses, and the fear of pain and death, among others, and all that and more in a climate that Cadwell has identified as unique to work with HIV patients, the "unremitting exposure to death and grief" (Cadwell 1989). The shock of diagnosis may give way rather quickly to avoidance, isolation, and denial, and perhaps to the search for stability in the professional arena when it is so lacking in the other aspects of an individual's life.

Literature Review

Value of Consultation

In effect, we have two issues to address in the literature: the first deals broadly with necessary and unnecessary disclosures, and the second one confronts the problems of incapacitation and planning for continuity of patients' treatment, including when it is time to close a practice and how that might be tackled. Both of these have been explored to some extent in recent articles (Philip 1993; Philip and Stevens 1992). In each of these articles the assumption was made that disclosure to a trusted colleague, peer group, consultant, or supervisor constitutes the first important, necessary step in deciding when, to whom, and how much to disclose. It is in the ensuing consultations that unnecessary disclosures, those that thin the power of the transference and distract attention from the patient's fantasy material by intruding the therapist's reality, are weeded out. It is in these more private discussions that the impact of a therapist's serious illness on the treatment frame is explored with the partnership of one who attempts objectivity and nondirectiveness and who respects confidentiality. It is also in these meetings that explicit plans can be made, long before the need to implement them arises, for absences resulting from temporary incapacitation or for eventual referral of an ill or dying therapist's patients. This amounts to support of a very basic, more universal kind. One hopes that the consultation process is supportive enough that the therapist does not feel that control over his or her practice is threatened as another consequence of the immense struggle to perform professionally with remaining energies. By being aggressively directive, the consultant could undermine the therapist's integrity.

Others have written on the benefits of consultation to private practitioners in the case of acute life-threatening disease (Alexander et al. 1989; Silver 1990) or in the case of terminal illness (Alexander et al. 1989). Both Alexander et al. (1989) and Philip and Stevens (1992) explored countertransference problems for the consultant in this process. Silver also described some of her experiences of coping with a terminal illness within an institutional environment where she received the valuable support of both patients and colleagues. However, not all institutions or agencies offer such a helpful or supportive holding environment. The practitioner in private practice must create such a helpful environment on his or her own. Some years later when she felt more certain of her cure, Silver seriously questioned the wisdom of not requesting supervision regarding treatment of her private patients during her recovery.

Potential for Betrayal

One extremely important matter appearing in the literature is the potential for the patient to experience a sense of betrayal when the therapist fails to explore then validate the patient's perception that the therapist is not well. There are countless stories afloat of poorly handled situations of this kind that leave one with the sense that too rigid an adherence to anonymity may serve the therapist's needs far more than the patient's. On the other hand, Abend (1982) held that giving the simple facts can relay implicit messages to the patient, and that these messages may also benefit the therapist more than the patient. For example, if the therapist were to say, "I'm not feeling well," he or she might illicit a sympathetic response that gratified the therapist's need, but possibly at the expense of the patient's work. The therapist would be getting in the way of the patient's material if he or she revealed material without addressing the patient's deeper psychodynamic meaning of the exchange.

Where do we make the choices, then, between these dangers? Morrison (1990) and Friedman (1991) both advocated that patients' perceptions of a therapist's illness demand validation, but these authors clearly continued to pursue the meaning of this content to patients in their clinical work, and Morrison in particular reminded us that the patient's ambivalence about knowing facts deserves focus as well.

Does this mean that the gay therapist who seroconverts must soon thereafter disclose this fact to patients? Does one wait until the illness becomes obvious (presenting a dramatic change, such as the visible presence of Kaposi's sarcoma), creates absences because of hospitalizations, interferes with a general sense of well-being, or attracts complications such as infections and so forth? Can we distinguish between the presence of HIV antibodies and the actual diagnosis of AIDS in our recommendations for changes in psychotherapy practice? Should different criteria be applied to the therapist working in the institutional or agency format from one working in the private practice format? I do not think at the present the answers are very clear, but there are some guidelines worth considering. Because denial is so persistent in each case of life-threatening illness, we need to consider these questions on an individual basis.

Friedman (1991) used her cancer diagnosis, combined with a prospective patient's history of significant loss, as the criteria for informing prospective patients of her illness, but did not use these criteria to justify telling her existing patients. Should this model be applicable to gay therapists treating gay patients? Should the gay therapist inform prospective gay patients of his HIV-positive status? Would nongay patients deserve the same consideration only if they had experienced significant loss? Should the therapist weigh these matters against remaining life expectancy? When in a state of remission, the therapist might feel a reduced sense of obligation to disclose his or her illness if the prognosis is not definitively bleak. In doing just that, Friedman (1991) admitted to succumbing to denial in failing to foresee the possibility that her time to work with new patients might become limited by the illness. I remain concerned about disclosure to only selected patients (whether depending on how long they have been in treatment or other circumstances), especially when the therapist in all probability will have to undergo treatment with potentially lethal medicines and will likely go through periods of debilitation, and when, of course, the prognosis for the long term is not good.

Some Benefits of Disclosure

In my own experience there were some clear benefits to disclosing my health status to all patients. The rich opportunities such disclosure presented for exploring universal life and death issues, the particular losses of each patient, the meanings attached, and also the meaning of the relationship with the therapist in the reality sense—all of these were used to promote growth, a growth in which the therapist shared. The downside of such disclosure involved feelings of self-exposure, the potential for patients to feel their own issues were being trivialized, a variety of uncomfortable and difficult countertransference feelings on my part (e.g., worry over income loss as a consequence of abandonment by patients), my loss of composure by showing the depth of my grief, and my guilt feelings for having withheld information. However, following disclosure I felt relief from having regained what I felt was an honest footing with my patients. My own tension lessened as I shifted focus onto the tasks of both continuing treatment and preparing for its premature ending.

When I had told my patients I was ill and would work with them as long as I could if they wished, I gave them the understanding that we would both be alert to whether or not I was able to continue at any point to meet their therapeutic needs. In other words, they were given some control over the process of letting go. My patients were able to work on their own issues and our shared issue of loss of one another for a year and a half before I closed my clinical practice in the face of complications that left my health too unstable to provide the constancy they needed. I was able to conclude that feelings of deception and betrayal can be short-circuited and grief and mourning can be more appropriately worked through when the therapist helps the patients anticipate the loss of their therapist and are made partners in providing for continuity of treatment.

Compartmentalization, Attunement, and Decathexis

Within the literature there are those (Friedman 1991; Morrison 1990) who felt a keener attunement to the patient and were capable of compartmentalizing their personal struggles. Others (Alexander et al. 1989; DeWald 1982; Halpert 1982), including myself, spoke more of a fading of attentiveness and a decathexis in relation to the patient. This disengagement is a phenomenon that consultation can particularly monitor. Therapists who are ill but who can legitimately hope for wellness are likely to recover their capacity to become affectively involved with a patient in the therapeutic relationship, but those who face death and its antecedent terrifying conditions will eventually need to conserve their psychological energies for themselves. Because there really is not a clear guideline for the exact point at which an ill therapist's capacities are so severely compromised as to represent an impairment that would bar practicing, regular consultation makes sense.

Alternatives to Direct Clinical Practice

Rosner (1986) addressed the alternatives to direct practice, suggesting pursuits such as writing, teaching, lecturing, or consulting. For any therapist, well or otherwise, diversification of practice is a net to cast out early in one's career. As the net becomes fuller and fuller with possibilities, one can draw it in when needed. For the gay therapist at risk for HIV infection, this early planning might be even more essential. Today numerous institutions and organizations are in need of AIDS education and consultation, and this might be a direction for a group practice to pursue. It might well also be possible for a therapist in an agency or institutional environment to do brief or service-oriented work when psychotherapy no longer is a viable choice. The confrontation with both psychosocial issues and economic losses in private practice is probably less cushioned. It would seem that the time to anticipate financial and insurance needs and the value of diversification in practice is when we are well.

Anticipating Termination and Continuity

When illness approaches a terminal stage, the need for decisiveness is clear. The anticipatory work should be as complete as possible: the therapist has engaged patients in a lively partnership for planning the continuity of treatment if necessary, thereby conveying a profound sense of concern; informed colleagues have had time to find a role both in the supportive sphere and in the afterwork with patients and among themselves; and the real separations are accomplished with a minimum of confusion and anger, however great the grieving.

The Patient's Perspective

The following two long-term cases illuminate the importance of focusing on the meaning patients assign to their therapists' illnesses. That meaning changes the impact of the illness on the treatment frame.

Case 1

I had seen Ms. A, a middle-aged "slow learner" with anxiety neurosis and depression, for supportive therapy regularly for 14 years prior to my hospitalization and consequent disclosure of illness. In the latter years, sessions were scheduled twice monthly; recent sessions had included Ms. A's steady male companion, a man also of some limitations who frequently experienced profound anxieties about losing her. For both of them, uncertainty about the imminence of my death remained on the surface for the year and a half before I closed my practice. Ms. A pondered whether she would be wise to transfer to another therapist before I showed signs of serious deterioration (i.e., more or less immediately) in order to avoid the contemplation of loss. Thus her ambivalence became acute. Enormous guilt developed as she felt the urge to abandon me as someone to whom she was deeply attached despite her characteristic obsessive doubts. In the transference this entirely reflected her struggle with dependency on her mother. Ms. A's partner worried whether the loss of our therapy would be so damaging to Ms. A's mental state that she would leave him and return to her family, reflecting his lifelong struggle with fears of abandonment and institutionalization. I provided every opportunity for this couple to meet with another therapist whenever I was away during the last year and a half. They both needed to test and debate their feelings, as well as process the loss and, particularly for her, the change.

Old material regarding fears about the inevitable death of parents came to the forefront. Both Ms. A and her companion had counted on my outliving her parents and being available for caring and for offering the wisdom of my experiences. Over and over, their doubts about the planned new therapist's essential wisdom, experience, capacity to understand, and reputation were raised as the first threads of a new clinical relationship were woven. Difficulties, as would be expected, were often expressed in concrete terms, such as office locations, the presence of other therapists in the office suite, and so on. Ms. A and her companion could only disguise their feelings as disappointment; pursuing whatever anger lay beneath their disappointment would have been shattering to them.

When the time of parting arrived, both Ms. A and her companion were able to express hopes and concern for me in the real context of life and death, to show appreciation and grief, and to indicate that a transitional phase in therapy felt relatively secure.

The case of Ms. B illustrates by contrast why it is important to keep in mind the patient's perspective when monitoring the effects of a therapist's serious illness on the course of treatment. The patient will stay in character; the transference will reveal this.

Case 2

Ms. B, who was in her early 40s, had been working for a number of years with me on learning to trust her observations both of her family of origin and of her husband within their troubled marriage. She had well-developed compulsive defenses against feelings of worthlessness and loneliness, a history of accomplishment from which she often failed to derive satisfaction, and a healthy perseverance in getting help for herself. Her ambivalence in general made the process of learning to trust her observations a long one.

One year after the disclosure of my illness to her, Ms. B told me her devastating news that an important woman friend of hers had leukemia and was scheduled for a bone marrow transplant some months hence. She was able to express much anguish and grief and some hope. This friend was especially rare, someone with whom she could identify. As much as she suppressed feelings in general, her grief reemerged in the thought that her friend could die during the transplant process. I probed her absent ideas about my own illness by inquiring whether she had thoughts about it she was not revealing. She said she did not see herself discussing it in treatment, but sometimes talked to her husband about it. In her view, the therapist is not supposed to be 100% herself or himself (i.e., does not reveal who she or he is). Ms. B trusted I would tell her what she needed to know at the appropriate time. The case with her friend was different: the friend clearly revealed that she was not well over the phone, whereas I appeared well week after week and did not talk about being ill.

Ms. B characteristically looked to others to define what she should think or feel, not having much faith in her own observations and not easily seeking validation; with the disclosure of the potential loss of an important friend coming after disclosure of my illness, her growth in this area was again slowed. In early July, she came to a session remarking how the shrubs at the front seemed to have flourished again after a really heavy pruning a year and a half ago (the time of my disclosure to her, I noted to myself) and that it took guts to take such a risk. Here was a gift of connection, disguised, between my having survived a year and a half and her friend's risk of death during the rapidly approaching bone marrow transplant process. I used the material to help her see her underlying concerns; at first she met my interpretation with denial and then with no protest.

It was shortly thereafter that I was informed that my condition had worsened dramatically and that I would have to go out of town for a highly experimental treatment. In the light of this news, I determined that it was the right time to close the practice. This meant that Ms. B, who had not kept this possibility on the surface of her thoughts, had only a short time to prepare for the premature termination of her treatment in a doubly difficult context. She expressed profound sadness at the further loss of her supports, but what she actually did reflected her strengths: she dug in and met all the challenges that life dealt her that autumn, and she found some new supports.

Summary

The generic aspects of health crises and their disclosure—potential loss of anonymity, changed assumptions about the therapist's honesty and good health, the meaning attributed to content by the patient, vulnerabilities and impairments engendered by illness—compel stricken therapists to acknowledge that they need guidelines and colleagues' help, both with monitoring the effects of serious illness on the treatment frame and with planning for continuity of treatment. Many, if not most of us, as clinicians, have gone through periods when compartmentalization of personal difficulties was both necessary and possible to achieve. It is axiomatic, however, that our patients detect our distress to an amazing degree despite our attempts to keep it hidden. As Silver (1990) stated, "The analyst who thinks she is being effective in keeping her own precarious physical (and by extension, mental) incapacities and uncertainties secret from the patients is operating with considerable denial" (p. 172). The professional family or community of which she speaks has a definite preventive role when terrible illness strikes; it is often in the absence of its concern, whether through not knowing or through distancing, that we find illustrations of chaos and disaster—cases in which the therapist has finally become so overwhelmed that things can barely be set right again. For myself, the professional family came to help when I requested it. How careful we must be not to take over for our colleague who is still able to perform professionally, nor to fail to help our colleague who is alert to the patients' therapeutic needs and his or her inability to provide for them but does not know how to proceed.

References

Abend SM: Serious illness in the analyst: countertransference considerations. J Am Psychoanal Assoc 30(2):365–379, 1982

Alexander J, Kolodzieski K, Sanville J, et al: On final terminations: consultations with a dying therapist. Clinical Social Work Journal 4:307–323, 1989

Cadwell S: Issues of identification for gay psychotherapists treating gay clients with HIV spectrum disorder: special vulnerability and its management. Unpublished Ph.D. dissertation, Smith College School for Social Work, Northampton, MA, 1989

DeWald P: Serious illness in the analyst: transference, countertransference and reality responses. J Am Psychoanal Assoc 30:347–363, 1982

Friedman G: Impact of a therapist's life-threatening illness on the therapeutic situation. Contemporary Psychoanalysis 27:405–421, 1991

Halpert E: When the analyst is chronically ill or dying. Psychoanal Q 51:372–389, 1982

Morrison A: Doing psychotherapy while living with a life-threatening illness, in Illness in the Analyst. Edited by Silver A, Schwartz H. Madison, CT, Madison International Universities Press, 1990, pp 227–250

Philip C: Dilemmas of disclosure to patients and colleagues when a therapist faces life-threatening illness (or dying). Hlth Soc Work 18:13–19, 1993

Philip C, Stevens E: Countertransference issues for the consultant when a colleague is critically ill. Clinical Social Work Journal 4:411–420, 1992

Rosner S: The seriously ill or dying analyst and the limits of neutrality. Psychology 4:357–371, 1986

Silver A: Resuming the work with a life-threatening illness—and further reflections, in Illness in the Analyst. Edited by Silver A, Schwartz H. Madison, CT, Madison International Universities Press, 1990, pp 151–176

Chapter 26

Therapists' Disclosure of HIV Status and the Decision to Stop Practicing: An HIV-Positive Therapist Responds

Michael Shernoff, C.S.W., A.C.S.W.

One of the most significant issues for psychotherapists is how to make the most disciplined use of themselves while remaining empathically connected to the patient. The literature is full of discussions about how not to allow the therapist's countertransference harm the treatment. However, issues of countertransference become more complicated when therapists treat patients with whom they may easily identify.

Following the development of gay- and lesbian-affirmative psychotherapy, the professional literature has continued to address the impact on therapy of a gay or lesbian patient knowing that his or her therapist is also gay or lesbian. When both therapist and patient are dealing with virtually identical life crises at the same time, the potential for therapeutic mistakes is enormous. Extraordinarily skilled therapeutic interaction is necessary between therapist and patient to avert these mistakes.

I am an openly gay psychotherapist. The majority of my patients who seek treatment with me know this prior to calling me for an initial consultation. After 15 years of practicing I was faced with a new situation, the urgency of which caused me to feel challenged professionally in ways I had never before experienced. In 1986 I decided to take the human immunodeficiency virus (HIV)–antibody test. Not surprisingly, the test results showed that I had been exposed. Although my health was perfect I became more depressed than I had ever been before or since.

In late 1989 my T cell count plunged and in, 1990, on my 39th birthday, I began to take zidovudine (AZT). The side effects of AZT left me feeling chronically sluggish, tired, cranky, and generally flulike for several months. I no longer had seemingly endless energy, and I felt as though I had suddenly aged 15 years. I had to learn to time my dosages to make sure that my medicine timer did not go off during a session with a patient, and I napped frequently in order to remain alert during all of my sessions.

Understandably during this period I found that I was often preoccupied with my own health concerns and with my fears that this was the beginning of a progression to a full-blown acquired immunodeficiency syndrome (AIDS). These thoughts intruded into my consciousness while I was working with patients who already had AIDS. Is that going to be me in a few months or years? I wondered.

I began to reflect on the appropriateness of sharing my health status with my patients. If I was to share it, how could this be accomplished in a manner that was most beneficial to the patients' treatment? Discussions about this issue with both my therapist and supervisor led to the painful question, How would I know if and when I should stop practicing? I began to grapple with these complementary issues. What follows are some case examples that illustrate the challenges inherent in attempting to provide competent treatment while living and practicing under the shadow of HIV and AIDS.

A Patient's Anxiety
About His Therapist's Health

The following case illustrates how the HIV status of the therapist can emerge as an important clinical issue.

Case 1

Once when I injured one of my hands and had to go to the emergency room, I had to cancel several patients' sessions. One of my partners telephoned the patients and told them that I had an emergency and would call them later to reschedule the appointment. One of the men I was scheduled to see was Mr. A, a 32-year-old man referred to me by his Alcoholics Anonymous (AA) sponsor. Mr. A's last two therapists had died from AIDS-related illnesses within 2 years of each other. Mr. A was seronegative and, in addition to wanting to work through his feelings about the deaths of his previous therapists, he wanted to explore his own fears of intimacy with other men that were making it difficult for him to form romantic relationships.

I telephoned Mr. A the evening after I had missed his session and left a message on his answering machine offering him a choice of times to reschedule the session the following day. Knowing that his last two therapists had both died of AIDS, I assumed that he might have been made anxious by the phone call canceling our session. With this in mind, I felt it was important that Mr. A either speak with me in person or hear my voice on his machine rescheduling the appointment I had to cancel.

When I saw Mr. A the next day, my hand was bandaged and my arm was in a sling. He began the session by telling me that when he received the phone call telling him that I had to cancel his appointment because of an emergency, all he had really heard was that I was in the emergency room. He immediately began to panic that I too had AIDS and was going to leave him. While he was telling me this, I was thinking that I hoped I did not get sick any time soon so as not to provide one more reason why he should not trust other gay men.

Mr. A went on to say that the phone call from my colleague had reawakened all the feelings he had about the deaths of his previous therapists as well as of several close friends who had also recently died. He told me that he realized that he did not even know what my serostatus was and felt that perhaps he was holding back from telling me everything out of the fear that I, like his last two therapists, might die. He then quickly said that of course he did not want me to get sick, but his feelings at this point were mostly about how he would be affected if I were to become permanently disabled. He then asked how I would react if he asked me what my serostatus was.

I began by telling him how glad I was that he had been able to share all of those feelings with me. I told him that at the present time I was not sure how I would respond to a request from him about my

HIV status. Before answering him I would want us to spend time exploring all of his feelings, and what it would mean if I was seropositive and what it would mean if I was seronegative. I also said that before I made any decision about whether to answer this question, I would spend time thinking about where we were in his treatment. I explained that I would want how I chose to respond to be in the best interest of his therapy. I then asked him how he felt hearing this response to his hypothetical question.

After thinking for a few moments he told me that he was very comfortable with my response and that it made him feel well taken care of by me. He had been afraid that I would not tell him my HIV status because of my concerns about confidentiality. He then said that he was not even sure that he really wanted to know what my HIV status was. I then asked if he felt that any other incident had prompted his reaction to my emergency.

Although blocking at first, he shortly began to discuss the fact that his sponsor in AA had moved away from New York 2 weeks ago. This man had been instrumental in Mr. A's achieving sobriety and they had become close friends. He said that a few nights earlier he had heard himself sharing the news of his sponsor's leaving in an AA meeting. We then proceeded to discuss his feelings of loss and abandonment related to this, something he had been having difficulty doing in previous sessions.

Although I felt that I handled this session with sensitivity for Mr. A's feelings, this was a difficult session for me, because it raised some anxieties and questions on which I had not previously spent much time reflecting. Suppose that Mr. A had insisted on knowing my HIV status. Did he have a right to know this information? What if he refused to continue treatment with an HIV-positive therapist? This would not have been paranoia, but a simple avoidance of intimacy and resistance to treatment on his part. This session precipitated my worries about who would want to begin long-term therapy with a seropositive therapist. Would I have to limit my practice to AIDS-related cases? This was not something I wanted to do.

Because Mr. A worked for one of the gay and lesbian social service agencies in Manhattan, we had already discussed his feelings about his coworkers, who were friends and colleagues of mine, talking to him about me. After this session I began to think about the consequences of Mr. A discovering my HIV status from someone other than myself, and how I would clinically handle this situation.

The Therapist's Own Narcissism

When I tune a patient out during his session, my own narcissistic injuries are being triggered and I regress to a less-developed way of being. I am not able to put aside my own reactions in order to be present for my patient, encouraging him to share his feelings. In part, I would rather not have to listen to his feelings, as they are so similar to the ones against which I struggle to defend myself. An incident occurred that illustrates the impact of these issues on another therapist's practice.

Case 2

A colleague of mine, Mr. B, had been in practice for over 10 years. He was an intelligent and committed therapist whose patients were all gay men. He developed Kaposi's sarcoma and lost weight over a 2-year period before spending a month in the hospital for an AIDS-related condition. He then resumed seeing patients.

When Mr. B returned to work he told all of his patients that he had AIDS and asked them if they wished to continue working with him. Shortly before he told me this he mentioned that he was now so short of breath that he was winded by the few steps he had to walk to let patients into his apartment. It was obvious to me that he was quickly approaching death. He told me that none of his patients had chosen to stop seeing him once they knew he had AIDS. In addition, because he was now collecting disability income, he was asking each of his patients to pay him in cash at reduced fees because he could not declare the income or fill out insurance forms. I became very angry when he was telling me this. Mr. B's decision to remain in practice under these conditions provided a clear example to me of a therapist's narcissistic needs interfering with the provision of good treatment to his patients. I asked him how he expected his patients to make the decision to leave him while he was dying. His patients obviously felt much gratitude to him for all the help he had provided to them over the years. Now, however, he was asking them to take care of him.

I felt that Mr. B should have told his patients that he could no longer guarantee the same quality and consistency of therapy that he had always provided. After telling them this he should have seen each of his patients for another four to six sessions to facilitate terminations and transfer to other therapists. Had he accomplished this, he would have maintained his primary commitment to the well-being of his patients. His inability to maintain this commitment was a sign that his own life crisis intruded into the treatment of his patients. After a final hospitalization, Mr. B died. It was left to Mr. B's friends and grieving lover to notify his patients of his death.

The way Mr. B handled his illness raised several questions for me. First, was it ethical for him to continue practicing when he was so ill and clearly unable to prioritize the needs of his patients? I found his conduct unprofessional. A mutual colleague countered that Mr. B provided his patients with the opportunity to give something back to him and to take care of him. He asked if I was so certain that it could never be a positive therapeutic experience for any of Mr. B's patients to be caring for him. I remained skeptical, for it is my belief that in order for therapy to work, patients must trust that they do not need to take care of their therapist.

Second, should Mr. B have told his patients his health status earlier? I do not have any clear opinion about this. My concern was that, had he done so, it might have changed the focus of the psychotherapeutic work from the patients themselves and their issues to their concern for the therapist. Some discussion of this would certainly have been appropriate, especially if it preceded termination. Third, at what point did Mr. B become unable to make astute clinical decisions about how to conduct his practice? I do not know if Mr. B was receiving clinical supervision, consultation, therapy, or some other form of professional feedback at the time.

A Therapist With AIDS
Stops Practicing

After I have shared the story of Mr. B with colleagues and friends, I often hear that I am being hard and unfeeling. "Why do I take the moral high ground with this friend and colleague?" I am asked. On one level I do believe that it was simply unprofessional for him not to have made the painful decision to discontinue his practice. But I asked myself, when and if the time comes, will I be able to behave any more professionally? My model for handling this difficult situation was Mr. C.

Case 3

Mr. C was progressively symptomatic for a year before he was diagnosed with his first bout of Pneumocystis carinii pneumonia (PCP). Although he did not seem to be in any denial about the deterioration of his health, he had not formed any plans for taking care of his patients in the case of a medical emergency. Mr. C's first bout of PCP had a dramatic onset, requiring that he be rushed to an emergency room from a training session on AIDS he was conducting at a local hospital.

The day Mr. C went to the emergency room I canceled his patients for the next 2 days and told them that Mr. C was ill. The following week I again called each of Mr. C's patients, informing them that he was still ill and would not be working the rest of that month. I asked them if they wished to make an appointment with me to discuss their feelings about this. None of Mr. C's patients asked whether or not he had AIDS, and I did not volunteer this information.

When Mr. C returned to work 2 months later he told each of his patients that he had AIDS and he explored their feelings about this. He explained that, based on the likelihood that other medical emergencies would prevent him from guaranteeing the consistency of their treatment, he had decided to discontinue his work as a therapist. Mr. C worked with his patients for eight more sessions, during which time he wrapped up their treatment, terminated their work together, and facilitated their transfer to another therapist.

Mr. C was in the midst of moving into full-time private practice when he developed PCP. He shared with me how angry he was that his dream of being a full-time therapist was being denied to him just as he was reaching his professional goal. Although this was a painful decision to make, he felt that it was the only responsible way to handle his practice having become so seriously ill.

Conclusions

Although the literature contains a few articles about the illness or imminent death of the therapist (Abend 1980; Chernin 1976; DeWald

1980; Rosner 1986), literature on the therapist and patient sharing the same life-threatening condition appears to be just emerging. There are certain unique factors in this situation that may prove troublesome for the gay therapist and detrimental to the treatment he provides if left unaddressed. For example, how does the therapist cope with the constant reminder of his own health status and impending death when his practice is full of patients facing identical issues? The therapist's access to and use of clinical supervision, consultation, and psychotherapy, and his ability to remain self-examining during his personal crisis will largely determine whether or not he is able to continue to provide good treatment during so stressful a period.

The therapist's level of acceptance of his own condition and possible death will determine how emotionally available he is to work with patients needing to discuss their struggles and feelings about the same illness. A therapist who is in a great deal of denial about his own physical condition will most likely not be able to help patients who need to initiate discussions about their situations. If the therapist is in denial about his own illness he is certain to reinforce any denial that his patients may be experiencing, and will not be able to confront the patients' denial when it would be best to do so.

The question, How much time do I have left before I get sick or before I die? has a powerful influence on both the therapist and the patient. The therapist has to be able to assess if and when it is appropriate to bring the patient's thoughts and feelings about this into the open for exploration. The HIV-positive patient enters therapy wanting to be "healed" emotionally before he becomes too debilitated to do this difficult psychic work. The HIV-positive therapist also feels the pressure of having limited time to accomplish the healing before he, himself, becomes too to continue working. It takes great skill to acknowledge the therapist's illness without intruding into the patient's treatment.

Much has been written about the concept of living with AIDS or with HIV. People with AIDS have felt it crucial to their own sense of empowerment not to be viewed simply as "victims" or "patients." If the therapist believes that he is *living with* HIV or AIDS and not *dying from* HIV or AIDS, he is more likely to try to help patients restructure their own experience of the illness to conform to this belief system.

Although the above-described intervention is often useful, there are people with AIDS who clearly are dying from the illness and need simply to be able to discuss their experience.

The gay therapist's experience of death and dying can shape his work with patients susceptible to the same illness he has. Does the therapist believe that death is the end of it all, or does he envision some kind of life following death? If the therapist is not able to understand his own beliefs and feelings surrounding death, he will not be able to initiate discussions about this with patients. A therapist's inability to discuss these issues creates a sense of secrecy or shame in the patient who may not have anyone else with whom to discuss these feelings.

One of the interesting questions is whether the countertransference issues that arise from being HIV positive and working with HIV-positive gay men are in fact any different from those every therapist faces during the course of his or her daily work. There is the potential to view the feelings and concerns of many of these patients as having an urgency that must be responded to immediately. Any tendencies the therapist has towards grandiosity can be highlighted by the apparent urgency of the impending mortality of both the patient and therapist. Even if the urgency does stem from the patient, is it good treatment to respond to and thus validate a patient's urgency rather than explore it? Does the fact that the issues being explored, defended against, denied, or acted out are connected to the patient's and therapist's responses to illness and mortality justify conducting the treatment any differently than if the presenting problem were different?

Guntrip (1969) said that the therapist needs to know from his own experience what the patient is experiencing. Yet the potential for the therapist to make clinical mistakes is enormous when he or she is simultaneously experiencing many of the identical situations and feelings as the patient. I have learned that just because my patients are experiencing very similar situations to the ones that I am living through, I cannot assume that they will or should react in the same ways that I do.

I used to confront a patient's defenses quicker and push him more if he was symptomatic with an HIV-related illness than I would have if I felt I had more time to work with him. When I explored this in supervision I realized that this came from my need to feel that something tangible was occurring during the treatment and not from what was the soundest clinical decision for the individual patient. It became clear that it was neither fair to my patients nor good therapy not to customize the treatment to meet each particular individual's needs, defensive structures, and psychodynamics. My sense of life's fragility was causing me to view my work as the contribution I would make that might help ensure my own immortality after I died.

Terminal illness usually causes individuals to regress, at least in some areas of their lives. Thus the therapist who is dying or living with a life-threatening illness has to work with patients who are regressing. Perhaps the patients' regression mirrors the therapist's own struggles with regression. I have observed that sometimes a patient's regression will serve as permission for the therapist to regress in a similar fashion.

When a gay man begins therapy, he does so expecting to continue the process and relationship with the therapist until the goals for therapy have been met. The patient with a life-threatening illness must be willing to embark on the therapeutic journey with the knowledge that this process could be abruptly terminated by his own death. The therapist with a life-threatening illness has the obligation to evaluate realistically whether or not the issues a new patient is presenting can be worked on effectively within the uncertain amount of time he has left. Correspondingly, the therapist must be able to know when he is reaching the point of not being able to continue to practice. Thus the gay therapist with a terminal illness must be able to distinguish between his own narcissistic needs to deny the severity of his own condition and his needs to continue working and what is in the best interest of his patients. Knowing when to let go of one's career, patients, and identity that have been so significant a part of one's life and when to refer patients to a respected colleague is difficult and yet crucial. It is a clear indication of both the personal and professional development of the therapist and of the quality of the professional assistance he is receiving. It is improper for the therapist to place the decision of whether or not to continue working together in the hands of patients. For many patients it may be impossible to place their own needs for ongoing treatment above the needs of the "helpless, dying, and beloved" therapist who has helped them so much.

So what I am left with is once again the need to bind my own anxieties during my work with patients. My increasing success with not having my own needs determine what I say or do not say during therapy has resulted in my having an increased sense of control in other areas of my life outside of work. Although I acknowledge how difficult it can be for any of us, patient or therapist, to face the reality of our own death, being forced to confront this on a daily basis in both my work and personal life has helped me demystify death and dying and move these issues from the abstract into the concrete realm. I have been able to shift my focus from the inevitability of my death, which I cannot control, to what I can to a considerable extent control, namely, how I live and how I work. This lesson is invaluable and one that I attempt to help my patients grapple with in their own therapy, when appropriate.

References

Abend S: Serious illness in the analyst: countertransference considerations. Paper presented at the fall meeting of the American Psychoanalytic Association, 1980, pp 365–379

Chernin P: Illness in a therapist-loss of omnipotence. Arch Gen Psychiatry 33:1327–1328, 1976

DeWeld P: Serious illness in the analyst: transference, countertransference, and reality responses. Paper presented at the fall meeting of the American Psychoanalytic Association, 1980, pp 347–363

Guntrip H: Schizoid Phenomena, Object Relations and the Self. New York, International Universities Press, 1969

Rosner S: The seriously ill or dying analyst and the limits of neutrality. Psychoanalytic Psychology 3:357–371, 1986

Chapter 27

The Process of Closing a Practice When the Therapist Has AIDS: A Case Study

Linda E. Hutton, Psy.D.

When a professional psycho-therapist faces the implacability of an escalating human immunodeficiency virus (HIV)–related illness within himself, for a time he struggles to continue as the caregiver. Eventually he must become caregiver to himself and give up his professional life. This chapter is about a bisexual-identified psychotherapist who had to cope with the realities of advancing HIV-related illness while he tried to continue to earn a living and work skillfully in a valued career. Deciding when and how to tell his patients that he was HIV positive was complicated by his difficulty accepting new symptoms that caused serious changes in his health. When his health began to deteriorate and several patients learned of his seropositivity from other sources, the need for an orderly disclosure of his HIV status to all his patients could not be postponed. For months after he told his patients, he struggled to keep working in his private practice. Eventually, despite planning and the best intentions, he was forced to terminate with his patients precipitously and end his professional life.

The material for this case example was collected from September 1990 to April 1991 in over 100 hours of meetings, supervisory sessions, and conversations with the psychotherapist, members of his supervision group, and his friends. The psychotherapist's thoughts and feelings about the process are the focus of the chapter. His patients' reactions, thoughts, and feelings were accessible only through his reporting. Confidentiality restrictions mitigated any desire to find out more about how the patients experienced this difficult time, although hearing from them directly would surely enhance our understanding of the disclosure and termination processes. What the therapist did share were issues that he felt required supervisory consultation and patient material that he felt was elucidating for the research study. Usually the material was an account of manifest content and actions (i.e., what the patients actually said and did, and some speculation about what they did not say).

Case Example

History

Mr. A was a licensed social worker who had been in private practice since 1978. Although he considered himself a bisexual man, Mr. A's sexual orientation had been gay since his divorce over 25 years ago. He was well known professionally and within the gay community as a specialist in psychotherapy for bisexual and gay men. Mr. A also had done psychosocial hospice work, had 5 years' experience working with end-stage acquired immunodeficiency syndrome (AIDS) patients, and was an AIDS activist. Diagnosed HIV positive in 1986, he showed no symptoms of any related illnesses until late 1989. Early in 1990 he had moderate symptoms and by the end of the year was diagnosed as having AIDS. He knew that his increasing symptomatology meant the beginning of a life focused predominantly around surviving this rapacious illness. He knew he would eventually have to tell his patients that he was seropositive to prepare them for changes that might occur.

Chronology

Worrisome symptoms, which began late in 1989, persisted intermittently through the winter and were fairly constant by the spring of 1990. Throughout the spring and summer, Mr. A tried to assimilate what was happening to him. He was tired all the time and had constant diarrhea. He felt terrified about these changes in his health. For a long time he could not believe that they were solely disease related or that they were permanent. By September 1990, he was more debilitated. The fatigue was extreme and constant, and the diarrhea was chronic. He continued to lose weight. He felt increasingly panicked, eventually certain that he had moved into a more dire stage of the disease. Later, a diagnosis confirmed he had AIDS.

For over a year, Mr. A's decision to disclose his HIV-positive status to his patients had been pending. He postponed telling them earlier because he had experienced his symptoms as transient and remitting and his overall health as manageable. He continued to ruminate about disclosing his seropositivity to his patients until he could no longer deny his worsening health. Realizing that his condition might precipitously force an interruption in his work, he decided he had to tell his patients that he was HIV positive. At the time, he was working 4-day weeks, seeing 14 individuals in weekly psychotherapy, and leading three psychotherapy groups. He saw an additional 5 patients as needed for consultation and support about issues surrounding their bisexuality.

During this same time, he joined a psychotherapy group for male psychotherapists who were HIV positive, and he arranged to meet for peer supervision with three other social workers whose areas of expertise were loss, death and dying, and bereavement. He continued working with his psychotherapist of many years. He also asked his friends to organize themselves formally to meet with him each month for support as he coped with his deteriorating health.

At the first meeting of his friends (who included several psychotherapists), he talked about his severe fatigue and the difficulty he had getting through his workdays. He also talked about how nourished he continued to feel in the psychotherapy sessions with his patients. A theme that emerged in this meeting and that remained central for him throughout the research project was how to manage his workload, maintain his income, and continue doing the work he loved doing while adjusting to the changes in his health. At this point, ending his life's work was not something Mr. A entertained, nor was quitting suggested by anyone around him. Those he asked, including his psychotherapist, supported his effort to continue working. For Mr. A, the question became how to restructure his work life so he could give himself the time he needed to rest and care for himself, while continuing to earn a living doing psychotherapy without being unfair to his patients or himself. Mr. A contemplated several options to accommodate the changes in his health: cutting back his practice by terminating a number of patients, refusing to take new patients, or waiting for attrition to trim his practice.

Among myriad unknowns, one thing was certain: Mr. A needed to inform his patients about his seropositive status to ensure that there was a context within those therapeutic relationships for understanding changes necessitated by any sudden health crises. After considering how and what to tell patients, he decided to tell the group members together and tell the individuals in their sessions, all in the space of a week. He decided he would tell some patients simply that he was HIV positive and include in the disclosure to others that he was also experiencing some health changes. He realized he could not give his patients a prognosis for his illness because he did not have one himself. He could not give nor suggest an end date for therapy if asked because he had no idea if he was going live months or years.

What was most important to Mr. A was that he felt he still had a contribution to make through his work. He felt that the circumstances of his seropositivity did not mitigate his talent nor his desire to do psychotherapy. Further, he felt his spiritual and emotional struggle with the illness had enhanced his understanding of life and changed his work by adding a perspective and sensitivity that he felt would be valuable to his patients. Work was, and continued to be, a central piece of his identity and sense of self. He had no idea when his illness might overtake his need and desire to contribute. There were many variables to consider. Would he continue to be plagued with diarrhea and constant fatigue? As he was learning to live with his current symptoms, perhaps he would be able to continue working for a long time. Perhaps he would be struck down with Pneumocystis carinii pneumonia, for example, and be in and out of hospitals. If so, would he emerge from those stays relatively well and manageably energetic or would he be debilitated and require long recovery periods? With HIV-related illnesses, many scenarios were possible.

He also had to face the realities of his finances. He had a private disability plan that he had purchased when he began practice; it would pay $2,000 per month. Initially he questioned whether he should simply go on disability, quit work altogether, and avoid the prolonged uncertainty. But he also wondered whether that was fair. Was he really sick enough? And he wondered whether he could live on only the money provided by his insurance. His regular income was almost four times that offered by the disability policy. All these considerations were postponed by his need and desire to keep working.

The core issue, the subtext for making all the decisions necessitated by his seropositivity, was his imminent death. Mr. A and all the people around him had to accept that he was terminally ill with an indeterminate future. The challenge was to make decisions that supported his living while he was actually beginning to die. The necessity and difficulty of accepting impending death were central to the disclosure of his seropositive status to his patients and to negotiating his work life. He alternated between denial and hope, naturally pivotal elements in the process, with each suggesting different possibilities, imperatives, and actions.

Disclosure

In the middle of October 1990, Mr. A began telling his patients about his HIV infection after a series of incidents pushed the disclosure process into motion. One patient, a man in group therapy with Mr. A, had found out a year previously that Mr. A was HIV positive because he worked at the health care center where Mr. A was treated. He had confronted Mr. A earlier and Mr. A confirmed what his patient asked him: "I told him I was [not] ready to reveal to the group. If he was not comfortable with that information we should talk about his leaving. Or if he was, then we should [have] some private [individual therapy] work sessions just to process what that was like for him. And he pretty much handled it okay." Mr. A asked this patient to keep the information secret, which he did. Mr. A realized his request created a collusive relationship between them, but he decided this was the only way to handle the dilemma.

Mr. A continued to think about when he would be ready to disclose his status to his other patients. His chance to contemplate the right time ended abruptly in early October when another patient told him he had learned from mutual acquaintances that Mr. A was HIV positive. Mr. A confirmed his status to this patient whom he saw individually and in another therapy group. He realized that until he disclosed to this second group, he and a patient were again colluding in another potent and possibly deleterious secret. Mr. A did ask this second patient to withhold the information from the group until he could tell them himself in the next session. Within the same week, a third patient asked Mr. A if he was HIV positive. This patient had simply guessed that Mr. A was HIV positive because of Mr. A's thin and haggard appearance. Mr. A was very surprised to be confronted but felt a therapeutic and personal obligation to con-firm his patient's suspicions. The concurrence of events forced the disclosure process from contemplation to action.

Within a week, Mr. A had told all of his patients he was HIV positive. He ended up telling each of his patients essentially the same thing. If a patient asked questions, he answered them. He tried to focus on telling the truth, not alarming the patient unnecessarily, and monitoring the disclosure process carefully within the session.

"I told them I was positive. I told them, in a general way, what my symptoms were and how long I'd been positive, and I shared with them the process of why I waited to tell, and the struggle that that was about. I informed them about how much supervision and consulting and thinking I'd done about this and that it felt time now. That it was never a question of if I would tell them, but when, and it felt like it was 'when' now because there were some slight changes [in my health] and also that I needed to step in and start taking better care of myself. And also I wanted to prepare them for a shock or a surprise . . . and give them choices about whether they wanted to stay with a therapist under these conditions or not. And that, from my perspective, I could see that the therapy was changing and how I do therapy was changing, and if they were looking for a traditional therapist-[patient] . . . relationship that I wouldn't be the best per-son to be with right now because I'm changing my sense of bound-aries, how I'm working, and how long I might, you know, whether I'm going to be here or not be here. So I told them, 'there's going to be a certain instability here from your point of view I would imagine and you need to know whether you can tolerate that or not. And we both need to figure out whether it makes, whether that's good for you or not.'"

Mr. A covered the dimensions of the dilemma for the patients when he enumerated the risks of instability in the treatment: his newly announced fragility, his possible unavailability, important changes in the way he wanted to conduct therapy, and the open question of whether the patient's interests were being best served by him. The holding environment created by the truthfulness and con-cern Mr. A shared was offset by the threat of the unknowns he out-lined. The burden of this disclosure was the uncertainty that created a tension for and between both him and his patients. For psycho-therapist and patient, the great period of not knowing began.

Because Mr. A's patients knew he was bisexual, the disclosure was limited solely to his seropositivity. The manifest reactions of most of his patients were responsive yet contained. All of his patients asked some questions about him—how he was feeling and how long he had known—and some asked questions about HIV and AIDS. Several asked how the disclosure would affect their therapy beyond what he had mentioned in his standard speech. In Mr. A's groups, the reactions were similar to those of his individual patients. According to Mr. A, the groups focused only briefly on his announcement of his HIV status after their usual check-in. They asked the same kinds of questions about how he was feeling and how long he had known. One patient, in his longest running group of 5 years cried and told Mr. A that he had felt something was wrong.

Mr. A had expected that the initial responses to his disclosure would be mitigated, in part, by some protective denial, so he was only somewhat surprised at the paucity of manifest content about his disclosure in his patients' reactions. But he had expected more emotional expressions of concern about himself and he felt disappointed and angry about what he experienced as his patients' lack of empathy. Examining his reaction, he realized that his anger was derived from the free-floating rage he felt about the unfairness of his illness, a rage that previously he had not felt so clearly. He was angry that he was ill, that he had to cope with increasing debilitation, that everything in his life seemed so difficult, and, most uncomfortably, that many were well and not facing what he was facing.

The self-examination occasioned by the disclosure was characteristic of Mr. A and helped him understand himself at this stage of his illness. At this time, he needed the gratification of knowing his patients cared for him and that they recognized their therapeutic work with him as an important part of their lives. To the extent that he was struggling to keep working, he needed to be appreciated for those efforts by his patients, even though they did not know how difficult working had become for him. He could understand and tolerate his need as an acceptable wish but it conflicted with his view of good psychotherapeutic treatment. He did wonder, beyond his own reactions, how much his patients had taken in about the reality of his illness and whether the portent of its effect on their treatment had been obvious to them.

About this time, two group contracts came up for 12-week renewal. Mr. A told the Monday night group that he did not want to work on Monday nights anymore. There was grumbling, but several members agreed to switch into the Tuesday group. The Wednesday group, down to four members, did not reconstitute itself. The manifest reason was their small number. One man, who was ambivalent about staying on, kept bringing up the issue of Mr. A's health: "Why are we planning another group when Mr. A is sick? I'm not sure I want to commit myself to something like that. Group is a long process and how do we know we will be able to go on as long as we need to?" Mr. A thought this was an excellent question, one that he answered by saying that he really could not guarantee how long the group would continue but that he felt renewing the contract for 12 weeks was reasonable. No other patients had questioned him about how long he would be able to continue working and Mr. A became annoyed when this man persistently returned to the issue of his health. Mr. A was irritated at being questioned rather than praised or cared for when he was feeling so vulnerable. His patient's doubts dovetailed with his own questions about his ability to continue working. Feeling he could not answer the man truthfully because he did not feel comfortable with the anger he felt and the uncertainty he could not resolve, Mr. A told his peer supervision group how he really wanted to answer the question of why the group should renew their treatment contract: "Because I'm still able to work and I can function and be useful as a therapist. It's just that there's this unknown here that's . . . out in the air. It doesn't seem to be bothering most of my other groups but . . . I'm also beginning to think, God, what am I doing, why am I doing this?"

The Realities

By mid-November 1990, Mr. A had reduced his work week to 3 days, but there was more deterioration in his health. Despite his conscientious attempt, the cutback to 3 instead of 4 days was not enough. At the second meeting of the support group of friends later that month, Mr. A said, "I'm so tired and I have to keep working to pay all the bills." He stopped and was silent. "I really don't know what to do about work and everything."

The group started discussing different options when several financially astute members of the group offered to help him review his finances and develop a plan that would allow him to see fewer patients yet continue to meet his financial needs. He was pressed by one friend of many years, also a psychotherapist, to set a date for ending his practice. He seemed relieved, as if his friend's insistence had freed him to consider quitting. To the surprise of all, he chose a date that evening. He decided he would end his practice after he returned from a vacation in Mexico on March 21, 1991.

The friends who helped him devise a financial plan asked him to outline his goals. They felt that by identifying his current priorities, they could help Mr. A with a financial plan that freed him from supporting a life-style that reflected a different time in his life and open up the possibility to him that he did not have to continue everything as he had been doing. His primary goal was to have more free time to meditate, be with friends, work as a volunteer caregiver for infants with AIDS, and also have unstructured time. The result was Mr. A decided to work 2 days a week and, instead of ending his practice on March 21, he would cut back a number of patients by that date.

The complexity of planning a different work schedule was highlighted by an inability to gauge how much time was left before Mr. A would be debilitated by his illness, questions about the quality of that time, and the difficulty everyone had in voicing these concerns. Everyone wondered whether Mr. A would be better to continue working simply to check his anxiety and increasing depression or if he would need to be free of all his obligations to meet the demands of declining health. Mr. A wondered too. No one knew. No one could know. Members of the support and supervision groups calculated and recalculated, guessed and second-guessed. Which was the correct plan? What was the most realistic timetable? Underlying all the questions and organizing differing points of view at particular times was the ability of each person, including Mr. A, to accept the truth: Mr. A was dying. The process of articulating goals and making a financial plan highlighted for Mr. A and his friends the fact that the insidious changes in his health were now permanent. The financial and work plan that Mr. A finally developed served as Mr. A's quiet announcement that there had been a serious and permanent shift in the course of the illness and that Mr. A's ability to work was irrefutably diminished.

The Second Round

The new plan to cut back his practice made it necessary, in Mr. A's view, to tell certain patients that he would be continuing to work with them, and tell others that he would not continue with them and that he would need to terminate with them on March 21. We called this the second round and it had come quickly.

"I realize what I'm doing here is a selection process. . . . [My reasons are because of] where the therapy is, and also financial— who'll pay me, who is seeing me regularly, who I feel is going to stick this out long term. So there are those considerations; but mostly the main consideration is where they are and the impact of my, saying, 'I can't see you anymore.' . . . If I'm coming from an honest place as a therapist, I've got to let people know."

Among those patients whose therapy he decided to continue, there was some confusion and honest doubt in their reactions to the second round.

"A patient asked me something the other day that blew my mind. We were working on whether he should stay or not. He . . . [said], 'I don't know whether it does makes sense. Do I need something? I don't know what to do. Tell me.' He continued, 'I know you don't want to manipulate me and I know that you want to sit back there and help me find my answer, but it's okay, I can deal with that if you manipulate me a little. I want to know what you think. Would you stay with you?'"

Mr. A met with his peer supervision group and they cautioned against continuing to tell certain patients that he was choosing them to work with in therapy. They felt the potential for misunderstanding was great. In fact, he later realized, one of his female patients thought he was inviting her to be a friend, which naturally distressed and confused her. He announced his decision to only the three patients whom he had chosen to continue working with, but not to those whom he had planned to stop seeing. He stopped saying anything about March 21 to his patients and, eventually, to his friends. He decided to let natural attrition trim his practice and to schedule all his patients into 2 days when he returned from his vacation.

Mr. A continued to see his patients and he also took on two new patients after he explained to them that he was HIV positive and could not guarantee how long he would be working. The decision to take on new patients reflected Mr. A's deep ambivalence about working at this time. He was tired but still able to work. He was frightened about how he could survive without the money and identity his work provided. None of his colleagues or friends challenged him about taking on new patients.

Mr. A related the comment one of his patients made in his fourth session about choosing to work with Mr. A after knowing that he was seropositive:

"[He] told me last night the reason he chose me is because death is happening, because death looms in my background, and [because] it's going to help him get it together so that he can work harder because he doesn't have time to waste." Mr. A laughed. "I don't know what to do with that one. That was like, . . . " Mr. A laughed again, "I'm going to die so he better use me quick." Mr. A laughed once again. "I was furious for a moment. . . . It made me wonder what I am doing . . . with new [patients]. Did it make sense to be taking on new [patients] and saying I have HIV and I might be dying? . . . I'm beginning to question the value and the appropriateness of putting myself and [patients] in that position."

He continued to see a range of reactions from his patients, including expressions of abandonment, guilt, the wish to merge, sadistic aggression, rejection, and concern.

Early in February 1991 Mr. A made more changes, eliminating whatever he could from his schedule because he needed all his energy to continue working. He discontinued his peer supervision because of exhaustion. He had only been able to meet with that group twice. Partially for health and financial reasons, but primarily because he believed the work of psychotherapy had been completed, he terminated his individual psychotherapy with his therapist's concurrence. He felt the group of HIV-positive psychotherapists was dynamically and interpersonally oriented and did not support his primary need for spiritual understanding, so he withdrew from that group. The spiritual crisis of death was one that he believed he had to face alone. His need for spiritual reconciliation and self-care became his priorities.

Early in March 1991, Mr. A took his vacation in Mexico. While he was there, all of his symptoms resolved and he felt perfectly healthy again. He thought about work and realized he still had energy and a need for his work. At the same time, he said he felt like he was going crazy: "I feel like I am waiting for something and I don't know what it is. Friends don't quite do it now. Work doesn't quite do it. I feel restless. Something is going on in my body, I can feel it and yet I feel fine."

Within a week of returning, he was exhausted and demoralized. He was shocked at the sudden reappearance of all his physical symptoms. He cut back to 2 days of work per week as he had planned and he found the difference enormously helpful. A natural attrition of patients helped to make the change.

Several patients had terminated by the end of March, although none had manifestly terminated because of Mr. A's disclosure. One patient, the man who had learned about Mr. A's HIV positive status from mutual friends, had planned to terminate well in advance of the disclosure in order to take a trip of several months' duration. Mr. A reported nothing unusual about the termination. (When the patient returned and called Mr. A to resume therapy, Mr. A had to tell him that was no longer possible.) Another patient, a bisexual man in group and individual treatment, felt he had resolved his presenting issues in therapy. Mr. A also felt that this termination was appropriate. There was no mention of Mr. A's illness in the termination although Mr. A believed the disclosure of his illness had affected this patient as, he believed, it had affected all of his patients, whether they spoke of his illness or not. This latter patient was one of Mr. A's patients who had not asked about the possible effect of Mr. A's illness on the psychotherapy when it was disclosed to him.

Another patient terminated with a month and a half of notice. Mr. A agreed with the patient that he had accomplished his therapeutic goals. Mr. A described him as "biting at the bit" to be on his own and try out what he had learned in therapy. He had been in treatment with Mr. A since the summer of 1987. This patient had always had trouble expressing his feelings but he was able to tell Mr. A how much he valued their work together and what an important person Mr. A was to him. He expressed concern about Mr. A's status and said he felt sad because Mr. A was seropositive. Mr. A said, "As Mr. A the therapist, I felt it was a very good termination. As Mr. A, just myself, I would have wished for a deeper good-bye." He felt that he wanted a more emotional expression of the man's appreciation for their journey together in therapy and a greater acknowledgment of concern about Mr. A's struggle for his life.

A fourth patient, in individual and group therapy, terminated several months after Mr. A's disclosure. He left group because of a mandatory business commitment that conflicted with the group meeting time. Shortly after this, he left individual treatment (begun in 1988) because he said he was feeling better and he was tired of his long commute to therapy. He also had become involved in an intimate relationship, which was going well. This patient had had a life-threatening illness when he was a teenager and most of his therapeutic work had been about the feelings surrounding this experience. Mr. A regretted the termination because the patient had been abused earlier in his life and had not yet worked on his abuse issues. Mr. A did feel the man had done important work and that he was not ready to deal with his severe childhood abuse. The termination session went well. Mr. A felt very close to this patient and was especially aware of the poignancy of the termination in light of his own illness and the patient's past experience with death.

"I did something I have never done before and I have questions about it because I think it came more out of my own neediness and . . . this is important. . . . There's a need, . . . I wouldn't see this [patient] anymore. I've worked a long time with this [patient], done good work and he's ready to leave. . . . He's tired of the commute. . . . A lot of the goals got accomplished and it felt good. I didn't want him to leave without asking him if he wanted to know how I was doing when, if things got bad. And I'd never had that thought before and I thought, Is this an appropriate question? Do I wait until he brings it up? So I decided I was going to wait until almost the end of the session to see if he brought it up and, if he didn't, I would, because until the end, one models as a therapist. He didn't bring it up, and I said, 'I need to know whether, if down the road I should become ill or hospitalized, do you want to know that?' And then I thought about that and I said, 'Well, that's true, that's a valid question, and, what I'm not telling you is I would like you to know that.' And he got all, . . . I could tell he had been thinking about it. He said, 'Oh yes, please.' And then I got teary and started to cry." Mr. A laughed. "I had to hold it back though because it would have blown him away too much to see me that emotional. So, that did make me think, You've got to be careful here because your own needs come up."

Personally, Mr. A felt good about what he had done but questioned whether it was within the boundaries of good psychotherapy. Instinctively, he felt he had done what he needed to do and believed his patient had been relieved by his offer.

Ending the Practice

By the end of March 1991, Mr. A had 12 individual patients and one group of 9 men. Four patients had terminated, none manifestly because of the disclosure. He had not had to cancel any therapy sessions because of his illness although he continued fighting diarrhea and exhaustion. His weight loss of 30 pounds combined with exhaustion had changed his appearance, although none of his patients commented on this. One day in early April 1991, Mr. A became disoriented. Although he was at home, he did not know where he was and telephoned friends for help. His period of disorientation lasted only a day but he was physically and emotionally depleted for the next 5 days. He saw his patients that week but the episode terrified him and prompted him to request neurological and neuropsychological testing. Within 2 weeks he decided to end his practice. His illness was now stronger than his desire to work. Once he realized that he was vulnerable to future episodes of disorientation, he believed continuing with patients would be irresponsible. He was frightened about how fast other debilitating changes might occur and thought that limiting stressors, of which his work was now the most serious, would decrease the chances of deterioration. He was able to give his patients 2 weeks' notice. By May 9, 1991, Mr. A had terminated with all his patients. Once he made the decision to quit, he felt deeply relieved.

In the final therapy sessions, each of his patients told him they had felt sad, angry, and relieved when he had told them that he had to terminate their treatment. They all said that since October they had, each in his own way, been holding their breath, wondering as one patient put it, "when the ax would fall." Mr. A said he was surprised at first to hear this but then realized, he had, at some level, been aware of their anxiety. He felt some immediate relief from the burden of work but knew he would need time to understand fully what ending his work life meant for him.

Conclusions

If we think of an HIV-positive gay psychotherapist's disclosure of his seropositive status to his patients as happening under better or worse circumstances, we must assume that the realities of Mr. A's personal and professional life created possibly the best scenario one can expect for initiating this particular disclosure. When he told his patients, they already knew he was bisexual so they did not have to assimilate the disclosure of both his sexual orientation and his HIV status. He had direct care experience with end-stage AIDS and hospice patients so he knew the magnitude of changes that were in his future. A supportive professional and personal network allowed his process to be an open one in which he shared his questions, doubts, and fears. He had a full array of clinical resources to support and guide him as he continued to work and comprehend his situation: a psychotherapy group of peers who were HIV positive, ongoing individual psychotherapy, and a peer supervision group composed of experienced psychotherapists who specialized in death and dying work. A private disability insurance policy gave him some financial security and therefore more freedom to make choices about work. At age 52, Mr. A had the background of age and experience to help him make sense of his illness. He was a religious man with a lifelong belief in God. He was able to draw on his faith for support and guidance as he struggled to accept his illness.

Everything in Mr. A's training directed his attention to the welfare of his patients but nothing in his training prepared him for attending to the impact his own crisis had on them. He recognized the collusion when he asked his patients for their silence just as he recognized the fears and doubts triggered by his disclosure. The range of his emotions frightened him but he continued to try to manage them appropriately within the therapeutic boundaries. He questioned himself when he saw his needs competing with those of his patients. Each new reality brought by his illness set up a confrontation between his needs and those of his patients: when he realized that his patients had to be told about his health status, when he told them he was HIV positive, when he became sicker, and when he had to face his financial situation.

Ultimately, Mr. A's welfare emerged as his priority and the basis for his decisions. When he took on new patients, he rationalized to himself and to his friends that his illness had deepened his awareness and rendered him more capable as a therapist. He also knew financial concern and denial of his illness were part of his decision to continue. His colleagues, caregivers, and friends, to the extent they knew about his decisions and had access to him, questioned and challenged him about his possible denial of his condition. Just as often, they needed to deny changes in his health. They easily shared his anxieties about finances and the future. Often it seemed that to puncture the denial was to eradicate the hope. Given only two supervisory sessions, compassionate and skilled colleagues did not have the opportunity to continue to suggest different perspectives in his choices about his work. Early on, his psychotherapist urged him to continue working. Later, Mr. A left therapy and this avenue of counsel was also foreclosed. In the end, Mr. A could give his patients only 2 weeks' notice of termination, which was not an ideal scenario by any theoretical standard. When his work's life was over he realized that he had known from the beginning that his patients were frightened when he told them about his illness.

When one reviews the small body of literature that focuses on dying psychotherapists, what emerges is how unusual Mr. A was in being able to continuously entertain concern for the welfare of his patients and, at the same time, face his impending death with openness and awareness of the process of dying.

Being a psychotherapist with a life-threatening illness is not only a challenge one man faced but a challenge the profession must face. Had there been ongoing professional discussion about this dilemma, Mr. A's experience might have been different and he certainly would not have been so alone as he negotiated these difficult junctures. In hindsight, there are things all HIV-positive psychotherapists can do to mitigate the difficulties of working while they are ill and to make ending their practices smoother. As mental health professionals, we need to illuminate this topic. We too may face this problem either as the ill psychotherapist or as a supervisor or patient of an ill psychotherapist. Several issues must be considered, as follows.

Possibility of contracting HIV.   We need to recognize that the possibility of having a life-threatening illness exists for all of us in the profession. Specifically, an HIV-positive diagnosis, must be seen as a marker beginning a phase in the working life of a psychotherapist that necessitates the initiation of mechanisms for support and guidance.

Importance of supervision.   Individual or group supervision is a vehicle for the gay psychotherapist to question, discuss, and manage the changes in his psychotherapy practice that accompany the crisis of being terminally ill. The supervisory contract must be clearly defined, articulated, and maintained because there will be tremendous pressures on all parties to veer from the work of examining clinical material. The supervisor needs to be the ballast for the psychotherapist while he negotiates his turbulent emotions and needs and those of his patients. Between the supervisor and supervisee, there may be a need and a wish for a collusion that prioritizes the personal and professional needs of the psychotherapist over those of his patients, denies his waning health and abilities, and diminishes the awareness of imminent death. Supervision can greatly assist the HIV-positive psychotherapist when it is guided by an experienced supervisor who is aware of the specific and, to some extent, predictable pressures that emerge in relationships conducted under the specter of a life-threatening illness and imminent death. Obtaining personal support, which the HIV-positive psychotherapist will need, is not the most efficacious use of supervision but this may not be obvious when supervisor and supervisee are working under such horrifying circumstances.

Need for individual psychotherapy. Psychotherapy is strongly indicated for the HIV-positive gay psychotherapist for many reasons, including those that are helpful for all people with HIV-related or life-threatening illnesses: to help assimilate changes in physical health, to help discover the meaning the illness has for him; to explore emotions surrounding the crisis (particularly those about dying and death), and to express feelings and thoughts that others may judge or react to negatively. In addition, the HIV-positive psychotherapist may be helped in assessing his need to be in the caregiving role and eventually in giving it up. In psychotherapy, the ill therapist may set aside his professional role, his expertise in HIV-related illness, life-threatening illnesses, and dying and death and the persuasiveness of previous treatments and allow himself to acknowledge the emotions attending the unique phase of life he has entered. As in supervision, there will be pressures for collusions and denial on the part of both parties. The treating psychotherapist will need to be skillful enough to focus the work on the wrenching issues of impending loss and strong enough to tolerate and work with the powerful emotions that arise when life is threatened.

Countertransference issues may be more potent for the treating psychotherapist as he witnesses the struggle of a colleague. To the extent the treating psychotherapist shares other aspects of identity with the ill psychotherapist, vigilance about his countertransference and noncountertransference responses will be helpful. The patient will be a professional under the terrible pressure of his illness and, for that reason, the treating psychotherapist may find himself more challenged than usual to maintain control of the treatment. Failure to provide the essentials of good treatment may keep the ill therapist from important personal work.

Work-related issues.   Unless he quits work immediately upon being diagnosed HIV positive, the gay psychotherapist must expect the related illnesses to affect his work. How extensively his work is affected will be determined by the extent to which the therapist is known by patients, colleagues, and friends to be a member of a high-risk group for HIV-related illnesses; the rapidity and severity of changes in his health; the meaning of the illnesses to the therapist; the status of his finances including the availability of private health and disability insurance; the personal and professional support that surrounds him; and the role and meaning of work in his life. Once the therapist has been diagnosed HIV positive, he must assume that his work will be framed, from that time on, within the context of the diagnosis and all the uncertainty that it implies.

Although the uncertainty of HIV disease is pervasive, the therapist can exert control by continuously identifying his needs and planning for them in the best possible way. Supervision can be augmented by a careful review of each of the therapist's cases, the goal being to have clinical dispositions ready for each patient when the therapist is no longer able to work. The psychotherapist can consider which patients need continued treatment, who are appropriate referral clinicians and when the referral should be made. As he reviews his cases, the therapist should consider that referrals can be made and new treatments begun while the therapist is still well. Transfers may be more efficacious if the referring therapist either participates in a transfer session or sees the patient once after the new treatment has begun. At a minimum, the HIV-positive therapist can develop written treatment plans for each patient.

If the therapist becomes disabled in the course of practice, it can be invaluable for him to have identified a colleague whom he trusts clinically to manage these plans. The same person may be willing to serve as a clinical barometer for the psychotherapist. The therapist can review for himself and his colleague the ways he will be monitoring his therapeutic work to ensure that quality is not sacrificed unwittingly. Asking himself how he will recognize whether his patients are having difficulty working with him once they know he is HIV positive or ill may help him negotiate these junctures in the therapies. Similarly, if he thinks about how he will be able to recognize times when his needs and the needs of his patients become competitive, he can better develop therapeutic strategies to manage the conflicting needs. With the help of a colleague, a supervisor, and his psychotherapist, the therapist will ensure that he is supported in continuing to work as effectively as possible.

Financial and practical challenges.   As with any person who is HIV positive, the gay psychotherapist with HIV needs to compile a financial inventory that includes current income and expenditures, including ongoing professional expenses and future commitments (e.g., leases, answering services, health care coverage). The therapist needs to consider what his financial picture will look like if he has to stop or drastically cut back his working and he needs to generate different financial options. Knowing what public resources are available and the details of how and when they can be obtained may expand options about work. If the therapist is feeling well and can maintain a full workload, he may design an accelerated savings plan as backup financial support later. Considering his future, the therapist may find it helpful to think about how he would ideally like to end his working life and the choices that would entail. For example, if there were no financial constraints, would the therapist continue working, reduce his workload, or quit?

Disclosure of serological status.   HIV-related illness does not lend itself to a predictable enough course for the therapist to plan his disclosure of his illness around a particular physical milestone. The dramatic physical vicissitudes are perhaps the most difficult aspect of living with HIV-related illness. The timing of the disclosure of an HIV-positive status to one's patients is best carefully thought out. Even so, variables other than the therapist's acceptance of his illness or his determination of when his patients need to know, can set the disclosure in motion. For example, patients who are members of social or professional networks, who are employed in health care work, or whose life history has attuned them to the keen observation of others may inquire about the therapist's health and trigger the disclosure process. Focusing on how, what, when, and how much to tell patients is critical. Each patient may not need to know the same things. Personal history may dictate the amount of information individual patients need. Some may need more and others may need less.

Specific consideration of each patient's treatment can affect the disclosure: the type of treatment (e.g., supportive psychotherapy, psychoanalytically oriented psychotherapy), the length of treatment, what the psychotherapist would expect patients would want to know, what the therapist can tell them about the future at the time of disclosure, and any treatment options he would like them to consider. If the disclosure of seropositivity accompanies the disclosure of an identity of the therapist that hitherto was unknown to the patient (e.g., high-risk group member, gay or bisexual man, intravenous drug user), patients will be absorbing a dual shock. Mr. A's case indicates that patients are not likely to take in the magnitude of what the therapist tells them, but, to the extent the therapist can be clear with them (even about what is not known) and to the extent he feels confident within himself, the disclosure process can be a therapeutic holding environment.

Thinking about the kinds of questions patients might ask may be helpful in preparing the therapist. Preparation may allow the therapist to consider the range of responses encouraged by the desire to be truthful, his wish for privacy, and the value of both to the treatment. The psychotherapist has the right to refuse to answer questions, but the manner in which he does so will have an impact on the future of the relationship. A disclosure session in which the therapist explores the patient's responses before providing any information other than the fact of his seropositivity would have to be done with extreme deftness in order for this technique not to be experienced as at best unempathic and at worst sadistic, because the disclosure itself is nontransferential, noncountertransferential material. Again, this one case example suggests patients will press far fewer questions on the therapist than he may wish. Even patients who seem to have a sophisticated understanding of HIV may not realize the implications of the therapist's HIV status for their continued treatment.

It is the therapist's responsibility to make patients aware of the possible effects on their therapy so they can make informed choices about whether or not to continue treatment. Relying on informed, supportive professional colleagues can be helpful in the disclosure process. If a patient has multiple providers whom one has permission to consult, the psychotherapist should consider informing the other providers and enlisting their collaboration as part of the HIV-status disclosure in order to provide the patient with extra support.

Disclosure of one's HIV-positive status is an introduction or expansion of the therapist's identity in the treatment relationship; the relationship will change as a result of this intrusion, particularly to the extent the work is conducted on the principle of limited personal disclosure by the psychotherapist. There may be changes in the therapist's social and professional networks as his disclosure becomes more public. When deciding on the timing of the disclosure, the therapist would do well to consider what advantage there is to having maximum control over the information by an early disclosure as opposed to the benefits of delay. The psychotherapist may want to continue to keep whatever advantage there is in managing the public disclosure of information about his health. Keeping referral and professional networks up to date about what work he is accepting, what new work he wants to do, and his availability for other work (e.g., public service speaking engagements or workshops) can be advantageous for the therapist and can check any misinformation or misunderstandings about his willingness and ability to work.

Deciding to end his practice is an extremely painful decision and surely a great loss for a psychotherapist. There are many factors to consider. The key may be to monitor oneself in supervision and in individual treatment. When the preponderance of energy and concern is directed toward his survival, the psychotherapist must face ending the part of his life that has been about helping others and refocus his caretaking on himself.

The psychotherapist who shared his experiences for this project did so faithfully, despite illness and his own burdens, in the hope that his experience would be helpful to others. He died in April 1992, surrounded by his closest friends.

Epilogue:
Where We Are Now

Steven A. Cadwell, Ph.D.
Robert A. Burnham, Jr., Ph.D.
Marshall Forstein, M.D.

and the dark fell anyway and all our people
sicken and have no rage the Feds are lying
about the numbers the money goes for toilet
seats in bombers the State of the Union
is pious as Pius washing his hands of Hitler
Jews are not a Catholic charity when is
enough enough I had a self myself
once but he died when do we leave the mirror
and lie down in front of the tanks let them
put two million of us away see how quick
it looks like Belsen force out all their hate
the cool indifferent genocide that locks up
all the pills whatever it takes witness
the night and the waste for those who are not yet
touched for soon the thing will ravish their women
their jock sons like in rows in the empty infield
the scream in the streets will rise to a siren din
and they will beg us to teach them how to
bear it we who are losing our reason

Paul Monette
Manifesto in *Love Alone*

As gay psychotherapists, we are immersed in the acquired immunodeficiency syndrome (AIDS) epidemic. We are deeply affected and forever changed. In compiling this book, we as editors have struggled to comprehend and integrate our rage and sadness as gay men and our responsibility as therapists. We too struggle with unremitting loss. We must find the stamina to stay with those who are dying, struggling to learn to let go, and with those who are living, struggling to make sense of going on.

Regardless of background, ethnicity, or sexual orientation, we have to face the limits of our relationship with each of our patients. Some will accept our offer and let us journey with them. We may offer some guidance, some perspective, some company. But then we come to the end. In a normal course of treatment, this is the negotiated juncture in therapy when termination occurs. The patient steps out into his own autonomous life, and it is hoped he is more free of neurotic unhappiness and better prepared to engage in relationships with others and deal with the inevitable disappointments in the life ahead.

Therapy with gay men is always fraught with the stigma of being different as gay men or as men infected with the human immunodeficiency virus (HIV). In therapy with a gay man in the terminal phase of illness, the treatment relationship may be prematurely and suddenly ended by death. The therapist's expectation of the work must shift from consolidating the patient's identity in preparation for death rather than life. For the therapist working with a gay patient with HIV, being able to let the patient go in death may be the ultimate challenge.

Over the past 2 years of our labor on this book, we have reviewed the meaning of the first decade of the epidemic for us. The voices we have brought together to witness these years are only a few. Many more must be heard. In the beginning it was difficult to find a voice to speak to the overwhelming grief in the gay community. Where is our wailing wall? The chapters on grief in the earliest versions of the table of contents went unclaimed, unwritten, and only resurfaced when we realized their absence in the later stages of the book's development. Like the rest of our community, we depended on other forms for expression of this grief: the AIDS quilt, the poets of this plague, the political activism of our community, and the extraordinary volunteerism that sustains those who are experiencing illness and works to prevent others from becoming infected. We are aware of our own resistance and difficulty in processing and managing our individual grief. We struggle to simultaneously acknowledge and deny our personal grief so that we might be available to support others through their experience of past, present, and impending loss. In retrospect, we realize that, throughout this volume, we have chronicled our personal and professional struggle with death, grief, and loss from the beginning of the epidemic.

Often in this work, we must be able to help our gay patients die, and stay with them up to that point of death. We must be vigilant that we do not let them go prematurely lest we abandon them. A critical experience for most gay men has been their earlier abandonment by the nongay culture and often also by their families of origin. For the therapist to disengage too soon would be to recapitulate to these earlier experiences and confirm the gay man's internalized sense of rejection, worthlessness, and shame. What we offer most powerfully is the potentially healing relationship to offset that earlier abuse and trauma. Thus death and dying might be experienced for what they are: sad, sometimes tragic, but an inevitable part of life, like breathing, holding the air in, and letting it go. We have much to learn about attaining this acceptance of death, and yet we continue to rail against it in ones so young. We have much to learn about building our stamina to stay with our patients through this difficult passage.

The AIDS epidemic is different from any other epidemic because of its cultural, social, political, medical, religious, and spiritual context. For all its differences, ultimately what we find in AIDS is universal: the reality of death for us all. As therapists who choose to work with gay men, we choose to care for those who are dying and to deal with the pain of living as one is dying. We also choose to care for those who are surviving and to reaffirm the meaning of living in the midst of devastation. We are a part of the family that supports the survivors of this assault and trauma. We must perpetually rediscover affirmation in the face of despair. More than once we have been awakened to the essential wonder of existence by our patients who know only too well the fleeting preciousness of life.

A large part of our ongoing work is to bear the deaths of our patients, our colleagues, our lovers, and our friends: the first generation
of openly gay men in America who dared to speak the name of their
love, served as role models, claimed a place in the larger society, and
defined what being gay in America could be. Much of this generation
has been decimated with virtually no acknowledgment by the larger
society. Because of that denial and devaluation of the human spirit
simply because of their sexual orientation, newer generations of gay
men as well as others will continue to be decimated. Thus we need to
prepare ourselves for this unremitting loss and manage our own lives
and affirm the lives of those surviving and of generations of gay men
to come.

Our capacity to deal with death and dying is critical, but this is
only one piece of the work with gay men. As Erikson (1950) so well
framed it, as we face our death we are challenged to find the integrity
in our lives and to not languish in our despair. Our work is to understand what AIDS may represent to each gay man, regardless of serological status; to help him overcome guilt and shame in order to define
the purpose, meaning, and celebration in his life. To the HIV-infected
gay man, diagnosis defines an irrevocable aspect of his life. With the
gay man who is not infected, we work to understand that to be gay
does not mean that he inevitably must become infected. His right to
an uninfected life needs continual affirmation in his own thought and
behavior. Therapy has a mission to signal the dangers of lost integrity,
to comprehend despair, and to sound the hope and opportunity of life.

Our work in the next decade is to search for the voice of each of
our gay patients, and to create a unique relationship with those who
are dying as well as those who are living, in whom we affirm gay identity and gay sexuality. We will pray that scientific breakthroughs will
enhance each individual's ability to live longer and with less debilitation, truly making HIV infection a chronic, but manageable condition.
But for now, each will have his personal story about what it means to
be gay, his personal meaning of AIDS, and his own constructions of
what it means to be sick, to be dying, and to die. We will continue to
learn from their experience in order to work more effectively with
those gay men who continue to live.

The dilemma as survivors is not simply to tolerate the life some gay men are fortunate enough to preserve, but to forge actively a cel-ebrated life and create meaning and purpose amid such devastation. The resiliency of the human spirit is in the commitment to freedom of the true self and our love for others. In such freedom begins our re-sponsibilities. This is the legacy future generations of gay men require of us.

> The story that endlessly eludes the decorum of the press is the death of a generation of gay men. What is written here is only one man's passing and one man's cry, a warrior burying a warrior. May it fuel the fire of those on the front lines who mean to prevail, and of their friends who stand in the fire with them. We will not be bowed down or erased by this. I learned too well what it means to be a people, learned in the joy of my best friend what all the meaningless pain and horror cannot take away—that all there is is love. Pity us not.
>
> Paul Monette
> *Love Alone*

Reference

Erikson EH: Childhood and Society. New York, WW Norton, 1950

Index

DATE DUE
